'Here is a book whose authors immerse themselves in the histories and discourses of psychoanalysis and the forces of cultural and political ideologies to offer reflective and critical analyses of the psychoanalytic "treatment" of queerness. These insightful and at times provocative essays reflect on the quotidian aspects of queer lived lives, the fragilities of the contemporary era, and how they can meaningfully interact with a discipline of psychoanalysis fit for the 21st century.'

Eve Watson, *Psychoanalyst and Writer, Dublin*

'Psychoanalysis will be queer or it will not be. Against dismissals of psychoanalysis as outdated, biased, patriarchal, heterosexist, transphobic, racist, colonial, and bourgeois, every essay in this book challenges prejudice, debunking myths and assumptions about psychoanalysis while reorienting it brilliantly.'

Patricia Gherovici, *Psychoanalyst and author*
of Transgender Psychoanalysis, *Philadelphia*

'*The Queerness of Psychoanalysis: From Freud and Lacan to Laplanche and Beyond* is a collection of papers that works to provoke, deepen and broaden our psychoanalytic thinking, to take seriously the views of queer subjects, scholarship, psychoanalysts and philosophers. These papers pushed me to learn psychoanalytic and philosophical ideas and schools of thought beyond the limits of my training and exposure. The interdisciplinary scope of the collection offers a unique challenge to curious, expansive readers of psychoanalysis. Raising the voices of queer, trans and gender non-binary people is a welcomed gift and urgent necessity for psychoanalysis at a time when the field still clings to views that pathologize and devalue queer people and seek to marginalize and exclude our input.'

Jack Pula, *MD, New York*

W0234908

The Queerness of Psychoanalysis

The Queerness of Psychoanalysis: From Freud and Lacan to Laplanche and Beyond is an exploration of psychoanalysis' often complicated and fraught history with thinking about queerness, as well as its multifaceted heritage.

Throughout the chapters, the contributors write about psychoanalysis' relationship with queerness, the ways in which queerness is represented in the psychoanalytic archive, and how that archive endures in the present and creates various disruptive effects both within and beyond the clinic. Each chapter from the global cohort of contributors approaches queerness from a different angle: they consider the literary aspects of queerness' presence in the analytic world; the clinical complexities of working with queer and trans people; metapsychological inclusion and exclusion of queerness, and many other subjects. Taken together these contributions constitute a decisive intervention into the psychoanalytic canon. They are an unabashed demand for accepting and furthering the representation and inclusion of queer, and in particular trans, people within psychoanalysis. It is a call for action to utilize and deepen psychoanalysis' enormous explicatory powers and bring together voices that have so far been denied a unity of expression, while critically reevaluating psychoanalysis' historical relationship to queerness. Each chapter proposes different ways of thinking and writing psychoanalytically, with many of the papers queering the format and forms of expression commonly found in academic writing, through their use of dialogues, conversations, or other experimental forms of writing.

Written almost exclusively by analysts, scholars, and activists who identify as trans and/or queer, this important volume puts theory into practice by centering queer and trans voices.

Vanessa Sinclair is a psychoanalyst based in Sweden, who works with people internationally. She is the host of Rendering Unconscious Podcast and a founding member of Das Unbehagen: A Free Association for Psychoanalysis. She sits on the International Advisory Board of the journal *Psychoanalysis, Culture & Society* and is an Editorial Advisor for *Parapraxis* magazine. Dr. Sinclair is the author of *Scansion in Psychoanalysis and Art: The Cut in Creation* (Routledge, 2021) and the editor of *Psychoanalytic Perspectives on the Films of Ingmar Bergman:*

From Freud to Lacan and Beyond (Routledge, 2023) and *On Psychoanalysis and Violence: Contemporary Lacanian Perspectives* (Routledge, 2019) with Manya Steinkoler.

Elisabeth Punzi is a licensed psychologist and a lecturer at the Department of Psychology at Gothenburg University, Sweden. She leads a project concerning heritage and health at the Centre for Critical Heritage Studies, Gothenburg University and teaches psychoanalytic theory, psychology of religion, qualitative research methods, and many other topics.

Myriam Sauer is a PhD candidate at the Latin-America Institute of Freie Universitaet Berlin, Germany, as well as a writer and poet. Her primary academic interests lie in the fields of psychoanalysis, queer studies, literature, and sociology.

The Queerness of Psychoanalysis

From Freud and Lacan to Laplanche and Beyond

Edited by
Vanessa Sinclair,
Elisabeth Punzi, and Myriam Sauer

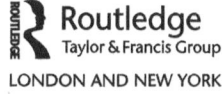 Routledge
Taylor & Francis Group

LONDON AND NEW YORK

Designed cover image: Phantom of Dreams (1992) – Collage by Artist Val Denham

First published 2025
by Routledge
4 Park Square, Milton Park, Abingdon, Oxon OX14 4RN

and by Routledge
605 Third Avenue, New York, NY 10158

Routledge is an imprint of the Taylor & Francis Group, an informa business

British Library Cataloguing-in-Publication Data
A catalogue record for this book is available from the British Library

Library of Congress Cataloging-in-Publication Data
Names: Sinclair, Vanessa, editor. | Punzi, Elisabeth, editor. | Sauer, Myriam, editor.
Title: The queerness of psychoanalysis : from Freud and Lacan to Laplanche and beyond / edited by Vanessa Sinclair, Elisabeth Punzi, and Myriam Sauer.
Description: Abingdon, Oxon ; New York, NY : Routledge, 2025. | Includes bibliographical references and index. |
Identifiers: LCCN 2024027154 (print) | LCCN 2024027155 (ebook) | ISBN 9781032603827 (paperback) | ISBN 9781032624105 (hardback) | ISBN 9781032624129 (ebook)
Subjects: LCSH: Psychoanalysis and homosexuality. | Sex (Psychology) | Sexual minorities—Psychology.
Classification: LCC RC451.4.G39 Q44 2025 (print) | LCC RC451.4.G39
(ebook) | DDC 616.89/1708664—dc23/eng/20240911
LC record available at https://lccn.loc.gov/2024027154
LC ebook record available at https://lccn.loc.gov/2024027155

ISBN: 978-1-032-62410-5 (hbk)
ISBN: 978-1-032-60382-7 (pbk)
ISBN: 978-1-032-62412-9 (ebk)

DOI: 10.4324/9781032624129

Typeset in Times New Roman
by codeMantra

Dedicated to Cecilia Gentili (1972–2024)

Contents

Notes on Contributors

Elisabeth Punzi, PhD (she/her) is a licensed psychologist and a lecturer at the Department of Psychology at Gothenburg University. She leads a project concerning heritage and health at the Centre for Critical Heritage Studies, Gothenburg, Sweden, and teaches psychoanalytic theory, psychology of religion, and qualitative research methods, among other topics. Her research concerns clinical practice, critical psychology/psychiatry, and the importance of expressive arts for health and recovery, as well as Jewish identity, heritage, and congregational life.

Myriam Sauer (she/her) is a PhD candidate at the Latin-America Institute of Freie Universität Berlin, Berlin, Germany, as well as a writer and poet. Her first novel, entitled *Eine Passage durch den reißenden Strom* (*A Torrential Passage*), came out in Fall 2023 with Querverlag. Her primary academic interests lie in the fields of psychoanalysis, sociology, queer studies, literature, and philosophy.

Vanessa Sinclair, PsyD (she/her) is a psychoanalyst based in Sweden, who works with analysands internationally. She is the host of Rendering Unconscious Podcast, which was awarded the 2023 Gradiva Award for Digital Media by the National Association for the Advancement of Psychoanalysis. Her books include *Things Happen* (Trapart Books, 2024), *Psychoanalytic Perspectives on the Films of Ingmar Bergman: From Freud to Lacan and Beyond* (Routledge, 2023), *Scansion in Psychoanalysis and Art: The Cut in Creation* (Routledge, 2021), *Outsider Inpatient: Reflections on Art as Therapy* (Trapart Books, 2021) with Elisabeth Punzi, *The Mega Golem: A Womanual for All Times and Spaces* (Trapart Books, 2021) with Carl Abrahamsson, *On Psychoanalysis and Violence: Contemporary Lacanian Perspectives* (Routledge, 2019) with Manya Steinkoler, and the *Rendering Unconscious* book series (Trapart Books).

Gila Ashtor, PhD, LP is an assistant professor of clinical psychoanalysis at Columbia University, New York, NY, where she teaches undergraduates and graduate students, as well as a faculty member of the Columbia University Center for Psychoanalytic Training and Research, where she teaches and supervises candidates in training. She is the author of *Homo Psyche: On Queer Theory and*

Erotophobia (Fordham University Press, 2021), *Exigent Psychoanalysis: The Interventions of Jean Laplanche* (Routledge, 2021) and *Aural History* (Punctum, 2020). Her book, Contemporary Theories of Masochism is forthcoming from Routledge. Ashtor is an assistant adjunct professor of psychoanalysis (postdoc) at New York University, New York, NY. She is on the faculty of the Institute for Psychoanalytic Training and Research, New York, NY, and in the MFA program where she teaches writers. Her primary areas of academic and clinical expertise include identity, trauma, sexuality, and masochism. She is in private practice in New York City.

Ken Corbett, PhD is a professor at New York University, New York, NY, teaching in the Postdoctoral Program in Psychotherapy and Psychoanalysis. He is the author of *Boyhoods: Rethinking Masculinities* (Yale University Press, 2009) and *A Murder Over a Girl: Gender, Justice, Junior High* (Henry Holt, 2016).

Griffin Hansbury, LCSW-R (he/him) is a psychoanalyst and social worker in practice since 2001. He has also trained in eye movement desensitization and reprocessing (EMDR), an effective therapy for trauma, and is certified in Imago Therapy, a helpful method for improving communication between partners and family members. As an internationally recognized expert on gender identity, he was the first psychoanalyst to publish as openly transgender. His writing on the subject has advanced the field, appearing in several peer-reviewed journals, including *The Journal of the American Psychoanalytic Association, Psychoanalytic Dialogues, Studies in Gender and Sexuality, The Psychoanalytic Review, Journal of Gay & Lesbian Mental Health, International Journal of Transgenderism*, and *TSQ: Transgender Studies Quarterly*. His widely read article "The Masculine Vaginal: Working With Queer Men's Embodiment at the Transgender Edge" has been translated and published in several countries, including Argentina, Germany, and Italy.

Geoffrey Hervey (they/them) is a community organizer, mental health professional, and professional drag artist. They have a master's degree in clinical mental health counseling from Vanderbilt University and are currently pursuing a PsyD at George Washington University, Washington, DC. Their clinical interests center the mental health of marginalized groups of people from a collective liberation framework. As Sin Clair, they have performed in the Southeast U.S. to audiences of thousands and created the Lipsync Legend Tournament to benefit local community mental health organizations.

Esther Hutfless (they/them) is a philosopher and psychoanalyst in Vienna, Austria, and adjunct lecturer in philosophy, psychoanalysis, gender studies, and queer theory at the University of Vienna, Vienna, Austria, and Sigmund Freud University, Linz, Austria. Hutfless gives lectures, seminars, and workshops on psychoanalysis in diverse higher education institutions. Hutfless' research areas include psychoanalysis, deconstruction, poststructuralist philosophy, feminist theory and Queer Theory.

Luce deLire is a ship with eight sails, and she lies down by the quay. As a philosopher, she publishes on the metaphysics of infinity but also on queer theory, anti-racism, postcolonialism, and political theory. In her performances, she embodies figures of the collective imaginary. For more (including booking), see getaphilosopher.com.

Simone A. Medina Polo (she/her) is a philosopher and PhD candidate at the Global Centre for Advanced Studies, Dublin, Ireland, for philosophy and psychoanalysis.

Molly Merson, LMFT (they/them, she/her) is a psychotherapist and psychoanalyst in full-time independent practice in the Bay Area, California, practicing on Lisjan Ohlone, Patwin, and Coast Miwok unceded territories. Molly is a clinician, supervisor, author, and instructor, offering interdisciplinary courses for clinicians on psychoanalysis and race, queerness, class, decoloniality, and liberation. Molly facilitates and participates in groups that invite discussions of the entanglements between""the social" and clinical life. Molly is the author of "The Whiteness Taboo: Interrogating Whiteness in Psychoanalysis", published in the journal *Psychoanalytic Dialogues* in 2021, and in the same year authored *Purposive encounters with lack in strength sports and diet culture*, published in the journal *Psychoanalysis, Culture and Society*.

M.E. O'Brien, PhD (she/her) writes and speaks on gender freedom and capitalism, and is a practicing analytic clinician in New York City. She is an associate editor of *Parapraxis*. She is the author of *Family Abolition: Capitalism and the Communization of Care* (Pluto Press, 2023), and co-author of the speculative novel, *Everything for Everyone: An Oral History of the New York Commune, 2052–2072* (Common Notions, 2022). She is also on the editorial collective at *Pinko*, a magazine on gay communism. She completed a PhD at New York University, New York, NY, where she wrote on how capitalism shaped New York City's LGBTQ social movements. She is currently a psychotherapist, a licensed clinical social worker, and in formation as an analyst. She is a candidate at Pulsion, a psychoanalytic institute in New York City.

Avgi Saketopoulou, PsyD is a queer psychoanalyst based in New York City, and faculty member of New York University's Postdoc Program in Psychotherapy and Psychoanalysis, New York, NY. Her books include *Sexuality Beyond Consent: Risk, Race, Traumatophilia* (NYU Press, 2023) and *Gender Without Identity* (UIT Books, 2023) with Ann Pellegrini.

Lara Sheehi, PsyD لارا شيحا (she/هي) is an assistant professor of clinical psychology at the Doha Institute for Graduate Studies, Doha, Qatar. She is the founding faculty director of the Psychoanalysis and the Arab World Lab and works on decolonial and anti-oppressive approaches to psychoanalysis, with a focus on liberation struggles in the Global South. Lara is the president of the Society for Psychoanalysis and Psychoanalytic Psychology and of the advisory board for the USA Palestine Mental Health Network. She is co-editor of *Studies in Gender and Sexuality*, co-editor of *Counterspace* in *Psychoanalysis, Culture and Society*, and a contributing editor to the Psychosocial Foundation's *Parapraxis* magazine. Lara is co-author with Stephen Sheehi of *Psychoanalysis Under Occupation: Practicing Resistance in Palestine* (Routledge, 2022) and is currently working on a new book, *From the Clinic to the Street: Psychoanalysis for Revolutionary Futures* (Pluto, 2025).

Tobias Wiggins, PhD (he/him) is an assistant professor of women's and gender studies at Athabasca University, Alberta, Canada. His federally funded research program centers transgender health and sexuality, queer and trans visual culture, clinical transphobia, arts-based research, and psychoanalysis. Broadly, Wiggins' work aims to address the continued pathologization of gender variance and to support trans-competent care and social advocacy. His recent publications appear in *Transgender Studies Quarterly*, *Studies in Gender and Sexuality*, *Psychoanalytic Study of the Child*, and the anthology *Sex, Sexuality and Trans Identities: Clinical Guidance for Psychotherapists and Counselors* (Jessica Kingsley Publishers, 2019).

Introduction

The Queerness of Psychoanalysis: From Freud and Lacan to Laplanche and Beyond

Vanessa Sinclair, Elisabeth Punzi, and Myriam Sauer (Eds.)

For more than a century, psychoanalysis has fostered a wealth of clinical work and theoretical insights, as well as literary and cultural criticism, including contributions to philosophy, film theory, women's and gender studies, and queer theory. However, the field has also faced various challenges and repudiations since its inception, from politically conservative divisions within the field, to detractors pointing to the cost, time commitment, and lack of empirically verifiable efficiency. While the uses of psychoanalysis have been diverse in theory and in practice, with many different schools – drive, ego, object, semiotic, self, and relational, to name but a few – having emerged since Sigmund Freud's death in 1939, the field itself lacks comprehensive organizational patterns. Sexuality was always at the forefront of Freud's theories, and sexuality and gender have been central points of reference for all psychoanalytic schools, yet their theories and relationships have varied wildly. Many schools of psychoanalysis – and individual psychoanalysts – have been outspoken in their pathologization of queerness, homosexuality, intersexuality, and/or trans* being (referred to collectively as the LGBTQI+ [lesbian, gay, bisexual, trans*, queer, questioning, intersex+] community), while others fight for the depathologization of non-normative sexualities and valorization of gender nonconforming ways of life.

Despite the spectral presence of queerness and transness, both remain hotly contested subjects within the realms of clinical and theoretical psychoanalysis; some question the usefulness of psychoanalysis to the theorization of queer or trans* matters altogether (Wark, 2022). Critiques directed at the overtly conservative, and at times reactionary, side of psychoanalysis are well-founded: there exists a long record of open pathologization of queer and trans* modes of being. And yet at the same time, psychoanalysis has from the beginning been a site of queer and trans* creation and resistance. Whether it is Freud famously writing to a concerned mother in 1935 that she ought not worry about her son's homosexuality (Freud, 1951), or Klein asserting in 1935 that "much love can be put into these [homosexual] relationships" (Klein, 1975, p. 331, fn1), or the more recent sustained metapsychological critiques formulated by critical theorists such as Lee Edelman (1994, 2004, 2011, 2023), Tim Dean (2009; with Oliver Davis, 2022), Kaja Silverman (2009), Jacqueline Rose (2005), David Marriott (2000, 2007, 2018, 2021), or

DOI: 10.4324/9781032624129-1

Hortense Spillers (1996), psychoanalysis is far from being inherently conservative or reactionary. Despite the stance some schools of psychoanalysis have maintained to remain apolitical – something that Derrida critiqued in 1981 in his work on *Geopsychoanalysis* (1991), and to which Ranjana Khanna added a forceful critique in 2003 – psychoanalysis persists as a powerful tool of interrogation, both within and outside of the clinic.

But whence this unresolved controversy over queerness and transness, and perhaps political questions more generally? Derrida's *Archive Fever* (1997) offers a trenchant answer to this question: because psychoanalytic thinking is premised upon the articulation of a double-bind of speech, it escapes unilateral condemnation as much as it escapes reductionist affirmation. Precisely because psychoanalysis is the discourse of the unconscious, which harbors contradictions and illogical figurations, psychoanalysis is a reflexive practice that can never be arrested on one particular belief or idea. As such, psychoanalysts have equally utilized Freud's thinking to develop theories to affirm or negate gender nonconforming people. In addition, the raw, unsettling force of queerness endures against all attempts at conceptual determination. What distinguishes psychoanalysis from many other protocols of reading is its steadfast commitment to particularism, to an *anti-hermeneutics of psychic life* (Laplanche, 1996), and to insisting on the breakdown of historically imposed representations.

There are few modes of thinking as relentless in their commitment to specificity as psychoanalysis, and it is here that psychoanalysis exudes an immense excitement. Psychoanalysis thus assumes a special relationship to questions of heritage, tradition, and inheritance. Although the discipline has its own complicated history of expectations, which is codified in the relationship between training analyst and analysand, it proffers a wide variety of tools for not merely limiting but engendering change and becoming. There exists, to invoke two of the contributors to this volume, a "more and more of gender," a playful and joyful exuberance of gender that can come alive in the clinic, rather than be oppressed by it (Hansbury & Saketopoulou).

This collection thus proposes a critical investigation into numerous questions related to queerness, transness, gender, and sexuality. It joins a slew of publications that have come out over the past few years (Gherovici, 2017; Gherovici & Steinkoler, 2022; Giffney & Watson, 2017; Hutfless & Zach, 2022, to name a few) that converge around these subjects and propose radically different approaches to queerness and transness through the lens of critical psychoanalysis.

Our contributors have been invited to write about psychoanalysis' relationship with queerness and representations of queerness within the psychoanalytic archive, and how that heritage perdures in the present and creates various disruptive effects both within and beyond the clinic, with the aim being nothing less than a transformation of psychoanalysis itself.

Taken together these contributions constitute a decisive intervention into the psychoanalytic canon. They are an unabashed demand for accepting and furthering the representation and inclusion of queer, and in particular trans*, people within psychoanalysis. It is a call for action to utilize and deepen the enormous explicatory powers of psychoanalysis, to critically reevaluate psychoanalysis' historical relationship to queerness, and to bring together voices that have so far been denied a unity, breadth, and depth of expression.

The Question of Heritage

A central concern of this volume is the question of the queerness of psychoanalysis historically. To what extent can one speak of a queer history or heritage of psychoanalysis? And to what extent do queer histories of psychoanalysis survive in the present? How are we to interpret heritage both in its material and symbolic dimension, given its manifold conservative and right-wing uses as a colonial artifice and means of creating a stable past? Christina Sharpe makes a crucial point in her recent work *Ordinary Notes* (2023), following Michel-Rolph Trouillot (1995), that pastness is a position, which is also linked to a constant effusion of the seemingly bygone into the present. This argument resonates with Lacan's famous claim about history and the past and present: the past exists precisely to the extent that it is historicized in the present (1988, p. 12), both through conscious acts of memorialization, but also unconscious identifications.

Heritage is a particularly complex name for the question of material forms of memory, and for particular struggles against collective forgetfulness. Yet, we must also ask: whose forgetfulness is being aided? Is it that of the colonizer, who erects statues to assert white supremacist dominance in the present? Or is it about reconstructing après-coup de longue durée of Black survival? To what extent are minoritized modes of being – and in particular those located at the intersections of these modes – at all assimilable into processes of historicization? Could this impossibility of being included in history not mark its own form of resistance, precisely to the degree that history can be its own form of captivity?

The tradition of psychoanalysis has been reticent on such matters, often either eschewing questions of race and class altogether, while utilizing its own language of sexual difference and Oedipality to discuss matters of gender and sexuality. The authors assembled in this volume pursue a different course: theirs is an outspoken interest in the structural elements of psychic locality. One of psychoanalysis' main questions – who speaks? – is taken here not in a decontextualized way as the expression of a universal subject; instead, the position of speech is disarticulated and understood as contextual. The elaboration of this contextuality in turn opens up a new mode of psychoanalytic speech altogether, one that is concerned with matters of justice, exclusion, and belonging.

Can one then speak of a psychoanalytic heritage? Certainly, to the extent that any heritage relies on reification, which – to borrow a concept by Bion (2014) recently reworked by Moten (2019) – revolves around mystics and the people gathering around them. To the extent that such reification is resisted, however, heritage reveals itself as a complex ideological artifice that may not be reducible to any particular conceptual status, yet nevertheless may be used – and often has been – as a means of bolstering oppression.

Included in this volume are contributions that critically examine the question of heritage and tradition, being mindful of its noxious effects, while further delving into and expanding the possibilities of a queer psychoanalysis. As such, they open up queer and trans* modalities of psychoanalytic expression through readings of the archive, including the Freudo-Lacanian tradition, the British school, the work of Jean Laplanche, and the American interpersonalist tradition.

A Map to the Text

The texts gathered in this volume, although united by certain political commitments, are diverse in scope, content, approach, form, and execution. Some chapters are explicitly clinical, while others approach psychoanalysis from a metapsychological perspective; some are more personal, while others are more theoretical. A wide range of thinkers are represented herein, including – but not limited to – Freud, Klein, Bion, Lacan, Laplanche, and the American relational tradition, as well as French philosophers, among them Derrida, Kristeva, and Deleuze.

The volume opens with an intervention by Tobias Wiggins, Assistant Professor of Women's and Gender Studies, who announces that "The Transgender Psychoanalysts are Coming!" In his contribution, Wiggins explores the history of psychoanalysis, in particular the institution, and its incessant pathologization of queer and trans* subjects since its inception, despite some of its most fundamentally queer and gender nonconforming premises and insights. Indeed, psychoanalysis has "girded its loins" against queer and trans* subjectivities for over a century, beginning with Freud and the earliest psychoanalytic institutes, and continuing till this very day. Early psychoanalytic theorists laid the groundwork for the pathologization of queer, trans*, and gender nonconforming subjects when they deemed the "fetishist, homosexual, and transvestite" as perverse. Trans* people were almost exclusively cast into the realm of perversion or psychosis, their particularities and subjectivities dismissed, degraded, or worse. Queer and trans* individuals have had to fight to be heard as authorities in the field of psychoanalysis, and thankfully more and more voices are coming to the fore, including those presented in this anthology.

In their article, philosopher and psychoanalyst Esther Hutfless engages with the work of Jean Laplanche, Julia Kristeva, and Jacques Derrida in order to interrogate the "cage of gender" and propose an "ethics of *sexual différance*." Questioning some of the core assumptions of clinical psychoanalysis, such as the presumption of a binary gender identity, they suggest alternative ways of understanding gender and sexuality that lie beyond binary sexuation. Hutfless takes up Paul B. Preciado's critique, presented in "Can the Monster Speak?," of pathologizing discourses within psychoanalysis, most of which tie back to a binary gender difference, and questions this binary thinking (2021). They draw on a neologism and – in contrast to concepts such as "gender difference" or "sexual difference" which ultimately remain trapped in a binary – refer to an ethics of sexual différance, which for Hutfless becomes the starting point of a queer, non-binary, and non-normative psychoanalysis.

Following this, scholar and novelist Myriam Sauer offers a sustained reading of Swiss Kleinian psychoanalyst Danielle Quinodoz, investigating the implicit manifold assumptions that underlie the construction of Quinodoz's own method. Sauer borrows numerous ideas from the work of Wilfred Bion and Jean Laplanche in order to foreground the pedagogical strictures of Quinodoz's approach. She draws particular attention to the limitations placed upon gender expression, while at the same time highlighting the centrality of openness and indeterminacy.

Next philosopher Simone A. Medina Polo presents her research on Tiresias as the patron saint of psychoanalysis. The blind prophet was described as such by Jacques Lacan (2014) and has recently been taken up as a figure of psychoanalytic trans-formation in psychoanalysis by Patricia Gherovici (2017), Bracha L. Ettinger (Cavanagh, 2023), Sheila L. Cavanagh (2023), and Geneviève Morel (2006), among other theorists and practitioners. Medina Polo posits that at the heart of Tiresias there is an irreducible excess with which psychoanalysis is struggling to keep up. This has proliferated discontents around and within psychoanalytic practice and discourse, referred to as the symptom of psychoanalysis. In response, Tiresias has been proposed as the *sinthome* of psychoanalysis, insofar as he represents a creative strategy for the reinvigoration of psychoanalysis as it comes to terms with this restless element and re-embodies or trans-forms itself.

Clinical psychologist Elisabeth Punzi presents her work on H.D. and Bryher, focusing on their encounters with psychoanalysis in general, and with Freud and Sachs in particular. Punzi highlights how their queerness, non-normative gender identifications and presentations, and polyamorous relationships were not pathologized by the psychoanalysts they encountered. In fact, Bryher was encouraged by Freud to pursue the path towards becoming a lay analyst, which shows that Freud did not find Bryher's gender identity to be an issue or hindrance to becoming a psychoanalyst in any way, something of which modern day psychoanalytic institutions should take note. Punzi also reflects on the queerness of Pallas Athena, since a statue of Pallas Athena from Freud's collection of antiquities was important in H.D.'s discussion of her analysis with Freud in the volume *Tribute to Freud* (1956).

In her chapter "Trans Childhoods and the Family Romance," scholar and psychoanalytic practitioner M.E. O'Brien explores the role of fantasy among trans*children, particularly of belonging elsewhere, as a form of what Freud called "the family romance." Using material from first person accounts by trans*and gender nonconforming people, with a focus on the experimental memoir of the late trans* activist and writer Cecilia Gentili, to whom this book is dedicated, the essay explores the use of family romance fantasies in trans* children reconciling their emergent experiences of gender with conflicting social expectations. O'Brien posits that the family romance offers a way of theorizing the subject's encounters with the symbolic order as articulated in questions of sexual difference and biological origins. This essay links three moments of provisional transition: in Freud's evolving theories of childhood sexuality, in these children's changing and conflicted knowledge of gender and sex, and in this essay's partial theoretical contribution towards an adequate account of sexual difference. In this way, Freud's conception of the family romance may contribute to understanding the self-articulation of trans* childhood experience and the complexities of gender identification.

In "Transsexuality at the Origin of Desire," philosopher Luce deLire examines Freud's reading of Schreber, asking: what would a psychoanalytic approach to gender and desire look like that takes trans* experiences as its point of departure? Pointing out how trans* and non-binary people, and trans* women in particular, have been exploited and mistreated by the psychoanalytic community since the inception of this practice, deLire proposes that trans* women have been constitutive to the discipline of psychoanalysis, though until very recently their presence has been all but repressed. She develops a theory of transsexuality that aligns with Freud's originary views on polymorphous perversity, understanding transsexuality, not as a minority issue, but a *common* issue shared by all subjects of patriarchal societies: cis, non-binary, trans, and others alike. One is not born cis but rather becomes cis by virtue of an original displacement of the traumatic organization of the human psyche. deLire posits that real social change starts with an emancipation of such corporeal indeterminacy.

New York City-based psychoanalysts Griffin Hansbury and Avgi Saketopolou engage in a dissection of the clinical practice of psychoanalysis and its fraught relationship to transness and queerness in "Sissy Dance $1: The More and More of Gender." Critiquing the field's tendency to attack rather than foster the indetermination of gender, Saketopolou and Hansbury draw attention to psychoanalysis' fear of excess, insisting that trans* forms of life are not exclusively marked by loss, rejection, or exclusion but instead are potential sites of spontaneous exploration and transformation, invoking as an example the case of a trans* feminine performer.

Continuing in this conversational style, in "Dragging Psychoanalysis" drag practitioner and performer Geoffrey Hervey (Sin Clair) and psychoanalyst Lara Sheehi stage an intervention into the canon of psychoanalysis by engaging with the art form of drag. Pointing out that psychoanalysis has had little to say or theorize about the queer subculture and practice of drag, this chapter showcases multiple conversations between a variety of drag artists facilitated by Hervey, a psychoanalytic doctoral trainee. The conversations are presented herein with a lead-in conversation by two clinicians, Sheehi and Hervey – a mentor and her former student, who facilitated these conversations. The chapter, in its form and collaborative creation, attempts to challenge this particular oversight of queerness, while also highlighting the psychoanalytic richness within the drag artform.

In "Erotophobia: Or, Isn't Everyone A Pervert?," Assistant Professor of Clinical Psychoanalysis Gila Ashtor challenges the queer theory currently imported into psychoanalysis, which she posits is often the *narrow* (sexuality is bodily sex) position championed by a few critics, rather than the *expansive* (sexuality is an unsettled realm) position elaborated by so many foundational queer theorists. Ashtor elaborates that this uncritical embrace relies on a superficial, problematic version of queer theory that discounts the dynamics of relationality in favor of concrete *embodiment*. She claims this is why recent psychoanalytic writing on queer theory often sounds like it is equating radical *sex* with a radical *psyche*, or makes simplistic claims about certain desires as inherently revolutionary. Ashtor posits that this is not only a misrepresentation of queer theory, but fundamentally opposes the expansion of sexuality that is central to so much queer thought. She therefore calls for further exploration and elaboration of Jean Laplanche's *enlarged* sexuality to remedy this.

Utilizing autotheory, queer theory, psychoanalytic theory and praxis, and an engagement with bodies of queer ecological knowing, clinician and scholar Molly Merson presents "Freud Would Not Be Queer Without Us," inviting a consideration of psychoanalysis as a living, breathing, sensory system through which queer life is engaged, invited, and shaped through retrospective meaning-making in the context of oppressive systems.

Finally, the anthology concludes with psychoanalyst Ken Corbett's "Credo," in which he proposes a general axiomatics of clinical practice that draws on various psychoanalytic and philosophical sources. He encourages us to rethink our psychoanalytic beliefs to include the potentials that are not in our consulting rooms, to include patients who remain outside the setting, and to reach toward modes of practice and care that we cannot yet imagine.

Bibliography

Bion, W.R. (2014). *Attention and Interpretation: A Scientific Approach to Insight in Psycho-Analysis and Groups.* Ed. by Chris Mawson. London and New York: Routledge.

Cavanagh, S.L. (2023). "Tiresias and the Other Sexual Difference: Jacques Lacan and Bracha L. Ettinger." In Gherovici, P. and Steinkoler, M. (Eds.) *Psychoanalysis, Gender, and Sexualities: From Feminism to Trans*.* London: Routledge. pp. 197–211.

Davis, O. and Dean, T. (2022). *Hatred of Sex.* Lincoln and London: University of Nebraska Press.

Dean, T. (2009). *Unlimited Intimacy: Reflections on the Subculture of Barebacking.* Chicago: University of Chicago Press.

Derrida, J. (1991). "Geopsychoanalysis: '...and the Rest of the World'." Trans. by Donald Nicholson-Smith. In *American Imago,* 48.2, pp. 199–231.

Derrida, J. (1997). *Archive Fever: A Freudian Impression.* Trans. by Eric Prenowitz. Chicago: University of Chicago Press.

Edelman, L. (1994). *Homographesis: Essays in Gay Literary and Cultural Theory.* New York: Routledge.

Edelman, L. (2004). *No Future: Queer Theory and the Death Drive.* Durham: Duke University Press.

Edelman, L. (2011). "Against Survival: Queerness in a Time That's Out of Joint." In: *Shakespeare Quarterly,* 62.2, pp. 148–169.

Edelman, L. (2023). *Bad Education: Why Queer Theory Teaches Us Nothing.* Durham: Duke University Press.

Freud, S. (1951). "Historical Notes: A Letter from Freud." In: *The American Journal of Psychiatry,* 107.10, pp. 786–787.

Gherovici, P. (2017). *Transgender Psychoanalysis: A Lacanian Psychoanalysis.* London and New York: Routledge.

Gherovici, P. and Steinkoler, M. (Eds.) (2022). *Psychoanalysis, Gender, and Sexualities: From Feminism to Trans*.* New York: Routledge.

Giffney, N. and Watson, E. (Eds.) (2017). *Clinical Encounters in Sexuality: Psychoanalytic Practice and Queer Theory.* Brooklyn: Punctum Books.

H.D. (1956). *Tribute to Freud.* New York: New Directions.

Hutfless, E. and Zach, B. (Eds.) (2022). *Queering Psychoanalysis. Psychoanalyse und Queer Theory: Transdisziplinäre Verschränkungen.* Munster: Edition Assemblage.

Khanna, R. (2003). *Dark Continents: Psychoanalysis and Colonialism.* Durham: Duke University Press.

Klein, M. (1975). "Love, Guilt and Reparation." In: *Love, Guilt, and Reparation and Other Works (1921–1945).* New York: Free Press.

Lacan, J. (1988). *The Seminar of Jacques Lacan I. Freud's Papers on Technique (1953–1954).* Ed. by Jacques-Alain Miller. Trans. by John Forrester. New York and London: Cambridge University Press/Norton.

Lacan, J. (2014). *The Seminar of Jacques Lacan, Book X: Anxiety (1962–1963).* Ed. by J-A. Miller. Trans. by A.R. Prince. London: Polity.

Laplanche, J. (1996). "Psychoanalysis as Anti-Hermeneutics." In *Radical Philosophy,* 79, pp. 7–12.

Marriott, D. (2000). *On Black Men.* New York: Columbia University Press.

Marriott, D. (2007). *Haunted Life: Visual Culture and Black Modernity.* New Brunswick: Rutgers University Press.

Marriott, D. (2018). *Whither Fanon? Studies in the Blackness of Being.* Stanford: Stanford University Press.

Marriott, D. (2021). *Lacan Noir. Lacan and Afro-Pessimism.* London: Palgrave Macmillan.

Morel, G. (2006). "The Sexual Sinthome." Trans. Roland Végső. In *Umbr(a): Incurable,* 1, pp. 65–83.

Moten, F. (2019). "The Mystic Group." In *Studies in Gender and Sexuality,* 20.2, pp. 101–105.

Preciado, P.B. (2021). *Can the Monster Speak? Report to an Academy of Psychoanalysts.* Trans. Wynne F. Cambridge, MA: semiotext(e).

Rose, J. (2005). *Sexuality in the Field of Vision.* London and New York: Verso.

Sharpe, C. (2023). *Ordinary Notes.* New York: Farrar, Straus and Giroux.

Silverman, K. (2009). *Flesh of My Flesh.* Stanford: Stanford University Press.

Spillers, H.J. (1996). "'All the Things You Could Be By Now, If Sigmund Freud's Wife Was Your Mother': Psychoanalysis and Race." In *boundary 2,* 23.3, pp. 75–141.

Trouillot, M-R. (1995). *Silencing the Past: Power and the Production of History.* Boston: Beacon Press.

Wark, M. (2022). "Dear Cis Analysts. A Call for Reparations." In *Parapraxis* 02. URL: https://www.parapraxismagazine.com/articles/dear-cis-analysts. Accessed: March 11, 2024.

Chapter 1

Gird Your Loins
The Transgender Psychoanalysts are Coming!

Tobias Wiggins

To "gird your loins" is a common idiom with a comical edge, a metonymic and thus anticipatory expression (Kövecses, 2016). As a declaration, it is meant to warn of an upcoming difficulty or strenuous undertaking. The saying can also be used to assign danger or menace to something external and felt to be encroaching, whether or not that proposed danger is truly real or substantive. In that way, this figure of speech generates an assumed peril before it arrives, while also undercutting that danger with hyperbole. In its biblical origins, loin girding was reserved for men and entailed the tucking of a long garment between the legs to enable physical action. These gendered and sexed ideologies were further coded to reinforce gentlemanly, colonial ventures such as war (Low, 2011). In tandem with protecting one's genitals then, discursively, the girdee protected specific virile boundaries of subjectivity and nation.

The institution of psychoanalysis has been girding its loins against transgender subjects since its inception,[1] despite some of its most fundamentally queer and gender nonconforming premises (Freud, 1905/2011; Butler, 1990; Dean, 2000; Edelman, 2004; Gherovici, 2010; Giffney & Watson, 2017; this volume). Through a pronounced attention to genitality, binarism, and a dense history of homo- and trans-phobic cases, clinical psychoanalysis has almost exclusively cast transgender subjectivities into the realm of either perversion (Wiggins, 2020, 2022) or psychosis (Hansbury, 2017b; Salah, 2018). Indeed, by way of the now bygone theoretical trifecta fetishist/homosexual/transvestite, those with wayward gendered convictions were seen to be the *worst* regressed and *most* attached to a "too close" mother (Bak, 1953). These early, well-supported psychoanalytic perspectives have laid a sturdy groundwork for assorted clinical dismissals, or outright degradation, of gender nonconforming subjectivities and these theories have evolved over time. Echoing our opening expression's antagonism between danger and dismissal, transgender people have been treated as a serious threat to the various gender-based Western normativities embedded within psychoanalytic organizations, while simultaneously being painted as inconsequential and humorous given their assumedly profound psychological deviance.

Within contemporary clinical psychoanalysis, a growing body of scholarship has endeavored to correct and challenge such transphobic legacies (Gherovici &

DOI: 10.4324/9781032624129-2

Steinkoler, 2023), which, although notably dampened, still do hold an authorita-tive anachronistic foothold in some parts of the field (see, for example, Bell, 2020; Miller, 2021). As of late, however, we have also witnessed a significant uptick in concerned psychoanalytic debates and dialogues about clinical work with this population (Blass et al., 2021; Gozlan et al., 2022). A slew of fresh psychoanalytic articles, special issues, and conference panels have cropped up, all examining the contours of trans life and potential therapeutic approaches to work with transgen-der, nonbinary, and gender nonconforming identifications. Frequently framed as a benevolent or curious exploration, this recent influx mirrors the current inunda-tion of similar dialogues accompanying anti-trans moral panics in the mainstream imaginary[2] (Elster, 2022). Additionally, in some cases, it seems that professional psychoanalytic communities may have actually been the instigators of these more sweeping, anxious public controversies that have ultimately resulted in repres-sive laws and restricted trans healthcare services (Osserman & Wallerstein, 2022). These emergent tensions have been especially heated in relation to transgender and gender creative youth, whose more tenuous agency makes them a prime vector for unmetabolized and newly tabooed transphobic affects.

This chapter engages with these prevalent contentions from the under-considered, yet consequential, issue of transgender people's systemic exclusion from the pro-fessional status of "psychoanalyst." This notable gap is further amplified by insti-tutional psychoanalysis' minimal, if not altogether absent, engagement with the wealth of rich, intersectional transgender studies scholarship – even that which travels in psychoanalytic thought (see, for example, Prosser, 1998; Awkward-Rich, 2017; Salah 2017; Israeli-Nevo, 2019; Breslow, 2021). Institutional psychoanalysis' girding against trans subjects has, thus far, been primarily challenged by cisgender clinicians who have labored arduously to address the overarching essentialization of gender and sex, and the possibility of non-discriminatory clinical work with this underserved population. Their efforts have been instrumental in a setting where it has been impossible for transgender people's perspectives to be heard otherwise; and if they are permitted to be heard, they may only be experienced as monstrous (Preciado, 2021). However, as important disruptions of long-worn norms begin to take hold and rouse change, the most rudimentary move of meaningful profes-sional inclusion has not taken place. To be clear, trans people do notice this glaring omission. As McKenzie Wark (2023) writes in her open letter to cis analysts as a call for reparations: "Dear Psychoanalysts, I'm going to assume nearly all of you are cis, even though you may have trans patients. There's so few trans analysts. And why is that? And what are you doing about it" (p. 38)?

With such a stark statement, some readers may feel an impulse to defend the gains that have taken place or innumerate the transgender, nonbinary, and gender nonconforming people they know in the psychoanalytic field. There have surely been perceptible institutional shifts and some public attempts at repair. For ex-ample, the American Psychoanalytic Association (APsaA) and the psychoanalytic division of the American Psychological Association (APA) have both recently issued formal apologies for harms caused to LGBTQ+ communities through pathologization and conversion therapies.[3] Over the past ten years, many institutes now periodically offer continuing education courses with titles such as *Emergent Gender-Sexualities* or *Trans in Transition*.[4] Institutional psychoanalysis has also been fortunate to receive contributions from three transgender psychoanalysts.[5] Griffin Hansbury's prolific writing (2004, 2005a, 2005b, 2017a, 2022) includes a highly cited piece which addresses psychotic countertransference in a century of psychoanalytic writing (2017b) and another unprecedented contribution on the trans-trans analytic dyad (2011). Jack Pula (2015) made a critical intervention with his personal narrative of undergoing a psychoanalysis as an analyst-in-training while he was transitioning. In this troubling case, his analyst could not make sense of his gender transition outside of pathology, which created an impasse, ending the treatment.[6] Finally, although not explicitly connecting his identity to his work, Oren Gozlan has written extensively (2008, 2011, 2015, 2018, 2022) on gender's enigmatic qualities, retroactive meanings, and the implications of its constant push for settlement: "everyone is duped by gender's apparent obviousness" (2018, p. 6). Turning to art, literature, and aesthetics, Gozlan unearths novel and generous openings into some of the most divisive issues within psychoanalysis, such as transsexual surgery and hormone blockers.

Given the increasing visibility of cisgender allies and accomplices within psychoanalysis, there is also no doubt that more transgender people are involved in training institutes than ever before, who have not yet begun to present or publish.[7] And without question, there are many others who, for various reasons, cannot or will choose not to bring their identity to the fore. Homonormative narratives of being "out" are often framed as an agentic imperative for self-acceptance. They do not easily capture the complex fields of visibility and invisibility that many transgender people navigate. As Gossett, Stanley & Burton (2017) have emphasized, trans visibility under neoliberalism can function like a "trap door": it may open a pathway through which we finally access livable lives, while simultaneously aggravating our exposure to discursive or overt violences, extractive/exploitative representations, and the disproportionate possibility of death, especially for trans women of colour. It is, of course then, not surprising that the very few transgender people who have been able to train and write in psychoanalytic journals are those who hold additional intersections of privilege: they are white, transmasculine, and practice in presiding North American cities such as New York, which is a Western colonial epicenter and veritable hub for institutes and critical psychoanalysis.

However, even with these, and perhaps other advances in mind, a chronic climate of anxiety and gatekeeping surrounding trans subjectivities within psychoanalysis persists. To put the number of visible transgender psychoanalysts into perspective, the International Psychoanalytic Association (IPA) includes more than 13,000 psychoanalysts as members and works with 70 constituent organizations (IPA, 2023). There are also numerous non-IPA-affiliated psychoanalytic institutes across the globe whose many alumni would not be included in those numbers. Given the sustained scarceness of transgender psychoanalysts, even the most reflexive clinical material inadvertently yet repeatedly assigns transgender people to the status of "patient" from whom the cisgender psychoanalyst may learn something about gender. If escaping the role of patient, trans people's supposed inherent gender subversion has acted primarily as cisgender inspiration for ethical debate, or fodder for opposing restrictive gendered conventions. In addition to these well-intentioned but nonetheless objectifying practical uses of trans subjects, this framing may contribute to a lasting difficulty in seeing transgender people as potential colleagues.

The apologies that have circulated thus far lump transgender people into the larger LGB acronym, a move that dilutes the specific barriers and perpetual medical violence that transgender people endure. Additionally, there are often many competing, politicized motivations behind public apologies that have more to do with the delineation of power than with genuine repair. When not matched with meaningful action, apologies can have contradictory effects, much like the Canadian government's 2008 apology to Indigenous peoples for the genocidal practice of residential schools, which has not led to an abatement of systemic colonial violence (Thobani, 2023). In fact, such practices of reconciliation often conversely re-establish the status-quo, by primarily making white people feel better about themselves and generating new "shape shifting" forms of colonization (Corntassel, 2012; Simpson, 2016). Public statements of remorse therefore often conceal and preserve aggression (Greenberg, 2012; Segal, 1973), acting as psychosocial relief for its perpetrators, which in turn brings about more insidious forms of harm.

Psychoanalysis' vast contributions to transgender pathology, including a distinctive archive of writing gender nonconformance into madness and its present manifestations in transgender debates, have not been adequately addressed by crucial governing bodies such as the IPA and APsaA. The lack of fulsome acknowledgement and an absence of transparent commitment to substantive change means that authentic reparations with transgender people in psychoanalysis are currently inconceivable. The insufficient or merely performative recognition of ongoing destructive impulses will lead only to repeated, yet uniquely disguised, expressions of prejudice. These often stealthier displays of transphobia can then be refolded into intellectual culture and institutional practices, appearing through curriculum, the content of publications in reputable journals, professional listservs, interpersonal microaggressions, low acceptance and completion rates of trans candidates, binary gender infrastructure and policy, and formal or informal supervision. Typically conducted with discretion, many of these practices further aim to muzzle dissident voices who present views on gender and sexuality that may still be experienced by the institution as ego-dystonic. One unmistakable example of such protective impetus recently materialized when the *International Journal of Psychoanalysis (IJP)* obstructed publication of the IPA Tiresias Award paper.

Avgi Saketopoulou and Ann Pellegrini's (2023) well-received book, *Gender Without Identity*, was born from this repression. The preface, titled "a book that was not meant to be" (p. vii), endeavors to summarize the shameful trajectory of impasses, enforced by the *IJP*, the oldest psychoanalytic journal, which was established by Freud. Their original paper, titled "A Feminine Boy: Normative Investments and Reparative Fantasy at the Intersections of Gender, Race, and Religion," won the inaugural Tiresias Award in 2021. The award itself was a monumental achievement. Inspired by polymorphism and ambiguity within the Tiresias myth (Posadas, 2023), it aimed to foster gender and sexuality diversity-based knowledge within the IPA and psychoanalysis more broadly. Their paper was formally accepted and thoroughly edited by the *IJP* to mutual agreement, but everything changed when the authors added a final, footnoted acknowledgement. The journal claimed that these statements were too political and requested that the following lines be removed:

> This project insists on welcoming "queer" subjects (patients as well as candidates and analysts) who have too often been treated as problems *for* psychoanalysts rather than as offering opportunities from which to think our metapsychology anew. Wresting such spaces is not easy nor always pleasant, but it is necessary and *critical to psychoanalysis' survival...* May future generations of queer and trans analysts and patients never encounter what many of us who are queer-identified have had to: that, more than anything, is the vision of our work in this paper (Saketopoulou & Pellegrini, 2023, p. xi, emphasis in original).

I cite this section in full to amplify its message, but also to consider more closely what, precisely, had imperiled the *IJP*'s political equilibrium. It is undeniable that these select lines were felt to be tremendously fraught, as the journal not only refused publication without their deletion, but further, aimed to suppress the publication of this work overall.[8] The article itself openly discusses widespread transphobia within psychoanalysis, proposes that trans people should be granted the "dignity of belief" (p. 54), and draws upon Laplanche to argue that gender subjectification is a process of "self-theorization" and a translation of trauma that all subjects undergo (including cisgender people). So, while all contentious notions within psychoanalysis, it was not these topics that were of concern to the *IJP*. Instead, the censored statement maintains that queer and trans people *should be invited into the profession of psychoanalysis*, not only as patients, "but also as colleagues, teachers, and analysts" (Saketopoulou & Pellegrini, p. xi). Bolstering this striking and anomalous call, the authors stress that these minoritarian subjects will offer pivotal contributions, yet to be seen, that may even save psychoanalysis. They invoke a future where queer and trans analysts can simply exist, unscathed by the unnamed encounters faced by their predecessors. The *IJP*'s wildly disproportionate response to this footnote highlights that moving queer and trans subjects away from mere conceptual inspiration and into the role of a valuable collaborator threatens to undermine something foundational within psychoanalysis.

As a queer and transgender scholar of Women's and Gender Studies, my interest in psychoanalysis originally bloomed through exposure to critical and nuanced interdisciplinary feminist scholarship. It was not until late in my PhD that I first ventured into what I now sometimes like to jokingly call "psychoanalysis proper,"[9] or its clinical and professional domains. At that time, I was quickly taken aback by the foreclosed thinking I encountered regarding marginalized identities and politicized topics, often hedged in analytic neutrality. From my non-clinical, humanities and university-based perspective, psychoanalytic thinking had produced some of the most inspired interventions to the knotted, unbridled social problems and violences of our time. How was it that these practitioners of dreaming, the unconscious, free associations, and polymorphous desiring had become so fixed and confined in their approach to difference? From my outsider standpoint, I had assumed that the innately deconstructive and non-prescriptive nature of psychoanalysis would garner expansive therapeutic approaches, and that they would be of distinct value to non-normative and minoritarian subjectivities.

After almost 15 years of laboring along the perimeters of psychoanalysis proper, I have fielded innumerable psychical assaults against my transness. The assorted extension courses I took within institutes repeatedly referenced and openly discussed overtly transphobic material without critical analysis. On a break during one such training course, I even had a highly regarded teaching analyst, who knew I am a transgender man, purposefully hand me the women's key when I enquired about a bathroom. Despite navigating such consistent aggressions, my abiding appreciation for psychoanalytic thought led to the eventual pursuit of a psychoanalytic training. However, the requisite training analysis[10] quickly erected additional, insurmountable barriers. When consulting with potential training analysts – all of whom were affluent, and also holding some combination of being white, cis, straight, male psychiatrists close to retirement – I was met with an abundance of creatively inappropriate questions about my gender transition, including fascinated inquiries about my genitals and clichéd assumptions about my sexuality. Even if I could bear their hegemonic positionalities and invasively uninformed clinical moves, after initial meetings, many of them found seemingly innocuous reasons to excuse themselves from the training analysis. Through their actions and inexperience, my access to training was indirectly shuttered.

As I carry the weight of these experiences and try to imagine what might be possible for psychoanalysis' trans-mutation or "sex change" (Gherovichi, 2011), lately I have found myself daydreaming about the queerly beloved film *The Devil Wears Prada* (Frankel, 2006). In one of the most memorable opening scenes, the fiercely driven and much feared editor-in-chief, Miranda Priestly (iconically played by Meryl Streep), steps a single suede heel out of her chauffeur's car onto New York City's streets. As she heads pointedly towards a fictional headquarters of the Vogue-inspired, high-fashion *Runway* magazine, her office erupts into an anxious, preparatory frenzy. "She's not supposed to be here till nine... Alright everyone: Gird your Loins!" shouts Nigel – the film's token gay best friend – as papers fly, unhealthy snacks are tossed in the waste bin, and comfortable clogs are swapped for Dolce pumps.

Like the alarm rising upon Priestly's impending office arrival, when it comes to gender difference, it feels as though many psychoanalysts are once again hyperbolically battening their institutional hatches, hunkering down on familiar dogmatic concepts, and tucking away their most precious professional parts for fear of a fantasized loss. Clinical psychoanalysis' loins, it seems, may be enduringly threatened by its own haunting legend of the perverse or psychotic transexual, one generated by a phallic woman or mother (Bak, 1968), and her fetishized, encroaching suede high heel. I have witnessed countless gutting examples of the appearance of this phantasm at conferences and public talks, yet one instance will forever stand out in my mind. Only a few years ago, at a large, esteemed event in Canada, a keynote speaker delivered a case study wherein his patient was troubled by an enmeshment with his purported "phallic mother." The concluding surprise kernel of the case was the analyst's enlightening discovery, one which uncovered the unconscious repetition of a relational perversion: delivered as a titillating punchline, the presenter finished his talk by revealing the patient's current partner happened to be a transgender woman. The patient, he implied, sustained this relationship due to his enmeshment with his "phallic mother" and thus suffered from a regressive, fetishistic illness.

The injury of this moment extended beyond its singular and quotidian transphobic enunciation – that is, one in which a trans subject is reduced to genital morphology, where nuanced psychoanalytic theories of gender have been collapsed into pejorative sexed essentialism, and finally, a trans partner is degraded to the status of a mere cisgender symptom. This single interpretation stretched even farther, across a whole psychoanalytic institution that had fostered and supported this analyst's line of thinking and his clinical interventions that, in turn, facilitated an entitlement to wield trans pathology for professional clout. The subsequent lack of reproach from the audience, save for a few concerned remarks primarily uttered from queer scholars, left me deeply unsettled. I certainly worried for my own psychological safety in this space, but I was also struck with a profound concern for the patient's psychic life and for his partner. And as a trans man, I felt a familiar rage well up for trans women who disproportionately face the brunt of overt and discursive transphobic violence based in transmisogyny (Serano, 2007). But finally, given my interest in training, in this familiar setting of a psychoanalytic lecture hall full of cisgender people unconscientiously volleying their fascinations about transgender subjectivity around the room, I wondered anew how any gender nonconforming person could ever feasibly become, or even desire to become, a psychoanalyst.

Rebuttals against transgender pathologization in clinical psychoanalytic writings have taken three primary forms; however, none of these have yet focused upon the dearth of transgender perspectives in the field, nor have they speculated on what such contributions may bring. First, a revisionist move has worked to showcase the queerer and more polymorphous, less rigidly materialist and binary interpretations of several canonical thinkers such as Freud (Salamon, 2004; Yadlin-Gadot, 2023), Lacan (Carlson, 2010; Cavanagh, 2018; Coffman, 2022), Winnicott (Gozlan, 2022), and, most recently, Laplanche (Saketopoulou & Pellegrini, 2023). Over the last decade, these authors have broadened the presiding hetero- and cis-normative psychoanalytic understandings of gender, sex, and the body; a heterogeneous intervention with notable consequence for all subjects, while additionally carving out a novel, less perilous space for those who are transgender. Second, and often overlapping, these amended theories have been applied to clinical vignettes with transgender patients, calling attention to their value and practical application in a potentially affirming[11] psychoanalysis (see, for example, Gherovici, 2017; Gozlan, 2011; Saketopoulou, 2014). However, given the over-saturation of professional fissures on the topic of transgender subjectivity, many published clinical vignettes also recount practitioners' unintentional, yet potentially damaging prejudices as they are enacted in the consulting room. Subsequently, a third and most recent wave of scholarship has focused more pointedly upon the clinician's trans-specific and/or transphobic countertransference, that is, the ways the analyst's unconscious gendered life and bias can be felt, acted out, and – depending on the school of thought – potentially used within treatment with trans people.

We must credit Hansbury's (2017b) instrumental piece here, which, in surveying the unthinkable anxieties of transphobia in written psychoanalytic history, has set the stage for contemporary analysts to candidly discuss their own countertransference reactions to their transgender and gender nonconforming patients. This emerging work, which now includes two special issues on the topic (Evzonas 2021, 2022), has considered a wide range of countertransferential affects and enactments. Analysts have explored typical anxieties and fears that arise in the face of transition-related desires such as, for example, gender-affirming surgery or hormones (Kloppenberg, 2021; Silverman, 2023), as well as more "rogue" countertransference feelings like excitement, envy, and disgust (Harris, 2022; Hansbury & Saketopoulou, 2022). Others have tackled the paradoxical clinical hindrances that arise when trying to be a "safe analyst" for transgender people (Porchat & Santos, 2021), of wanting to "do good" (Gherovici, 2022), or to be a supportive "transgender expert" (Offman, 2023).

Hilary Offman's (2023) relational-constructivist article "On Being an Expert-Enough Expert" dismantles the commonplace assumption that a therapist must hold a gender nonconforming identity or transpositive expertise to work effectively with transgender clients. When one of her long-term patients, Sam, decides to undergo a gender transition during treatment, he at first attempts to find a new therapist who is also trans. Offman professes that "at the time, this made complete sense to me" (p. 50). However, Sam eventually returned, explaining the trans therapist he visited was "too weird" and given the general lack of trans therapists, he was choosing to stay with her. Offman then began to doubt her previous discernment, wondering "why I had so readily assumed that a transgender expert, not a cisgender heteronormative like me, would automatically be the best... I had no idea, and still don't whether transgender analysts work differently from cisgender analysts or what their work might look like if they did" (p. 50). Instead of drawing upon a shared social location or specific trans competency then, she employed her dialectical expertise, revealing how her own cisgender identity and a "politically correct deference to the other's opinion" (p. 56) surfaced in the transference-countertransference matrix.

This expanding genre of clinical writing on the perils of being "transpositive," "good," or "safe" reveals a nascent psychical trouble for earnestly supportive psychoanalysts, who are not only rapidly learning about the lived experiences of transgender people but may be newly encountering these patients in their practice. Offman's intercession is significant, as she normalizes concerns about causing harm due to inexperience with this population, which could decrease clinician's avoidance of these issues. But this type of encouragement is also double-edged. On one hand, she reminds cisgender psychoanalysts that their distinctive expertise lays in an attunement to the unconscious, and thus any preconceived knowing (about gender transition or elsewise) could in fact impede the psychoanalytic process. As most psychoanalytic modalities value ambiguity and the overdetermined, any rigid approaches to being a supportive ally might significantly restrain insight and therapeutic action. Offman's framing thus challenges the taken-for-granted notion that specialized trans competency is required, or even an asset, which could accordingly improve analysts' confidence and willingness to take on transgender clients.

Yet on the other hand, although unintended, this stance could also problematically justify the psychoanalytic convention of disregarding even the most rudimentary transgender knowledges and clinical contributions. As the dogmatism endemic to professional psychoanalysis (Kirsner, 2000) continues to keep such perspectives at bay, Offman's bolstering of an innate clinical expertise may unfortunately work to further reconsolidate a cisgender hegemony within psychoanalysis. Consequently, it is more likely that many avoidable harms – and these harms extend far beyond the examples surveyed in this chapter – can be explained away as merely being proper psychoanalytic technique. Ultimately, even the humblest and most reflexive "expert-enough expertise" will be deficient if it is generated alongside the active, systemic, and largely unchallenged exclusion of potential transgender colleagues. While it is necessary for psychoanalysts to examine their countertransferential responses to transgender clients, particularly within our increasingly hostile political climate, we must also assess how this type of scholarship uncritically recenters cisgender voices and concerns. Moreover, when authors focus chiefly on the "restrictive" and "rigid" aspects of transpositive clinical approaches, these otherwise manifold and often trans-led interventions can be easefully split off as "not really psychoanalytic." Instead of theorizing innovative bridges between such purportedly disparate ways of knowing, many transpositive insights are cast as controlling or omnipotent politically correct discourse and are left outside of accepted criteria for an authentic psychoanalytic exchange.[12]

To be clear, I do not mean to imply that transgender psychoanalysts will necessarily be the best option for transgender analysands, nor that they would innately be the experts on those client's needs and experience. This understanding of identity-based therapeutic proficiency erroneously hinges upon first, the tacit reduction of transgender psychic life to some helpful underlying identitarian unity; and second, the idea that such a fantasized commonality will be innately therapeutically beneficial. The transgender psychoanalysts for whom we have not yet had the pleasure of encountering, if given the chance, will assuredly impart vastly divergent theories, perspectives, and interventions. As trans philosopher Penelope Haulotte (2023) has effectively argued, the idea that trans people share narrative coherence, or that there are harmonious characteristics within all trans life, necessarily "adopt[s] a cisgender orientation towards the question of trans identity" (pp. 36–37). In other words, when transgender studies scholars emphasize or try to find "resemblances between [trans] properties, bodies, or experiences" (p. 37), they enduringly rely on a cis-medicalized notion that there is something essential about transgender life to be uncovered. As an alternative, Haulotte sets a course towards transgender existentialism, which instead "sees the unity of trans people as essentially precarious" (p. 37). What trans people truly have in common is a *situation*, one in which we collectively face the multifaceted oppressive forces of a particular dominant gendered position, or the "alienation and unfreedom" (p. 37) that accompany cisgender society. In this collective situation, what trans people actually share is a contrary, or perhaps queer, responsibility towards dismantling their unity.

As I have shown throughout this chapter, within professional psychoanalysis this unified cis-tuation has taken many shapes, ultimately leading to the sustained, institutionalized omission of transgender psychoanalysts and their unique contributions, which, as Saketopoulou (2020) has emphatically stated, are "critical to building the knowledge base of psychoanalysis" (p. 1020). This continued absence is no accident. On an elementary level, it reflects a prolonged unwillingness to take meaningful accountability for a vastly destructive history of transphobic discourse and clinical practice. Our shared circumstance is also one of blatantly insufficient action on behalf of psychoanalytic institutions to directly address and curtail these still normalized and now diversified iterations of discrimination. Given this paucity, those transgender people who do attempt to venture across the girded boundary into psychoanalysis proper may find themselves isolated, vulnerable to injury, and without clear recourse against persistent gender-based aggressions. This risk is heightened if they hold additional intersections of marginalization or do not reside in a city center with a critical psychoanalytic community. While psychoanalytic writing that aims to disrupt the cisnormative status-quo has made essential intercessions, it simply has not yet been enough to pry open doors tenaciously shuttered to those very subjects. Which should leave analysts who "ha[ve] no idea, and still don't whether transgender analysts work differently from cisgender analysts or what their work might look like if they did," (p. 50) considering instead: how is it possible that this question is still being asked and what, precisely, are the implications of its rhetoric?

When Talia Mae Bettcher (2019) explored the question "what *is* trans philosophy?" (p. 2) in her field-defining article, she emphasized the importance of certain presuppositions, or starting points, that are necessarily built into its methodological commitments. While (cis) philosophy has been most fascinated by inquiries like "What is a woman?" or "What is a man?," and may correspondingly interrogate the nature of trans personhood or its validity, trans philosophy instead begins from the underlying premise that "trans self-identities are at least presumptively valid: It should be taken for granted, for example, that if a trans man says he is a man, he is, indeed, a man" (p. 10). In its liberation from such well-worn topics and speculations, trans philosophers place value and relevance in different inquiries. For example, Bettcher highlights that we may be more interested in a pressing issue like "why do people want to kill us? WTF?" (p. 8), which would otherwise not be investigated: "Alas, the fascinated philosopher may not even be aware of the host of other philosophical questions that arise for trans people—particularly as they are geared toward illumination in the WTF" (p. 14). Similarly, within professional psychoanalysis, the centering of a cisgender outlook has brought about a restriction on what questions are feasible as many trans methodological starting points have not yet been conceived.

I have established how the revisionist approaches to cis-heteronormative psychoanalysis still focus primarily on gender's meanings and etymologies, while clinical case studies have, with a few notable exceptions, drawn upon a cis analyst/trans patient dyad. The predominance of a cisgender standpoint in psychoanalytic writing about transgender people has allowed for only a particular set of questions to be asked, such as: "How can a cisgender psychoanalyst, with little to no knowledge about transgender lives, ethically and effectively work with a transgender patient?," or "Should I use my client's new pronouns without interrogation, especially if changed to something unfamiliar like *they/them*?," or "If I write a medical letter supporting my client's physical transition, am I stepping outside of the analytic frame to the detriment of the analysis?," and, finally, "Is it really a true psychoanalysis if I'm (trans)affirming?". These and other familiar starting points carry assorted connotations and can lead to disparate outcomes, depending upon factors like the analyst's unconscious life, the sociopolitical context, and institutional expectations. It is also possible for transgender scholars to become preoccupied with extinguishing the conceptual fires that this shared cis-tuation entails, which could result in a truncation of their other concerns.

Nevertheless, a transgender clinician may arrive to psychoanalytic theorizing with a set of presuppositions that stretch and overturn the very grounds from which we habitually begin. Since these transgender starting points have not yet materialized, it is impossible to foresee their various permutations. Following Bettcher (2019), however, we can surmise that many will be invested in an illumination of the WTF, both within psychoanalytic theory and perhaps too, as it arises for their clients within the consulting room. The WTF question "why do people want to kill us?" will take different shapes in this specific professional context. Beyond physical violence, psychoanalysis can account for the ways that trans people's life chances are starkly diminished through the institutionalized conditions that threaten their long-term existence (Spade, 2015). These circumstances could prompt a transgender analyst to illuminate the WTF by asking, for example: "What is the impact of a distinct lack of transgender therapists on transgender people's psychic life?," or "How does the recurrent denial of transgender healthcare and gatekeeping appear in the transference, especially when a letter supporting physical transition has been written without hesitation?," or "How does clinical psychoanalysis actively contribute to trans death, and how can psychoanalysis instead advance trans survival?".

Since these and other trans methodological starting points are still considered un-orthodox, they may be experienced as "too weird" or "not really psychoanalytic" by colleagues and clients alike. However, this eccentricity is precisely what should be pursued over any basic transgender "inclusion" within psychoanalysis proper.

As queer and critical race theories have established, the politics of institutional inclusion are rife with harmful concessions (Duggan, 2003; Puar, 2007; Ahmed, 2012). Acceptance is often predicated upon the homogenization of the previously excluded category (i.e. homonormativity), and to varying degrees, one must collude with an otherwise unchanged organization to be welcomed. These sacrifices for legibility often encourage the further peripheralization of transgender people who do not inhabit additional dominant subject positions, such as whiteness and hetero-sexuality, as well as pressure to separate from social justice issues still labelled as too radical, such as decolonial and Palestinian movements. Under neoliberalism, such representational justice (deLire, 2023) can satisfy extractive requirements to appear equitable by showcasing trans bodies and minds, while simultaneously per-petuating violence against them.

In this setting then, transgender people's biggest asset is their still unfaltering irreconcilability with clinical psychoanalysis in its present form. The profession's continued systemic girding against transgender people demonstrates that the ex-ploitative forces of inclusion, which primarily function to sustain existing power dynamics, have not yet fully established themselves within trans-psychoanalytic relations – however, those normalizing forces are surely knocking. Consequently, when cis interlocutors turn away from cis starting points towards the active and bold interventions that will bring transgender people in, they should be accompa-nied by a wish to erode other protective boundaries encasing the profession. They must welcome forms of transgender desire, pleasure, and suffering that exceed the containment offered by psychoanalysis proper, including its over-prescribed theo-ries and clinical approaches. To this end, transgender psychoanalysts certainly pose a real threat to professional psychoanalysis' loins. Our contributions have the capacity to alter the foundations of cherished institutional values, to overturn our shared cis-tuation, and to reshape a substantive expansion of the parameters which resolutely define "true psychoanalysis." While it may be disquieting to invite such a rupture, the field simply cannot advance without the unravellings brought about by our presence. Indeed, such an ungirding may leave the most harmful "private parts" of psychoanalysis helpfully exposed, so that the queers may finally, and unapologetically screw them: the transgender psychoanalysts are coming!

Acknowledgments

I want to thank Caitlin Janzen, Caty Monahon, Nina Paulovicova, Lara Sheehi, and Justin Shubert for their generous review and sharp feedback on drafts of this book chapter. A much earlier version of this work was presented at APSaA's 111th annual meeting through Shubert's initiative into "how views about transgender identities and queerness, both conscious and unconscious, become enacted in the field." Through this panel, I received invaluable support from my co-panelists and co-conspirators, Willa France, Ethan M. Grumbach, and Lara Sheehi. Such collaborations are the lifeblood of resistance and change, as well as fueling the laughter that tugs at my sleeves, nudging me to move beyond silence. I want to humbly acknowledge all the transgender, nonbinary, and gender nonconforming people with an interest in psychoanalysis that came before me, and all those who lived through a transphobic psychoanalytic therapy – whether visible or not, your existence makes mine possible. And of course, to my analyst, for whom a thank you will always be inadequate, you are a paver of ways in more ways than one.

Notes

1 Freud (1911/19585) did not provide any theory of trans identities, however, the topic was indirectly addressed in the famous Schreber case and then regularly returned to as an après-coup for later psychoanalysts who used Schreber to stigmatize trans people as psychotic. Furthermore, this book chapter chiefly addresses "institutional psychoanalysis," as it was originally conceived by Freud as a clinical practice, which has also been called "applied" or "professional" psychoanalysis. Although overlapping, institutional psychoanalysis can be differentiated from the wider use of psychoanalytic theory in various university disciplines in the humanities and social sciences.

2 Such anti-trans moral panics include the fueling hatred and imaginary fears surrounding trans people's use of bathrooms, trans women's participation in sports, detransitioning, hormone blockers, and more.

3 In June 2019, the APsaA issued an "overdue" apology to the LGBTQ+ community for the pathologization of homosexuality and transgender identities (APsaA, 2019). While APsaA did publish a news release about the apology, the whole text is not available to the public (at the time of writing, late 2023). Soon after, in December of 2020, Division 39 of the APA, the Society for Psychoanalysis and Psychoanalytic Psychology, offered an apology letter to the LGBTQ+ community which recognized the harms done by psychoanalysis, the compounding influences of additional intersections of oppression, and offered ten meaningful steps forward (LeRoy & Tummala-Narra 2020). They state: "We apologize for personal biases and prejudice that have often been couched in theoretical rationalizations used to justify conscious and unconscious discrimination and hate in interpersonal spaces and systemic attitudes and behaviour."

4 Many similar course titles have appeared in my inbox over recent years, and these two were hosted at the New York-based Institute for Psychoanalytic Training and Research (IPTAR) and Metropolitan Institute for Training in Psychoanalytic Psychotherapy (MITPP).

5 Permission has been sought to name transgender people in this book chapter who are not otherwise clear about their gender identity in published writing.

6 Pula provides formidable insight and personal vulnerability regarding his own psychic life and the analyst's countertransference: "In retrospect, I believe my analyst thought I was enacting a sadomasochistic dynamic in which I was forcing the analysis off track, away from analyzing my longing for and fears of deep, desirous love, in favor of a sexualized, gendered, bodily transformation as a way of acting out an erotic transference.... I was asking my analyst to do more than that analyst could fathom" (p. 813).

7 In 2022, I was invited to APSaA's 111th annual meeting in Boston for a panel on the theme of "Gender & Sexuality." Through this invitation, I made the acquaintance of Willa France, whose work I hold in high regard. She is a transgender woman currently undergoing training, who has begun writing and regularly presenting at conferences.

8 The *IJP* amplified its warnings to the authors through legal-sounding language and egregiously implied that publication of the piece in a different journal would break its commitments to the Tiresias Award committee. The underlaying message was that "either the *IJP* would publish their preferred version of the paper, or there would be no publication of the first Tiresias Award paper at all" (Saketopoulou & Pellegrini, 2023, p. xii).

9 Not only does this designation invoke an amusing tongue-in-cheek whitewashed, Austenian aesthetic, it speaks to the fantasy that psychoanalysis can have an esteemed, standardized form with appropriately regulated boundaries.

10 When undergoing an IPA recognized psychoanalytic training, candidates must also undergo a personal psychoanalysis with a specialized clinician called a "training analyst." Training analysts have been officially selected by constituent organizations as being qualified to analyze candidates (IPA, 2017); however, this process has been critiqued for its nepotism, autocracy, and as being marked by power struggles (Kirsher, 2000).

11 The word "affirming," although commonly employed within many queer and trans therapies, is much contested in psychoanalysis. For example, given psychoanalyst's work with the unconscious, it is assumed that any typical therapeutic affirmation – like the most standard trans affirmation "I believe you when you say you are X gender" – could foreclose that subject's exploration of the unconscious. That said, although I personally use the language of affirmation here, not all those cited would agree that psychoanalysis with trans subjects can or should be affirming.

12 I recently encountered such a split when taking part in a psychoanalytic dialogue on the topic of transgender children (Gozlan et al., 2022). The conversation eventually turned to the oft disputed question of writing letters that endorse trans people's access to surgery or hormones. The analysts in our discussion, although not sternly withholding such support, stipulated that there was no analytically "neutral" place from which to write such a letter, one elaborating that "…once we take up the position of advocacy and support and writing letters, *we are in a different position from an analytic one*" (p. 14, emphasis added). It may be advantageous instead, I would argue, to expand the parameters of "what counts" as a clinical psychoanalytic position, including theorizing on how a "real psychoanalysis" necessarily encompasses such politicized moments, especially when working with marginalized people.

Bibliography

Ahmed, S. (2012). *On being included: Racism and diversity in institutional life.* Durham: Duke University Press.

American Psychoanalytic Association (APsA). (2019). *American Psychoanalytic Association Issues Overdue Apology to LGBTQ Community.* Retrieved December 27, 2023 from https://apsa.org/wp-content/uploads/2022/10/StonewallApology.pdf.

Awkward-Rich, C. (2017). "Trans, feminism: Or, reading like a depressed transsexual." *Signs: Journal of Women in Culture and Society, 42*(4), 819–841.

Bak, R.C. (1953). "Fetishism." *Journal of the American Psychoanalytic Association, 1,* 285–298.

Bak, R.C. (1968). "The phallic woman." *The Psychoanalytic Study of the Child, 23*(1), 15–36.

Bell, D. (2020). "First do no harm." *The International Journal of Psychoanalysis, 101*(5), 1031–1038.

Bettcher, T.M. (2019). "What is trans philosophy?" *Hypatia, 34*(4), 644–667.

Blass, R. B., Bell, D., & Saketopoulou, A. (2021). "Can we think psychoanalytically about transgenderism? An expanded live Zoom debate with David Bell and Avgi Saketopoulou, moderated by Rachel Blass." *The International Journal of Psychoanalysis, 102*(5), 968–1000.

Breslow, J. (2021). *Ambivalent Childhoods: Speculative Futures and the Psychic Life of the Child.* Minneapolis: University of Minnesota Press.

Butler, J. (1990). *Gender Trouble: Feminism and the Subversion of Identity.* New York: Routledge.

Carlson, S.T. (2010). "Transgender subjectivity and the logic of sexual difference." *differences, 21*(2), 46–72.

Cavanagh, S.L. (2018). "Transgender embodiment: A Lacanian approach." *The Psychoanalytic Review, 105*(3), 303–327.

Coffman, C. (2022). *Queer Traversals Psychoanalytic Queer and Trans Theories.* London: Bloomsbury Academics.

Corntassel, J. (2012). "Re-envisioning resurgence: Indigenous pathways to decolonization and sustainable self-determination." *Decolonization: Indigeneity, Education & Society, 1*(1), 86–101.

Chiland, C. (2000). "The psychoanalyst and the transsexual patient." *The International Journal of Psycho-Analysis, 81*(1), 21.

D'Angelo, R. (2020). "The man I am trying to be is not me." *The International Journal of Psychoanalysis, 101*(5), 951–970.

Dean, T. (2000). *Beyond Sexuality.* Chicago: University Of Chicago Press.

DeLire, L. (2023). "Beyond representational justice." *Texte Zur Kunst, 129*(48). Retrieved January 13, 2024 from https://www.textezurkunst.de/en/129/luce-delire-beyond-representational-justice/.

Duggan, L. (2003). *The Twilight of Equality?: Neoliberalism, Cultural Politics, and the Attack on Democracy.* Boston: Beacon Press.

Edelman, L. (2004). *No Future: Queer Theory and the Death Drive.* Durham: Duke University Press.

Elster, M. (2022). "Insidious concern: Trans panic and the limits of care." *TSQ: Transgender Studies Quarterly, 9*(3), 407–424.

Evzonas, N. (2021). "Trans∗, France, and countertransference: Introduction to the special issue." *The Psychoanalytic Review, 108*(4), 373–385.

Evzonas, N. (2022). "Multivoiced dialogue, becomingness, and all-embracing countertransference: Introduction to the special issue." *The Psychoanalytic Review, 109*(3), 213–225.

Frankel, D. (Director). (2006). *Devil Wears Prada.* [Film]. Fox 2000 Pictures. USA.

Freud, S. (1958). "Psycho-analytic notes on an autobiographical account of a case of paranoia (dementia paranoides)." (J. Strachey, Trans.). In *The Standard Edition of the Complete Psychological Works of Sigmund Freud (SE).* London: The Hogarth Press. (Original work published 1911).

Freud, S. (2011). *Three Essays on the Theory of Sexuality.* (J. Strachey, Trans.). Eastford, CT: Martino Fine Books. (Original work published 1905).

Gherovici, P. (2010). *Please Select Your Gender: From the Invention of Hysteria to the Democratizing of Transgenderism.* New York: Routledge.

Gherovici, P. (2011). "Psychoanalysis needs a sex change." *Gay & Lesbian Issues and Psychology Review, 7*(1), 3–18.

Gherovici, P. (2022). "Beyond fear and pity." *The Psychoanalytic Review, 109*(3), 287–308.

Gherovici, P. & Steinkoler, M. (2023). "Introduction." In Gherovici, P & Steinkoler, M. (Eds.), *Psychoanalysis, Gender, and Sexuality.* (pp. 1–40). New York: Routledge.

Giffney, N. & Watson, E. (2017). *Clinical Encounters in Sexuality: Psychoanalytic Practice & Queer Theory.* Santa Barbara: Punctum Books.

Gossett, R., Stanley, E.A. & Burton, J. (2017). *Trap Door: Trans Cultural Production and the Politics of Visibility.* Cambridge: MIT Press.

Gozlan, O. (2008). "The accident of gender." *The Psychoanalytic Review*, 95(4), 541–570.

Gozlan, O. (2011). "Transsexual surgery: A novel reminder and a navel remainder." *International Forum of Psychoanalysis*, 20(1), 45–52.

Gozlan, O. (2015). *Transsexuality and the Art of Transitioning: A Lacanian Approach.* London: Routledge.

Gozlan, O. (2018). "From continuity to contiguity: A response to the fraught temporality of gender." *The Psychoanalytic Review*, 105(1), 1–29.

Gozlan, O. (2022). "Adolescent ruthlessness and the transitioning of the analyst's mind." *Journal of the American Psychoanalytic Association*, 70(3), 459–484.

Gozlan, O., Osserman, J., Silber, L., Wallerstein, H., Watson, E. & Wiggins, T. (2022). "Transgender children: from controversy to dialogue." *The Psychoanalytic Study of the Child*, 75(1), 198–214.

Greenberg, B. (2012). *Kleinian Reparation: A Psychoanalytic Exploration of Residential School Apology in Canada* (Doctoral dissertation, University of Toronto).

Hansbury, G. (2004). "Sexual TNT: A transman tells the truth about testosterone." *Journal of Gay & Lesbian Psychotherapy*, 8(1–2), 7–18.

Hansbury, G. (2005a). "Mourning the loss of the idealized self: A transsexual passage." *Psychoanalytic Social Work*, 12(1), 19–35.

Hansbury, G. (2005b). "The middle men: An introduction to the transmasculine identities." *Studies in Gender and Sexuality*, 6(3), 241–264.

Hansbury, G. (2011). "King Kong & Goldilocks: Imagining transmasculinities through the trans–trans dyad." *Psychoanalytic Dialogues*, 21(2), 210–220.

Hansbury, G. (2017a). "The masculine vaginal: Working with queer men's embodiment at the transgender edge." *Journal of the American Psychoanalytic Association*, 65(6), 1009–1031.

Hansbury, G. (2017b). "Unthinkable anxieties: Reading transphobic countertransferences in a century of psychoanalytic writing." *TSQ: Transgender Studies Quarterly*, 4(3–4), 384–404.

Hansbury, G. (2022). "Don't take up space: How the patriarchy works to undermine trans communities from within." In Petrucelli, J., Schoen, S. & Snider, N. (Eds.). *Patriarchy and Its Discontents.* (pp. 253–262). New York: Routledge.

Hansbury, G. & Saketopoulou, A. (2022). "Sissy dance $1: The more and more of gender." *The Psychoanalytic Review*, 109(3), 227–256.

Harris, A. (2022). "Transgender and analytic countertransference." *The Psychoanalytic Review*, 109(3), 277–286.

Haulotte, P. (2023). "Program for a transgender existentialism." *TSQ: Transgender Studies Quarterly*, 10(1), 32–41.

International Psychoanalytic Association (IPA), (2017). *Requirements for the Appointment of Training Analysts and Interim Training Analysts*. International Psychoanalytic Association. Retrieved January 6, 2024 from https://www.ipa.world/IPA/en/IPA1/Procedural_Code/Requirements_for_the_Appointment_of_Training_Analysts.aspx.

International Psychoanalytic Association (IPA), (2023). *IPA International Psychoanalytical Association: An IPA for all!* Linkedin. Retrieved November 22, 2023 from https://www.linkedin.com/company/international-psychoanalytical-association-ipa/?originalSubdomain=uk.

Israeli-Nevo, A. (2019). "May her memory be a revolution." *lambda nordica*, 24(2–3), 173–190.

Kirsner, D. (2000). *Unfree Associations: Inside Psychoanalytic Institutes*. London: Process Press Ltd.

Kloppenberg, B. (2022). "What happens when a trans patient happens." *Journal of the American Psychoanalytic Association, 70*(3), 525–546.

Kövecses, Z. (2016). "'Girding up the loins': A cognitive sematic analysis of humorous expressions." *Półrocznik Językoznawczy Tertium, 1*(1&2), 74–91.

LeRoy, M. & Tummala-Narra, U. (2020). *Letter of Apology to LGBTQ+ Communities and APA Division 39 Members (Past and Present) On Behalf of the Board of Directors, APA Division 39 – Society for Psychoanalysis and Psychoanalytic Psychology.* American Psychological Association Division 39. Retrieved December 27 2023 from https://div39members.wildapricot.org/resources/Documents/Apology%20Letter%20Final%20with%20disclaimer.pdf.

Low, K. (2011). "Implications surrounding girding the loins in light of gender, body, and power." *Journal for the Study of the Old Testament, 36*(1), 3–30.

Miller, J.A. (2021). "Docile au trans." *Lacan Quotidien.* 928, 3–18. Retrieved Dec 31, 2023 from https://lacanquotidien.fr/blog/wp-content/uploads/2021/04/LQ-928.pdf.

Offman, H. (2023). "On neing an 'expert-enough expert': Working psychoanalytically with transgender patients." *Psychoanalytic Perspectives, 20*(1), 49–64.

Osserman, J. & Wallerstein, H. (2022). "Transgender children: From controversy to dialogue." *The Psychoanalytic Study of the Child, 75*(1), 159–172.

Porchat, P. & Santos, B. (2021). "'Are we safe analysts?' Cisgender countertransferential fantasies in the treatment of transgender patients." *The Psychoanalytic Review, 108*(4), 411–431.

Posadas, M. (2023). "The staff of Tiresias: Resistance, revolt, ruptures, and repairing in psychoanalysis today." In Saketopoulou, A. & Pellegrini, A. *Gender without Identity.* New York: The Unconscious in Translation.

Preciado, P.B. (2021). *Can the Monster Speak?: Report to an Academy of Psychoanalysts* (Vol.32). Cambridge: MIT Press.

Prosser, J. (1998). *Second Skins: The Body Narratives of Transsexuality.* New York: Columbia University Press.

Puar, J. (2007). *Terrorist Assemblages: Homonationalism in Queer Times.* Durham: Duke University Press.

Pula, J. (2015). "Understanding gender through the lens of transgender experience." *Psychoanalytic Inquiry*, 35(8), 809–822.

Saketopoulou, A. (2014). "Mourning the body as bedrock: Developmental considerations in treating transsexual patients analytically." *Journal of the American Psychoanalytic Association, 62*(5), 773–806.

Saketopoulou, A. (2020). "Thinking psychoanalytically, thinking better: Reflections on transgender." *The International Journal of Psychoanalysis, 101*(5), 1019–1030.

Saketopoulou, A. & Pellegrini, A. (2023). *Gender without Identity.* New York: The Unconscious in Translation.

Salah, T. (2017). "'Time isn't after us': Some Tiresian Durations." *Somatechnics, 7*(1), 16–33.

Salah, T. (2018). "To Return to Schreber." In Gozlan O. (Ed.) *Current Critical Debates in the Field of Transsexual Studies: In Transition.* pp. 169–180. New York and London: Routledge.

Salamon, G. (2004). "The bodily ego and the contested domain of the material." *differences*, 15(3), 95–122.

Segal, H. (1973). *Introduction to the Work of Melanie Klein.* London: The Hogarth Press.

Serano, S. (2007). *Whipping Girl: A Transsexual Woman on Sexism and the Scapegoating of Femininity.* New York: Seal Press.

Silverman, S. (2023). "Who's transitioning? A cisgender analyst working with gender expansive patients." *Psychoanalytic Perspectives, 20*(1), 31–48.

Simpson, L.B. (2016). "Indigenous resurgence and co-resistance." *Journal of the Critical Ethnic Studies Association, 2*(2), 19–34.

Spade D. (2015). *Normal Life: Administrative Violence, Critical Trans Politics, and the Limits of Law.* Duke University Press.

Thobani, S. (2023). "What do apologies apologize for? Rearrangements of state violence." *State Crime Journal, 12*(2), 187–205.

Wark, M. (2023) "Dear cis analysts: A call for reparations." *Parapraxis. 2*, 38–43.

Wiggins, T.B. (2020). "A perverse solution to misplaced distress: Trans subjects and clinical disavowal." *TSQ: Transgender Studies Quarterly, 7*(1), 56–76.

Wiggins, T.B. (2022). "Do psychoanalysts dream of polymorphous sleep?: Clinical desiring with transgender subjects." *Studies in Gender and Sexuality, 23*(2), 146–162.

Yadlin-Gadot, S. (2023). "Freud: The First Queer Theorist?" *Psychoanalytic Perspectives, 20*(1), 4–30.

Chapter 2

On the Cage of Gender

Perspectives on an Ethics of *Sexual Différance*

Esther Hutfless, Translated by Anja Müller and Michael Holohan

I would like to preface my text with a quotation. It comes from the author, curator, philosopher, and queer theorist Paul B. Preciado. In a lecture published in English under the title "Can the Monster speak?," Preciado addressed an audience of about 3,500 psychoanalysts: "I speak to you today from this elective, refashioned cage of the 'trans man,' of the 'non-binary body.' Some will say that this, too, is a political cage: whatever the case, this cage is better than that of 'men and women' in that it acknowledges its status as a cage" (2021, p. 20).

My article will revolve around this cage of gender, which ultimately encloses us all, but which – and here I follow Preciado and queer theory – does not have to be a binary cage.

I would like to follow Preciado also in another matter. I, too, want to reveal the position of my speaking. Of course, I could leave you to your imagination, as we do in psychoanalytic practice.

Disclosing the position of my speaking as a philosopher and psychoanalyst who identifies as queer and non-binary I understand to be an important epistemological and political act.[1] Epistemological because I want to point out that the position from which we speak and develop concepts, theories, and terms is never neutral, but always interspersed with power structures and shaped by our situatedness (cf. Haraway, 1988);[2] and political because it is a position that marks an *other* to the binary norm in psychoanalytic discourse. This "other to the norm" is that which, according to the current theories of psychoanalysis, cannot become symbolic because the shared symbolic order of language is rejected, the symbolic order which we must enter starting from the recognition of castration and the need to symbolize constitutive lack. It is also that which psychoanalysis perceives as determined by fantasies of omnipotence and threatened by psychosis or already plunged by it into the abyss of the real – to use a term of Jacques Lacan's here (Evans, 1996) – as castration, death, and sexual difference are supposedly denied (cf. Millot, 1990). This is one of those common psychoanalytic theories that has led many psychoanalysts to refuse to advocate gender reassignment for trans people or to admit trans people to psychoanalytic training.

The thesis of the non-recognition of castration – others' or one's own – is shared by trans people in psychoanalytic theory to some extent with homosexuals,

DOI: 10.4324/9781032624129-3

although the latter were not usually considered psychotic.[3] Homosexuality has been depathologized for some time now, and the theoretical foundations of the former pathologization have been critically questioned again and again, yet this has not led to a comprehensive revision of psychoanalytic approaches. Instead, as Ilka Quindeau points out, these theories are now applied to trans people in one way or another (cf. 2017, p. 182).

The following questions guide my discussion here: Is the process of becoming a subject, as conceived in psychoanalysis, necessarily bound to the assumption of a binary gender identity and the submission to the simple game of identity and difference borrowed from a binary logic? Can the subject become speaking and signifying without reference to the concept of a binary sexual difference (Hutfless, 2022, p. 6)? To what extent do theories, concepts, and terms represent unchanging and universal foundations within psychoanalysis? Are new social developments understood exclusively as problematic deviations that psychoanalysis must oppose, or do they perhaps also enable us to get a little closer to the enigma of gender and the sexual?[4]

The topic of gender initially leads us into a whole thicket of terms and concepts: biological sex, social gender, sexual difference, psychological bisexuality, gender identity, and psychosexual gender. Again and again, we are tempted to clear this thicket, to make a breach into this known-unknown terrain of gender, to enclose and capture it with terms and concepts.

Gender and sexual difference are perhaps best understood – as Judith Butler once put it (2004, p. 178) – in the sense of a question to which there can be no clear, no fixed, and no ultimately valid answer. A recurring question, then, that addresses the problematics of the drive, the body, biology, the social, identity, culture, the unconscious, discourse, the sexual, etc., and searches for the references, connections, entanglements, and relations of all of these.

Before I venture with you into the thicket of gender, I would like to follow the traces into another, distant thicket. It is the West African, colonized thicket in which the story of the ape Red Peter from Franz Kafka's story *A Report for An Academy* begins. For it is this story by Kafka to which Paul B. Preciado refers in the above-mentioned, the full title of which is *Je suis un monstre qui vous parle. Rapport pour une académie de psychanalystes*, and which was delivered in November 2019 at the annual meeting of the École de la Cause Freudienne in Paris. In this talk, Preciado critiques the influence of ideologies in relation to gender, sexual difference, and identity in psychoanalysis. Ideologies that make monsters of all those who understand their gender to be fluid, queer, or trans. Ideologies and theories that exclude trans people from psychoanalytic training, just as homosexuals used to be excluded.

It is no coincidence that Preciado draws on Kafka's narrative about the ape who is supposed to speak about his past life as an ape to an unspecified scientific academy, just as Preciado is supposed to speak as a trans man at a psychoanalytical conference dedicated to the topic of "women in psychoanalysis" (Gherovici, 2023, p. 65).[5]

In Kafka's text, the ape Red Peter can hardly remember his imprisonment in a West African British colony. He then found himself crammed into a cage in the hold of a steamer bound for Europe. He had to find a way out of this oppressive fate, the ape reports (Kafka, 1983). The way out that he found for himself was not freedom, because being free is an illusion. The ape's way out of his cage was finally to imitate the humans and to transform into one of them himself. In this way, he managed to leave the real cage of captivity, but inevitably ended up in a new cage: the cage of human subjectivity (Preciado, 2021, p. 18).

By choosing Kafka's account of the ape's attempted humanization as the starting point for his lecture, Paul B. Preciado relates his own position to that of the ape: Preciado as a transgender curiosity, monstrous and uncanny as the humanized, trained ape from Kafka's narrative (Gherovici, 2023, p. 66). Just as the ape essentially says to his audience, "You invited me here as a talking ape, but see, I am like you, I am human," with his comparison, Preciado may want to say something like, "You consider me curious, monstrous even, but see, I am like you, I am of gender."

The remarkable thing about the account of the ape, according to Preciado, is "that Kafka does not present this process of humanization as a story of emancipation or of liberation from animality, but rather as a critique of colonial European humanism and its anthropological taxonomies" (2021, p. 18). According to Preciado, Kafka – perhaps similarly to queer theory and post-structuralist discourse-critical movements of thought – is concerned with a critique of the classification and differentiation of living beings into systematic categories which are always inscribed with a hierarchization. Starting from the issue of gender, this hierarchization also unfolds in psychoanalytical theories.

And yet another important moment can be found in Kafka's story of the ape Red Peter: the deconstruction of the boundary between the human and the non-human. And this deconstruction of a binary immediately leads to the construction and appropriation of a new identity. The ape, however, seems to know about the artificial and precarious status of the latter. The movement that Kafka traces here is also reflected in queer theories and psychoanalysis: the deconstruction, the *analysis,* inevitably leads to new constructions (Heenen-Wolff, 2018). Perhaps those constructions are better, more complex, more inclusive, less rigid, and more mobile. Perhaps they are constructions we can sometimes become aware of and suffer less from. In this sense, Griffin Hansbury also refers to the ambivalence that is evident in, for example, transgender identity, which deconstructs essentialized biological sex while at the same time embodying it in new ways which are sometimes essentialist too (2011).

But the ape from Africa allows for other associations as well: it also makes us think of the "dark continent of femininity" around which Freud once circled. Is trans identity the new, expanded "dark continent" of psychoanalysis, which is now viewed and colonized from a cisgender perspective, just like women from the male perspective and homosexuals from the heterosexual perspective? Or is the unknown perhaps *gender* or the *sexual* itself, whose enigmatic character is warded off via the construction of binary thinking and a threatening female, homosexual, transgender otherness?[6] Is this also the case in psychoanalysis?

Is there not something in the complementarity and difference thinking of the heterosexual gender binary that annuls alterity? Something that tries to protect itself from the effect of difference – a radical uncatchable difference even, something that ultimately tries to re-establish wholeness via the fantasy of union and thus denies castration, as Jean-Bertrand Pontalis suggests (1977)? To quote Pontalis: "Once recognized, sexual binarity is recognized everywhere, from biology to theogony. As a manifestation of totality, it itself demands to be total" (1977, p. 103). The fantasy of the gender binary includes, with Pontalis, "a positive fantasy aimed at ensuring full possession of a phallus – paternal and maternal –" and "fantasy aimed at guaranteeing against any separation-castration-death" (1977, p. 106).[7]

Interestingly, the gender binary is hardly ever critically questioned in psychoanalysis. It has a quasi-universal, ontological, almost metaphysical status, although it does not capture empirical reality or the unconscious. It represents an epistemology that not only offers answers to our questions, but retrospectively determines the questions that, according to this epistemology, we can even ask at all, while obscuring its own retrospective genesis (cf. Preciado, 2021, p. 46).

Gender, as I understand it, is not simply a fact. Ideas of gender vary in different cultural contexts[8] and change over time, as cultural and scientific historian Thomas Laqueur has shown in his book *Making Sex: Body and Gender from the Greeks to Freud* (1990).

Until the 18th century, the single-gender model was predominant in Europe, based not on biological differences but on metaphysical and energetic states, on vitalistic warmth and coldness, along an axis whose telos was the male form. From then on, however, gender was increasingly conceived based on biological categories, as a binary difference which progressively evolved into a difference of essence that applied down to the level of individual cells as well as to the psyche (Laqueur, 1990, p. 152). This essentialization of a binary gender became more and more entrenched, at a time when women began demanding equality, interestingly enough. From then on, it served as a biological justification for continuing to assign women a subordinate role in society. The context for the articulation of the model of a binary essentialist gender difference was, as Laqueur shows, not a scientific advance in knowledge, but political calculations that served to secure heteronormative patriarchal social structures (1990, p. 152 f.).

In several respects, psychoanalysis – emerging at the end of the 19th and the beginning of the 20th century – marks a focal point for new conceptions of subject theory as well as for a changing understanding of gender, even though older conceptions continue to be present in Freud's work.

Freud was, on the one hand, a thinker of 19th century biologism, which postulates two sexes with different organs and physiologies, as well as evolutionism, which guarantees the adjustment of the genitals to heterosexual sexual intercourse (Laqueur, 1990, p. 243). Although Freud rejects the notion of more than two genders – as conceived, for example, by Karl Heinrich Ulrichs and Magnus Hirschfeld

(1864) – he was nevertheless a thinker who attempted to grasp gender with an unprecedented degree of complexity and who allowed a simple and exclusively biological concept of gender difference to collapse like a house of cards. Let us think of Freud's idea of bisexuality, in which male and female parts are found in all subjects; of the libido, which is active in essence but nevertheless genderless; of unconscious homosexual or heterosexual identification in all the vicissitudes of the drives, and so on. Freud's theory attempts to clarify not so much what exactly gender is, but rather how it occurs and what it entails, although Freud considers this process of gendering to be an overdetermination in *The Ego and the Id*: it could be oedipal identification, it could be bisexuality – we don't know (1923).

Freud's subject theory is ambivalent in a similar way to his gender theory. On the one hand, Freud borrows from Enlightenment thinking – "Where id was, there ego shall be," (1933, p. 80) whilst on the other hand, he thinks of a subject whose identity is called into question by the unconscious and the drives and which paves the way for the thinking of the split subject of postmodernism, which ultimately influenced queer theory as well (Glocer Fiorini, 2017, p. 16).

Psychoanalysis and queer theory (the latter emerging, among others, from post-structuralist approaches) therefore share a certain subject position that can be described as decentered, conflicted, thwarted, and subjugated. Conceptually, *queer* is understood by many theorists as a moment of elusion, of the unrepresentable, as that which remains "to come" and is therefore deferred and does not solidify into identity, or as that which constantly decenters any recentering movements (Butler, 1993; Hutfless, 2017b).[9] *Queer* in its most radical reading does not actually denote anything, but represents a phenomenon *in the field of language*, a force that always already operates in processes of signification by not referring to a presence, i.e. to an object, an origin, but by becoming productive starting from the radically absent, from that which always eludes language – and which therefore constitutes language in the first place (Hutfless, 2017b, p. 33). Following chains of association, this conception of *queer* also makes us think of the unconscious, of the deferred drive or Jacques Derrida's *différance*, to which I will return at the end of this text (ibid. p. 35).

This perspective of thinking gender as processually deferred, as decentered, can also be found, as I will show in the following, in the work of Jean Laplanche (Hutfless, 2022).[10] It is therefore no coincidence that many colleagues who try to think gender beyond the binary, to do justice to the unconscious and the libidinal and at the same time to consider the social and cultural level of unconscious structures, turn to Jean Laplanche, since his conception of the *sexual* as something to be translated comes very close to queer and poststructuralist positions.[11] I, too, would like to turn to Jean Laplanche in this pursuit of the question of a non-binary theory of gender and sexuality.

Laplanche also represents an exciting psychoanalytic reference point in that he has also engaged with the developments and discourses of gender studies, especially the approaches of Judith Butler, who is considered one of the founding figures of queer theory. His undogmatic approaches and his critique of ideological positions within psychoanalysis can therefore serve as a productive starting point for thinking gender beyond the binary.

In his 2003 text *Gender, Sex and the Sexual*, Laplanche explores the complex interplay of and the differences between these three registers. He develops his own theory of sexuation and gendering with the *sexual*[12] at its center. This term derives from Freud's *Three Essays on the Theory of Sexuality* (1905) and does not refer to gender in the narrower sense, nor to sexual difference, but to the infantile, polymorphous sexuality that enters the child through the "primal situation of seduction." According to Laplanche, the *sexual* is implanted in the child through so-called "enigmatic messages" emanating from adults. The enigmatic messages represent those parts of the communication from the adult to the child that are compromised and "parasitized" by the unconscious of the adults – by their infantile *sexual* in which unconscious notions of gender are also inscribed. They are present in every caring relationship between adult and child – be it personal hygiene, nursing, feeding, grooming, rocking, or soothing. It is above all non-verbal and affective, but also physical messages that affect and stimulate the child and its body. These are not intentionally transmitted by the adults and therefore do not make sense to the child at first. They become a question, an enigma. These can be aggression, fear, special affection, attention, confirmation, rejection, etc., or also a contradictory mixture of everything that is unconsciously directed at the child.

The child who receives these compromised messages tries to translate them, and this attempt is bound to fail, since they are messages that also remain unconscious to the adults themselves, since they feed on their repressed infantile sexuality (Scarfone, 2013). The *sexual* thus becomes an internal foreign body that cannot be dissolved or eliminated. It becomes the source-object of the drive, that is, the object that triggers the drive or bodily arousal, but also constitutes the drive for perpetual translation.

Laplanche uses the *sexual*, which, according to him, lies outside of sex and outside of gender difference and constitutes the core of the unconscious, to add a third category to the dualist gender theories that are based on the conceptual pair of *sex* and *gender*. This category of the *sexual* can already be found within Freud in the form of *infantile sexuality*. At the same time, Laplanche introduces the concept of gender to psychoanalysis in a new, systematic way, embedded in his theory of subject genesis, and with it the social and political level of gender. The concept of gender had already found its way into psychoanalysis in the 1960s, starting from medical discourses and initially linked to the concept of identity (Stoller, 1968). As Wolfgang Mertens notes, the focus on gender identity in psychoanalysis went hand in hand with the increased reception of the approaches of self-psychology and the object relations theory, while classical drive theory approaches to psychosexual development tended to be pushed into the background (cf. Mertens, 1997, p. 23; Breen, 1993, p. 15). It is also noteworthy that the concepts of gender and identity enter the stage of discourse at a time when "transsexuality" is moving to the center of medical, psychotherapeutic, and psychiatric interest (Hutfless, 2017a, p. 141). Gender – as a term in psychoanalysis first coined by Robert Stoller (1968) based on his work with transgender people – became something that could be diagnosed. The concept of gender identity initially serves to secure the heteronormative binary (cf. Schütze, 2009, p. 80). Although masculinity and femininity cannot necessarily be explained in purely biological terms, the concept of binary gender identity succeeds in saving the gender binary and nevertheless integrating all those who transgress this system into it. Feminist psychoanalysts detach the concept of gender from these identity discourses, deconstruct it, and approach it as a complex phenomenon (Goldner, 1991; Dimen & Goldner, 2001; Harris, 1991 and 2005). Numerous works, which I cannot go into here, have been published on this topic in recent years and decades. What I would like to mention, however, is the contribution of feminist, lesbian, and gay analysts to the psychoanalytical gender debate.

Jean Laplanche places gender – that is, socially constructed sex – chronologically first, since the anatomical sex cannot be clearly perceived or experienced by the child in the first months of their life. According to Laplanche, gender – in relation to the use of the term "gender or gender *identity,*" he is quite critical – is neither a simple imprint of some kind nor a habit but is essentially based on attributions that are tied to the priority of the other and that initially remain enigmatic. Laplanche thus shifts the identification process depicted by Freud in the Oedipus complex (Laplanche, 2011d, p. 110). It is not the child that identifies "with" mother or father, but rather it has always been identified – Laplanche therefore speaks of the "identification by" adults. In this sense, the attribution of gender always precedes its symbolization in the individual. What is significant about Laplanche's concept – and here he also goes beyond the approaches of gender studies and queer theory – is that attributions of gender are not simple acts of naming or invoking, but also represent a complex and contradictory process consisting of actions, language, and behaviors through which unconscious messages from the close attachment figures are always inscribed.

Laplanche first establishes the following basic assumptions:

- *Gender [le genre]*, i.e. the social sex, is plural – although it is usually socially shortened to a binary form;
- *Sex [le sexe]*, i.e. the so-called biological sex, is usually understood in dualistic terms through reproduction and the human symbolization of anatomical difference or through a recourse to a "popular" anatomy;
- *The Sexual [le sexuel]* is multiple and polymorphic.

Based on these basic assumptions, Laplanche formulates the following thesis: "The *sexual* is the unconscious residue of the symbolization-repression of gender by sex" (Laplanche, 2011a, p. 159). Gender, which is enigmatic for the child from the beginning, is, according to Laplanche, translated and initially more or less fixed from the child's 15th month of life through the perception or symbolization of anatomical gender difference. Since the ultimately untranslatable, which constitutes the enigmatic messages, cannot be resolved or eliminated through translation, the process of translation is not to be understood as a one-off, but as a continuous, life-long process. As Ilka Quindeau points out, this makes it understandable why sexual orientation or gender identity is not fixed once and for all in early childhood but can also change throughout life because of ongoing translations (2017).[13]

Laplanche points out that the perceived sexual difference in humans is based on a single organ and not on the complexity of the biological sexual difference. This perceived difference follows the phallic logic or ideology of presence and absence and obeys the law of the excluded third.[14] In this sense, Laplanche understands both "supposedly biological sex" and the castration complex as modes that seek to repress the *sexual*: "Yet what they seek to repress is precisely 'the *sexual*.' What sex and, as one might say, its secular arm the castration complex tend to repress is infantile sexuality. Repress it or, more precisely, create it by repressing it" (Laplanche, 2011a, p. 179). Through the dynamics of repression and translation – the latter draws on the binary structure prevalent in society as a code, but also makes use of other cultural and individual codes – plural gender is shortened to a duality and the polymorphous *sexual* remains as a residue to be repressed (cf. Laplanche, 2011b, p. 220).[15]

The *sexual*, that is, the libidinous infantile sexuality acquired in childhood via the process of implanting enigmatic messages, precedes the instinctual hormonal sexuality that is only activated in puberty. The *sexual* is re-metabolized in puberty by the emergence of instinctual hormonal sexuality, and old translations are partially rewritten. Laplanche thus does not deny that there is an "instinctual," "biological" sexuality, but he emphasizes "that this sexuality, which is hormonal in origin, is *absent in man* from birth to the pre-pubertal period" (Laplanche, 2011c, p. 43). The *sexual* is foregrounded in precisely that period from birth to puberty. It is tied neither to specific zones nor to gender difference, but to fantasy, and chooses objects and targets randomly and variably (Laplanche, 2011c).

When instinctual hormonal sexuality occurs, it finds "its place 'occupied,' as it were, by the infantile drives already and always present within the unconscious" (Laplanche, 2011c, p. 44). Since instinctual-hormonal sexuality comes later and meets "the *drive* of intersubjective origin," i.e. the *sexual*, which had developed "autonomously" over a long period of time, "there emerges a serious problem of integration and cohesion between the two" (Laplanche, 2011b, p. 206). Humans therefore do not have a determining "biological" sexuality or gender that is present from the beginning, and the fact that hormonal sexuality, which only appears later, finds its "place" already occupied, so to speak, always already deconstructs its "natural character." Sexuality in the broadest sense is therefore to be understood with Laplanche as a contradictory and precarious concept.

With Laplanche, then, binary gender structures represent codes that function as translation aids for the enigmatically *sexual*. I quote Laplanche:

Sexuation – psychological sexuation, I mean, the castration complex – is a way of elaborating, of treating the question of gender; that is, treating the gender which is given, assigned. The subject has been assigned until now to two groups of people, male and female, and he or she has to elaborate or translate this. The phallic theory is one of the most useful ways of treating gender difference. The most rigid too! (Laplanche, 2000, p. 37).

It seems significant to me to point out that Laplanche is not talking about sexual difference here but explicitly about gender difference.

With Laplanche, the Oedipus myth or the castration complex, which function as translation aids for the enigmatically *sexual*, do not belong to psychoanalytic theory, but to psychoanalytic mythology and ideology (Laplanche, 2011b). Laplanche therefore also does not locate the Oedipus complex as the starting point of the unconscious, its contents do not form the repressed, but rather the Oedipus myth stands on the side of the repressive, "not on the side of the sexual but of that which organizes it, and finally desexualizes it in the name of the laws of alliance, of procreation, etc." (Laplanche, 2011b, p. 220).

Laplanche understands the Oedipus complex, which is based on the binary opposition phallic/castrated and which becomes the "classical" starting point in psychoanalytic approaches for thinking the sexuation of the subject and of object choice, not as universal but as a cultural and secondary process that arises from an unconscious already constituted by alterity. Since the Freudian unconscious does not know negation and opposites can coincide without contradiction, this consequently also means that there is no castration in the unconscious and no phallic binarity that would be organized by the proposition of the excluded third and in which there would only be having or not having. According to Laplanche, castration can therefore only belong to the realm of the ego and the secondary process and not to the unconscious; it can, for example, occur secondarily as the ego's fear of inner drive desires (Fletcher, 2000; Laplanche, 1980, p. 178).

The entry into the symbolic, the ability to symbolize is therefore, with Laplanche, not bound to the Oedipus complex and castration, but rather to relationships with the first attachment figures that are present from the beginning, relational, but also asymmetrical. It is through these relationships that implantations take place, and they also gradually offer codes for translation.

Taking Laplanche as a starting point, I would therefore like to propose a distinction between constitutive alterity, the radical priority of the other, on the one hand, and on the other, the mytho-symbolic, which is to be understood as a heterogeneous ensemble of social and cultural productions and includes social norms and familial and collective ideas, as well as ideologies. These cultural productions also include psychoanalytical theories such as the Oedipus complex and certain ideas of masculinity and femininity bound to binary gender conceptions and identities. The mytho-symbolic serves as an aid to translation, but it is never neutral; it can lead to productive or conflictual translations for the subject. I consider the distinction between a subject-constitutive alterity and the mytho-symbolic – together with the primary mechanisms of inscription and the secondary ones of defense described by Laplanche (for example, the castration or the Oedipus complex) – to be essential for critically questioning normative concepts in psychoanalytic subject theories.

The ideological consequences of the capacity for symbolization coinciding with castration can be seen in the pathologization criticized by Preciado, which turns gender queers and trans people into monsters from a psychoanalytic perspective. While in Lacan's universe,[16] a critique of the phallogocentric concept of castration is at the same time a rejection of the symbolic and leads straight to psychosis, for Laplanche to question castration is not to question the unconscious as an effect of symbolization (Fletcher, 2000). Laplanche thus turns Lacan's formula "no representation without castration" into the opposite: "no castration without representation" (Fletcher, 2000, p. 108). It is therefore not castration whose recognition leads into the symbolic, but castration itself that already represents a representation, a symbolization.

Laplanche assumes – and here I agree with John Fletcher and consider this approach central to thinking queer, non-normative, non-binary subject positions in psychoanalysis – a bi-temporality. Already via the process of implanting enigmatic messages, the subject emerges as split and the primally repressed emerges as the source-object of the drive – including the drive to translate – and thus also as the subject striving for symbolization. Laplanche thus distinguishes between this operation of implantation/translation/primal repression[17] that produces the subject and the later processes of defense that he ties to the ego, such as projection, repression, denial, foreclosure, etc. It is Laplanche's criticism of both Lacan and Melanie Klein that they collapse the two levels – primal repression and secondary processes of defense – and pass off the much later defense processes as constitutive of the structure of the psyche.[18] According to Fletcher, keeping these modes apart in their temporality can be an important starting point for thinking non-normative gender in psychoanalysis beyond pathologization. If, on the other hand, these two modes are thought of as coinciding, this inevitably leads to the pathologization of "deviant" outcomes of the Oedipus complex and to the assumption of psychosis or the monstrous in connection with queer, non-binary gender identities.

Starting from Laplanche's thinking about the implantation of enigmatic messages and starting from his approach to translation as an unfinished process, from his thinking that binary gender identities are based on ideological presuppositions, we can understand non-binary, queer, fluid, non-heteronormative conceptions of gender as equivalent – open and contingent – attempts to symbolize and translate the *sexual* (Laplanche, 2021, p. 720). The assumption of gender, as Patricia Gherovici notes, is the result of an engagement with difference in the broadest sense, a difference that is determined neither by an anatomical nor by a social sex (Gherovici, 2023, p. 74). There is, I argue, therefore no reason to exclude trans people from psychoanalytic training simply because they are trans.

The translation model, starting from Laplanche, is not only based on a very dynamic model of the psyche – for the translation process is never finished with Laplanche – but is an ongoing process that is constantly refueled by the *sexual* as the source-object of the drive. The implantation/translation model also makes it possible, for example, to consider the dynamics – often neglected in psychoanalysis – of how social structures and power relations penetrate the unconscious. Society and culture provide translation codes for these messages; new social and cultural developments may also provide new and different translation aids.

The *sexual*, which – as Laplanche notes – forms the core of psychoanalysis as well as the core of the unconscious, does not refer to biological or anatomical facts, but consists of traces whose origin is the unconscious of the others and whose meaning therefore necessarily refers to an enigmatic blank space and not to a signified. This void can only ever be filled provisionally in the process of translation. It keeps the subject open to infinitely more translations, and any return to an "origin" – and thus also to a final translation – remains postponed. Difference in this sense therefore does not refer to a binary gender difference nor to a simple distinction or to non-identity. The difference that can be thought based on the *sexual* is grounded in an uncatchable alterity – it consists of traces and differences that set in motion the process of an unfinished movement of signification and meaning via the postponement of a final translation that understands itself to be true.

It is this sense of difference that informs the subtitle of the present text "Perspectives on an ethics of *sexual différance.*" This title follows the ethics of sexual difference formulated by the philosopher and psychoanalyst Luce Irigaray in the 1970s and the concept of *différance* introduced as a neologism by the philosopher and founder of deconstruction Jacques Derrida (1982).

Irigaray stated in the 1970s that we are not yet able to actually think difference. Difference must first be thought in order to bring the feminine – which has so far in psychoanalysis been captured and devalued exclusively by male parameters – into the discourse and to recognize it as having its own value and voice. Irigaray's attempt to propose an ethics of the *différence sexuelle*, however, remains trapped in binarity, as has been pointed out many times in feminist philosophical discourses (Irigaray, 1985, p. 1993).[19]

Based on Derrida's dictum that the gesture of deconstruction also consists in writing on the margins of the history of philosophy, the margins of the history of psychoanalysis, etc., and that this writing on the margins always produces rewritings, I also undertake two rewritings (1982). They take place quietly, but not invisibly. They take place in the writing; perhaps they are only to be heard as nuances in the voice. Nevertheless, from my point of view, they are shifts that have an inherent transformative power.

So what do I do when I refer to Luce Irigaray's éthique de la différence sexuelle in a way that shifts meaning? In German, I replace an *e* with an *a* in two places: in this way, the sexual [*das Sexuelle*] becomes Laplanche's *sexual* [*das Sexuale*] and difference [*die Differenz*] becomes Derrida's *différance* [*die différance*], in which Derrida has already inscribed an *a* that refers to the moment of movement, of the changing of meaning, which is always already inscribed in language.

The *différence sexuelle*, which Irigaray says is perhaps the task of our time to think, is always in danger of being read and thought according to the pattern of binarity. Even in German or English, *sexual difference* is mostly used in the sense of a gender binarity and has established itself as a kind of synonym for it.

The concept of *différance*, which seems to me more promising here than that of *difference*, is developed by Derrida based on psychoanalytical approaches. In French, *différance* means both *difference* and deferment and refers to Freud's concepts of the trace, the trajectory and the deferment of the drive. With this term, Derrida distances himself from the psychoanalytic conceptions of lack and castration, because for Derrida these topologies repeat the metaphysical gesture of declaring *one* or *something* to be a transcendental principle.[20]

Derrida's notion of *différance* refers to a baseless or an unattainable cause, much as Jean Laplanche's *sexual* refers to the uncatchable enigma and the notion of queer as relating to something elusive. Like *différance*, the *sexual* in Jean Laplanche's approaches is that which makes meaning possible. Thus, in order to free the *différence sexuelle* from the register of binarity, an *a* in my spelling moves into both difference [*die Differenz*], making it *différance* [*die différence*], and into the sexual [*das Sexuelle*], making it the *sexual* [*das Sexuale*], because the *sexual*, with Laplanche, is also that which lies outside of gender difference.

The *a* in *différance* is thus a silent reminder that sexual difference, castration, and lack are not to be understood as the cause of the subject or the cause of language, but are already attempts at translation.

When I propose in this article to think gender, with Butler, as a question and, with Irigaray, as an ethics, I am not concerned with an ethics that would result secondarily from a gender difference that can somehow be determined, but rather with thinking an *ethics of différance*. This means, in the analytical sense, staying with the question, with the uncatchable, the enigma, the unrepresentable; staying with a question that addresses otherness, that addresses a radical difference (Butler, 2004, p. 178). My argument is not about creating a new binary, either: non-binary vs. binary, two genders vs. many. It is not about simply replacing two with many. Gender begins neither with one nor with two nor with many, but with the enigmatic, the *sexual*, the drive, with the trace, and the *a* of *differánce* (see also Zupančič & Terada, 2015, p. 203).

The knowledge of the cage of gender, of the fact that we cannot escape the enigma of the *sexual*, that we must translate it again and again, does not free us from the cage, but it enables us to expand the cage, to make it more flexible, more mobile, less rigid, to understand it as something that is not necessarily forged according to the system of binarity.

Notes

1 To reveal the position of my speaking as a philosopher and psychoanalyst who identifies as queer and non-binary is, I am aware, an ambivalent act that is aware of the irresolvable problem of claiming something like an "identity" for oneself in order to be able to take a position in the discourse while at the same time understanding this position of the speaking subject to be split and therefore "identity" to be, ultimately, a fiction and construction (cf. Hutfless, 2017a).

2 In feminist theory, gender, queer, trans, and intersectional studies, it has become quite common to reveal one's own position of speaking and thus to reflect both one's own

world of experience and one's own positioning in the discourse of power, one's own situatedness, to use a term from Donna Haraway (1988). Haraway's concept of *situated knowledge* reminds us that *how* we produce knowledge, but also *what* knowledge we produce, is always dependent on the respective social contexts in which we are situated as human beings and that this situatedness is always accompanied by a responsibility.

3 In the homosexual positions described in the Oedipus complex, the boy denies the castration of the other (the mother), while the girl denies her own castration and identifies with the father. So, according to this theory, the lesbian woman would be closer to the supposedly psychotic transgender position.

4 All these questions can also refer us, as Leticia Glocer Fiorini notes, to the old and difficult debate within psychoanalysis as to whether it is general structures we are describing and observing, or whether and to what extent these supposedly general structures are historical and cultural in their origins. So is the Oedipus complex a myth, a narrative, a model, a complex, or a general structure? Is it universal or historically and culturally conditioned (cf. Glocer Fiorini, 2017, pp. 12 and 35)?

Queer theory, trans studies, and the LGBTIQ movement, among others, challenge psychoanalysis to think gender in the 21st century differently, anew, and in more complex ways and to question traditional concepts and pathologizations. Newly developing technologies that connect to our bodies, reproductive technologies, various supplements and prostheses of virtual and material kinds, and biochemical substances also challenge our thinking of bodies and genders. Paul B. Preciado, who compares these extensions of the somatic apparatus to Freud's psychic apparatus, which is also more than consciousness, points out that gender and corporeality, starting from these couplings and externalized modalities, are always already more than an oversimplified biology (cf. Preciado, 2021, p. 35).

5 Cf. https://www.causefreudienne.org/journees/ecf-j49-femmes-en-psychanalyse/

6 … just as the racial theories of the Enlightenment served to repel, colonize, and exploit the other for the sake of one's own.

7 Both quotes were translated from French into English by the author. Pontalis is not so much referring to Freud's concept of bisexuality, although the French original speaks of "bisexualité", but rather to the gender binary that underlies heterosexuality. I have therefore decided to translate "bisexualité" into English as "sexual binarity".

8 Gender concepts often seem universally valid to us today. In this context, the influence of European colonialism should not be underestimated since it has been pathologizing numerous other conceptions of gender beyond the heteronormative gender binary and has largely caused them to disappear. On various non-binary conceptions of gender, see, for example, Baumgartinger, 2017, p. 59.

9 At the same time, within queer theory, alongside approaches referring to deconstruction and post-structuralism, other approaches which operate more strongly with concepts of identity have developed since the 2000s, influenced by Black feminism and queer of color critique.

10 Julia Kristeva's subject in process, which I have dealt with in more detail elsewhere, can be understood in a very similar way (Hutfless, 2017a; Kristeva, 1998). Jacques Lacan's psychoanalytic theory of the subject can be located in this context as well, although there is also a discussion here about the extent to which Lacan actually overcomes the structuralist binarity and can be thought in poststructuralist terms. Within queer theory, there are certainly some theorists who refer to Lacan, such as Tim Dean, Christopher Lane, and Lee Edelman (Dean & Lane, 2001; Edelman, 2004).

11 Cf. for example the work of Ilka Quindeau, Nicolas Evzonas, Avgi Saketopoulou and Ann Pellegrini or the conference "Laplanche in the States" held in New York in 2021 (https://www.laplancheinthestates.com/; Evzonas, 2020; Quindeau, 2004, 2017; Saketopoulou and Pellegrini, 2023).

12 Translators' note: Laplanche's neologism "*le sexual*" (in place of the more common French "*le sexuel*") has been written by his English translators in italics, i.e. "the *sexual*", to distinguish it from the common usages of sexual in English. We have retained this practice in this article.

13 The process of translation – which goes hand in hand with an increasing integration of the psyche but which at the same time does not exclude future changes and deconstructions of earlier constructions – also conditions, with Laplanche, an ego that increasingly structures itself and emerges via the first seduction situation, but nevertheless remains precarious (cf. Laplanche, 2001).

14 Laplanche thus also addresses what we understand as biological or anatomical sex difference and how this understanding is mostly shaped by illusion and ideology: "The perceptible difference of sex as sign or as signifier has practically nothing to do with biological and physiological male/female difference [...] The contingent, perceptual and illusory character of anatomical sexual difference, the veritable destiny of modern civilization" (Laplanche, 2011a, pp. 178 and 180). Furthermore, Laplanche also questions the universality of the logic of castration in *Problématiques II. Castration et symbolisations* (cf. Laplanche, 1980).

15 Laplanche understands gender or gender identity, although it comes first, and in contrast to the approaches from gender studies and queer theory, not as a mode that discursively "organizes" gender and sexuality, but conversely as that which is subsequently organized and therefore also inverted by our "illusory" perception of gender difference and of hormonal/biological sex as well as our symbolization of it (Laplanche, 2011a).

16 Based on a benevolent reading of Lacan, the phallus can be read as an empty or missing signifier in the sense of absolute negativity or pure difference. However, Lacan's concept of the phallus as a central signifier has repeatedly been criticized for ultimately making this signifier into a transcendental, metaphysical category or making it absolute, and for Lacan's approach not going beyond the simple dynamics of patriarchal conceptions of identity and difference (cf. Butler, 1993; Laplanche, 1998; Derrida, 1975).

17 Primal repression arises from the residue of the first attempts at translation.

18 In contrast to implantation, Laplanche uses the term "intromission" to refer to those inscriptions that lead to psychotic formations within the psyche. Intromissions elude attempts at translation because the enigmatic messages in this case are contaminated with something violent and there is a prohibition on translating these violent enigmatic messages that emanate from the sender of these messages, i.e. the adults.

19 While in "This sex which is not one" (Irigaray, 1985) Irigaray works very deconstructively, also deconstructing binarity, in later works there are more re-centering movements that tend to understand femininity as a complementary concept to masculinity.

20 https://web.stanford.edu/class/history34q/readings/Derrida/Differance.html, fn 5.

Bibliography

Baumgartinger, P.P. (2017). *Trans Studies. Historische, begriffliche und aktivistische Aspekte*. Wien: Zaglossus.

Breen, D. (1993). *Gender Conundrum. Contemporary Psychoanalytic Perspectives on Femininity and Masculinity*. New York: Routledge.

Butler, J. (1993). *Bodies that Matter*. New York: Routledge.

Butler, J. (2004). "The End of Sexual Difference?" In: *Undoing Gender*. New York: Routledge. pp. 174–203.

Dean, T. and Lane, C. (2001). *Homosexuality and Psychoanalysis*. Chicago: The University of Chicago Press.

Derrida, J. (1975). "The Purveyor of Truth." *Yale French Studies No. 52, Graphesis: Perspectives in Literature and Philosophy* (1975). pp. 31–113.

Derrida, J. (1982). *Margins of Philosophy*. Chicago: The University of Chicago Press.

Dimen, M. and Goldner, V. (2001). *Gender in Psychoanalytic Space*. New York: Other Press.

Edelman, L. (2004). *No Future. Queer Theory and the Death Drive*. Durham: Duke University Press.

Evans, D. (1996). *An Introductory Dictionary of Lacanian Psychoanalysis*. New York: Routledge.

Evzonas, N. (2020). "Psychoanalytic Transphobia or a Generalized Gender Trauma." *Research in Psychoanalysis*, Volume 30, Issue 2. pp. 103–112.

Fletcher, J. (2000). "Gender, Sexuality and the Theory of Seduction." *Women: A Cultural Review*, 11 (1/2). pp. 95–108.

Freud, S. (1905). "Three Essays on the Theory of Sexuality." *The Complete Standard Edition of the Psychological Works of Sigmund Freud (SE) VII*. London: Hogarth Press. pp. 123–246.

Freud, S. (1923) "The Ego and the Id." *The Standard Edition of the Complete Psychological Works of Sigmund Freud (SE) XIX*. London: Hogarth Press. pp. 1–66.

Freud, S. (1933). "New Introductory Lectures On Psycho-Analysis. *The Standard Edition of the Complete Psychological Works of Sigmund Freud (SE) XXII*. London: Hogarth Press. pp. 1–182

Gherovici, P. (2023). "The Monsters Within and the Monsters Without: Gender Dissidents and the Future of Psychoanalysis." *Psychoanalytic Perspectives*, 20:1. pp. 65–81.

Glocer Fiorini, L. (2017). *Sexual Difference in Debate. Bodies, Desires, and Fictions*. London: Karnac.

Goldner, V. (1991). "Toward a Critical Relational Theory of Gender." *Psychoanalytic Dialogues*, 1. pp. 249–272.

Hansbury, G. (2011) "King Kong & Goldilocks: Imagining Transmasculinities Through the Trans–Trans Dyad." *Psychoanalytic Dialogues*, 21. pp. 210–220.

Haraway, D. (1988). "Situated Knowledges: The Science Question in Feminism and the Privilege of Partial Perspective." *Feminist Studies*, 14(3), pp. 575–599.

Harris, A. (1991). "Gender as Contradiction." *Psychoanalytic Dialogues*, 1. pp. 197–224.

Harris, A. (2005). "Gender in Linear and Nonlinear History." *Journal of the American Psychoanalytic Association*, 53. pp. 1079–1095.

Heenen-Wolff, S. (2018) "Gegen die Normativität in der Psychoanalyse." Gießen: Psychosozial-Verlag. pp. 105–106.

Hirschfeld. M. (1905). *Mischungen Männlicher und Weiblicher Geschlechtscharaktere; Sexuelle Zwischenstufen)*. Leipzig: Verlag Max Spohr.

Hutfless, E. (2017a). "Die Zukunft Einer Illusion: Eine Queer-Psychoanalytische Kritik am Identitätsdenken der Psychoanalyse." In: Hutfless, E. & Zach, B. (Eds.): *Queering Psychoanalysis. Psychoanalyse und Queer Theory – Transdisziplinäre Verschränkungen*. Wien: Zaglossus. pp. 133–180.

Hutfless, E. (2017b). "Queer [Theory] Annäherungen an das Undarstellbare." In: Hutfless, E. & Zach, B. (Eds.): *Queering Psychoanalysis. Psychoanalyse und Queer Theory – Transdisziplinäre Verschränkungen*. Wien: Zaglossus. pp. 31–46.

Hutfless, E. (2022). "Von Identität zu Differenz zu Alterität. Jean Laplanche und das Denken Nicht-Normativer Geschlechtlichkeit in der Psychoanalyse." *Kinderanalyse. Psychoanalyse im Kindes-und Jugendalter und ihre Anwendungen*. 30. Jahrgang, 1. pp. 4–27.

Irigaray, L. (1985). *This Sex Which Is Not One*. Ithaca: Cornell University Press.

Irigaray, L. (1993). *An Ethics of Sexual Difference*. Ithaca: Cornell University Press.

Kafka, F. (1983). "A Report to an Academy." In: *The Complete Stories*. New York: Schocken Books.

Kristeva, J. (1998). "The Subject in Process." In: French, P. & Lack, R-F. (Eds.): *The Tel Quel Reader*. New York: Routledge, pp. 133–178.

Laplanche, J. (1980). "Problématiques II. Castration et Symbolisations." Paris: Quadrige/ PUF.

Laplanche, J. (1998). "Die Psychoanalyse als Anti-Hermeneutik. Psyche – Zeitschrift für Psychoanalyse, 52(7). pp.605–618.

Laplanche, J. (2000). "The Other Within. Rethinking Psychoanalysis. Interview with Jean Laplanche." https://www.radicalphilosophy.com/interview/jean-laplanche-the-other-within-rethinking-psychoanalysis.

Laplanche, J. (2001). "An Interview with Jean Laplanche by Cathy Caruth." http://pmc.iath. virginia.edu/text-only/issue.101/11.2caruth.txt.

Laplanche, J. (2011a). "Gender, Sex and the *Sexual*." In: *Freud and the Sexual*. New York: International Psychoanalytic Books.

Laplanche, J. (2011b). "Three Meanings of the Term 'Unconscious' in the Framework of the General Theory of Seduction." In: *Freud and the Sexual*. New York: International Psychoanalytic Books.

Laplanche, J. (2011c). "Sexuality and Attachment in Metapsychology." In: *Freud and the Sexual*. New York: International Psychoanalytic Books.

Laplanche, J. (2011d). "Starting from the Fundamental Anthropological Situation." In: *Freud and the Sexual*. New York: International Psychoanalytic Books.

Laplanche, J. (2021). "Mythos und Theorie in der Psychoanalyse." *Psyche – Zeitschrift für Psychoanalyse*, 75. pp. 710–736.

Laqueur, T. (1990). *Making Sex. Body and Gender from the Greeks to Freud*. Cambridge: Harvard University Press.

Mertens, W. (1997). *Entwicklung der Psychosexualität und der Geschlechtsidentität: Band 1, Geburt bis 4. Lebensjahr*. Stuttgart: Kohlhammer.

Millot, C. (1990). *Horsexe. Essay on Transsexuality*. New York: Autonomedia.

Pontalis, J.-B. (1977). *Entre le Reve et la Douleur*. Paris: Gallimard.

Preciado, P.B. (2021). *Can the Monster Speak?* London: Fitzcarraldo Editions.

Quindeau, I. (2004). *Spur und Umschrift: Zur Konstitutiven Bedeutung von Erinnerung in der Psychoanalyse*. München: Wilhelm Fink Verlag.

Quindeau, I. (2017). "Geschlechtervielfalt und Polymorphes Begehren: Queere Perspektiven in der Psychoanalyse." In: Hutfless, E. & Zach, B. (eds.). *Queering Psychoanalysis. Psychoanalyse und Queer Theory – Transdisziplinäre Verschränkungen*. Wien: Zaglossus. pp. 181–210.

Saketopoulou, A. and Pellegrini, A. (2023). *Gender Without Identity*. New York: The Unconscious in Translation.

Scarfone, D. (2013). "A Brief Introduction to the Work of Jean Laplanche." *International Journal of Psychoanalysis*, 94. pp. 545–566.

Schütze, B. (2009). "Neo-Essentialismus in der Gender-Debatte: Transsexualismus als Schattendiskurs Pädagogischer Geschlechterforschung." Bielefeld: transcript.

Stoller, R. (1968). *Sex and Gender*. London: Karnac Books.

Ulrichs, K.H. (1864). *Forschungen über das Räthsel der Mannmännlichen Liebe*. Leipzig: Heinrich Matthes Verlag.

Zupančič, A. and Terada, R. (2015). "Sex, Ontology, Subjectivity: In Conversation with Alenka Zupančič." *Psychoanalysis, Culture & Society*, 20. pp. 192–206.

Chapter 3

Emptiness is the Cure for Psychoanalysis

Myriam Sauer

Introduction

Can there be a queer psychoanalysis? Does queerness have a space in psychoanalysis? Clearly, psychoanalysts have studied queerness as an object. However, can we conceive of a queerness – or transness – that was inherent to psychoanalysis? I am pursuing these questions by studying the presence of the trans feminine in the work of Swiss psychoanalyst Danielle Quinodoz, who to my knowledge was one of the first to have written a trans affirmative case study. My central finding is as follows: implicit to clinical discourse is that the other be touchable. The complexity of trans embodiment yields a scenario in which trans feminine psyche-soma eludes the established forms of touch. If pursued against the grain of orthodox praxis, we can detect within psychoanalysis a repressed core of unfettered being that thinks of absence and presence of form as playful contingencies, rather than as necessities.

The Teachings of Danielle Quinodoz

There exist now a number of clinical psychoanalysts that work affirmatively with trans people, and these thinkers and practitioners have, as their works so forcefully suggest, greatly helped their trans and gender nonconforming patients. I have in mind here, above all, the works of Griffin Hansbury and Avgi Saketopolou (who also appear in this volume) or Patricia Gherovici (Gherovici, 2017; Hansbury, 2017; Saketopolou & Pellegrini, 2023). However, we equally have to recognize that psychoanalysis' response to trans existence has historically been severely oppressive and continues to be oppressive in many parts of the world. I will not be reviewing the vast literature of transphobic (or homo- and queerphobic) works here, because I believe that in doing so I would grant them a form of attention (and recognition) that their work does not deserve. However, I do not believe that the often oppressive history of psychoanalysis calls for its elimination or repudiation, because psychoanalysis, in spite of its shortcomings, is too good to be left by the wayside, where it all too often becomes a technique of pathologization, discipline and control.

In this paper, I would like to focus instead on the work of Danielle Quinodoz, who proposes an encounter with archaic and split-off gendered parts, the feeling of being different, and the slow excavation of these parts   .

DOI: 10.4324/9781032624129-4

In order to engage with these archaic parts, Quinodoz has developed her own technique. This technique is dependent on generating "words that touch." These words touch by eliciting a "vibration of the emotions," and by opening up a "vista onto the world of symbols" (Quinodoz, 2003, p. 38). This technique is particularly helpful for patients that present complex personality structures, for which she reserves her own concept, that of heterogeneity. This concept refers to people who carry within themselves a simultaneity of contradictory emotional states, including split-off parts. This concept is a critical alternative to the psychiatric diagnosis of borderline personality disorder (Quinodoz, 2003, p. 15). One example of such a heterogeneous patient is the trans woman, Simone, and a remarkably beautiful case study details their time together, though I must also note that in spite of its care, it is also a document of discipline and control.

Simone enters analysis struggling with the appearance of her body (Quinodoz, 2003, p. 139). She feels a deep "existential malaise" due to a lack of inner cohesion. Although she did have gender-affirming bottom surgery 20 years prior to the analysis, Simone struggles with her body. In Quinodoz's view, Simone exhibits both neurotic and psychotic behavioral patterns, which makes her "heterogeneous." Quinodoz addresses her patient as a woman thus giving her the "social status she wanted and actually had," though at the same time Quinodoz also has difficulties at times ascertaining her patient's femininity. Rather than dismissing this countertransference, Quinodoz allows this anxiety to exist.

Quinodoz's initial fear is that Simone might regret her decision to have undergone surgery, yet over the course of treatment it transpires that Simone's main difficulty stems from having an unclear sense of "primary identity" (Quinodoz, 2003, p. 140). Simone is at an impasse – neither can she go back to being a man nor can she be a "fully-fledged woman" (Quinodoz, 2003, p. 141). Both analyst and analysand share this rather disconcerting sentiment, and subsequent work revolves around accepting split-off male parts and accepting that a woman can "turn men on." Simone finds this frustrating, and struggles to accept her new role as a desirable object (Quinodoz, 2003, p. 142). A year before her treatment concludes, a session takes place that Quinodoz describes as an "earthquake." Simone relates to her analyst the desire to get a number of surgeries, relating to her Adam's apple, her knees, and her jaw. Quinodoz interprets Simone's interest in these surgeries as a rejection of the analyst, whom Simone replaces with that of the surgeon, who has the fantasized power to make her a "true woman." Quinodoz experiences this as abandonment, and as Simone's unwillingness to engage with her own psychic reality and instead privilege her physical appearance.

Quinodoz shares her view with Simone, and tells her that her desire to find a surgeon is about the disregard for psychic reality, and implicitly, the neglected inner world of her patient. Simone becomes silent for the rest of the session, misses the next one, and eventually returns after consultation with her surgeon. Simone concedes that her problem is not purely physical. She struggles rather with an internal lack of feeling like a whole person (Quindoz, 2003, p. 143). Quinodoz considers this a "vital discovery," and subsequent work leads to Simone learning to embrace herself as a "lovable extraterrestrial," and as a transsexual living as a woman, rather than being a woman (these are Simone's words). Ultimately, and Quinodoz views this as progress, Simone stops rejecting men altogether and relishes in the fact that she can be attractive to them (Quinodoz, 2003, p. 144). While in the past she believed that a woman was "against men," she now feels more at ease with them. Simone notes: "a transsexual can become a lovable extraterrestrial."

It is here that Quinodoz distinguishes three types of identity, which are of particular relevance to my subsequent argument:

1 A social identity;
2 An existential identity;
3 A biological identity.

Socially Simone is a woman, however, existentially she can be neither. Existentially, Simone is a transsexual, while biologically – and this is quite a clever gesture – "Simone must speak for herself" (Quinodoz, 2003, p. 145). These various identities revolve around a problematic relationship to the fundamental difference between men and women. Simone's access to a positive form of splitting, namely between men and women, enables her to understand the heterogeneity of her being, rather than repress it out of fear of going mad over it (Quinodoz, 2003, p. 147). Her transsexualism now has its foundation in the recognition that men and women are different.

The work that Quinodoz describes is quite touching, and seems to have brought her patient some real liveliness and joy. The treatment of Simone, however, also repeats a number of problematic assumptions, such as that an interest in surgeries is an essentially dysmorphic phenomenon based on the repudiation of psychic interiority. It is equally important to underscore that the persecution that Quinodoz observes is real, and that aggressive clocking of trans feminine people fuels these persecutory fears; and that any additional surgeries may well have provided her with real comfort necessary to sustain the complexity of her psyche.

Leaving these nuances aside, what interests me is Quinodoz's theory of identity. The social identity, Quinodoz claims, is either male or female; there can be no third option, which belongs to the existential tier of identities. Simone's basic conflict consists in the heterogeneity of her social womanhood, her existential transsexuality, and a biological secrecy (Quinodoz, 2003, p. 145), and an analysis should enable her to live with this conflict. The basic assumption that social identity is either male or female is not true, because sociality is historical, and as such can make room for hundreds of genders; outside of the West, more gender-diverse socialities have been commonplace for centuries (Heyam, 2023). However, her notion that transsexuality constitutes an existential identity has significant ramifications. It raises a question: if trans people have an existential identity, what about cis people? The notion of "cis" is not available to Quinodoz, of course, and the cisgender norm passes as unmarked in her larger argument. However, Quinodoz does lend representation to the existential nature of trans being. Trans being concerns the foundations of existence, because a transition fundamentally rewrites a person's life, and introduces an apocalyptic rhythm into it that weaves into a larger composition of movement and yearning.

Even more striking is Quinodoz's assertion that as for biological identity "she must speak for herself." This statement is surprising given psychoanalysis' often relentless drive toward omniscient knowing and explanation. Quinodoz thus introduces secrecy into her consulting room by granting her patient a right of refusing absolute revelation. One of transphobia's key elements is its demand for visibility. Klein once remarked that in the male unconscious there exists a synonymy between penetration and exploration (Klein, 1975, p. 240), an idea we may well generalize, as Klein's own phallic prose, replete with penetrative metaphors, indicates. Historically, psychoanalysis has marshaled a relentless penetrative screening of its gender non-conforming patients. This "diaphanoscopy," to use a medical term, has rendered certain structures visible and thus controllable. Quinodoz's insistence on secrecy enables a particular kind of holding. This holding cannot be measured empirically but only be felt in the particular non-communicative effects that suffuse mind and body and render it receptive to Quinodoz's vision of "words that touch and enliven" (Quinodoz, 2003, p. 170). Quinodoz's vignette is a great example of astute clinical work because of its affective and linguistic tenderness. I find here "vacuoles of non-communication," to utilize a Deleuzian expression (Deleuze, 2013, p. 238), moments where the communication that flows through observation and interpretation is interrupted, and a deeper connection that stems from being alone together becomes possible.

Quinodoz's work thus contributes to a cartography of trans being; it introduces clarity and understanding into a context of relative confusion. It also enables trans subjects to understand themselves better. This clarity does come at a price. Its inclusion into the conceptual nomenclature of capitalist and psychiatric control turns trans being into legible existentiality. Quinodoz asserts that Simone's existential identity is that of being "transsexual." However, what conversion processes contributed to granting her this "existential identity?" Does the possibility of an existential identity require an abjecting gesture? If transsexuality acquires morphological legibility, then the possibility of a "non," a suspension of morphic situatedness, becomes unsayable.

Trans being shares with intersexuality a problematization of gender dimorphism. This problematization has provoked considerable aggression and hostility, and reappears in the notions of monstrosity and alienness that Simone herself brings into the consulting room. Quinodoz's work, although mindful of the complexity of limiting creative expressions of gender, insists on the necessity of splitting, which she describes, without fully explaining why, as "good splitting." Here the psychoanalytic archive haunts Quinodoz's texts, because her work, despite a commitment to openness and abandonment of orthodox technique, now turns into an educative lesson in Freudo-Kleinian theories of the mind.

It is of fundamental importance that Simone relate herself to Freud's concept of psychic bisexuality. Equally, she must accept "good splitting" and move into the depressive position by recognizing good-enough internal objects. Should such differentiation not occur, this heterogeneous patient would plunge into a deeper psychotic pain. Heterogeneous people are "persons" who are afraid that the perception of their heterogeneity will make them go mad. Quinodoz's post-Kleinian interventions thus consist of enabling her patients to pass through the different positions, to protect them from falling into diffusion and psychotic immobility. This clever catachresis of borderline carries its own connotations, which Quinodoz never fully discusses. How free can a trans person be in a clinical encounter that is so burdened by metapsychological references?

If the clinic of the British school revolves around containing unbearable pain and holding someone, then this implies that touch be shared and received. First, the clinic must transform the "formless infinity" of trans being into a particular morpheme in order for it to enter this intersubjective realm. Only if she accepts the theory of psychic bisexuality can she then enter into a realm marked by the capacity for concern (Winnicott, 1985). The capacity for concern, of course, requires guilt over having hurt someone else. Guilt gives way to repair and to care for the other, and thus seals the child into the social bond. The integration of the child also de-radicalizes the child's absoluteness in expressing its needs. The child develops a sense it may reasonably be allowed to expect.

I want to emphasize that my concern does not lie with these theories' findings, many of which are profound, but rather with the surreptitious presence of the psychoanalytic heritage and its intrusion into the formative processes of the analysand's psyche. Simone enters Quinodoz's consulting room feeling sad and utterly bereaved, and what she receives is a "touching" instruction in gender norms. Quinodoz's clinical brilliance consists in granting her patient the right to secrecy, and yet, owing to her inability to name and articulate her own cisgender position, her countertransference – which she acknowledges – remains an "unthinkable anxiety" (Hansbury, 2017).

At least some of this anxiety stems from unsaid sociological aspects, such as the fear that comes with having to hide one's trans femininity to avoid exposure to catastrophic violence. The teachings handed down to Simone instruct her on what she can "reasonably" ask for – being a lovable alien. It is inherent to the trans feminine experience to encounter reality as the frustration of not merely need-fulfillment, but also of its own range of gendered expressions. Gender now requires identification – the internalization of persecutory superego voices, which delimit what can and cannot be said. The trans feminine child may dream to be an athlete one day, but only if she transitions before a certain age, only if she reduces her testosterone levels, only if… etc. Identification thus introduces control into trans femininity at a very early moment. This reality of control is hardly exclusive to the trans feminine child, or the trans child in general, but is rather an element of the control society. The analysis becomes explicitly reproductive and turns into a series of teaching moments. Trans femininity, however, is queer in the sense that it is a "bad education," to invoke Lee Edelman – it teaches nothing (2023). It has no doctrine that can be handed down, no program, no system, because it resists diachrony. Purely synchronic, it emerges in fleeting moments, which never turn into conceptually rigorous language. That is not to say that it is a purely sensual feeling. The queerness of trans femininity lies in its resistance to the various conceptual strictures that tie it to clearly definable, interminably repeatable symptoms, which hem in trans feminine jouissance. The knowledge of these symptoms through metapsychology may provoke transformation but it can also arrest one's becoming through synthetic accounts that tether a person to a certain narrative that we find in analysis, a book, or on a walk in the park.

The personal narrative is so addictive because it grants respite from the fleetingness of one's own existentiality; it inscribes a person into a larger kinship of shared narratives and dreams, such as that of the mentalizing society that acknowledges its guilt and engages in reparations. Implicit to this model is the presumption of a shared language. However, do we share such a language? Is there not a ruse of community at work that serves to force us into a cage? Are there not forms of violence that we cannot mend by way of reparation? Wounds remain that hegemony strives to hide through representation.

Quinodoz's study revolves around inherited forms of representation. Representation renders a subject legible to others, and the Freudian theory of psychic bisexuality accomplishes this as forcefully as do the British theories of social integration. Psychoanalysis, as a discipline of *analysis* – of disarticulating, distending, and breaking apart – opposes conceptual strictures that render a subject entirely localizable within a discourse. It enables us to become open to the otherwise, to speak with Barnaby Barratt – the realm that lies beyond textuality and that cannot become meaningful through imaginative or symbolic instruments (2017). There exists, if only in whispers, the possibility of being beyond the archives and heritages that we inherit. It requires a tremendous amount of work to understand all the baggage that we inherit from our ancestors, and it is a resistance to discipline itself.

The clinic introduces care and concern into the patient's life, and this shift enables growth. However, growth is never "neutral" or merely "positive," but also carries an implicit negation of the refusal to accumulate psychosocial capital. This refusal of accumulation and social legibility is problematic since it moves against the established forms of regulation of the control society. In order to think differently about this limiting factor of the clinic I want to follow Laplanche's reading of "Anlehnung" that revolves less around holding than the transformative force of the sexual. Instead of an endogenous development of sexuality, the child grows up in a context of generalized seduction. Its parents bombard the child with enigmatic messages that it needs to translate. This act of translation propels the child's eventual sexual development (Laplanche, 2007).

The Laplanchian intervention unsettles the British view of the clinic. In the British school, clinical practice entails teaching the patient to become more sociable by developing guilt over its aggressions. It is through guilt that reparation or concern for others becomes possible. These basic Kleinian or Winnicottian assumptions make up the British clinic's implicit political bedrock. The clinic, as a space of shoulders to lean on and nourishing breasts, enters the outside world by promising a model of intersubjective protection through guilt. This political model is powerful because it teaches us that we share a number of unconscious tendencies and identifications, which revolve around an unwillingness to recognize the other's ambivalence, our own solipsistic belief in manic omnipotence, and so forth. Clinical practice, to repeat a point made by Quinodoz, involves learning the "good" splitting to become a proper member of the intersubjective bond. This intersubjective bond is reliant on the acceptance of dimorphism as an essential and non-negotiable element of kinship. However, both intersexual and trans people directly undermine this notion, and resist the Oedipus complex's "coercive violence" (Freud, 1961, p. 262). Simone's privileged access to existential identity stems from her contesting these existential strictures. Simone's secret biological identity is a refusal of translatability. Her identity resonates with the queer intimacy of the darkroom. The expectation of forcing everything into symbolizable figurations turns into a resistance to representation and translation. This secret is not about the fear of being found out, but rather a form, the defiant assertion that deep joy suffuses the trans feminine subject as she passes through the streets. Her secrecy, however, establishes a complicated relationship to touch, both physical and verbal. Touch, as a sensual experience, draws upon morphological patterns. It is the "good splitting" of psychic bisexuality that situates subjects as properly homo- or heterosexual. Secrecy makes Simone's narrative irreducible, heterogeneous, and mystical, and endows her with a unique form of creativity and playfulness. Her being is inconclusive and escapes the psychiatric attempt at arresting her on clinical categories of transsexuality.

Consequences of history

I have belabored a rather short vignette with the greatest of attention and care, both because I am convinced of its sharpness but also because it comes short in certain key aspects. Simone's story is that of being capable of relating to the other and its desire for her. Quinodoz teaches her patient how to better love herself and others, by instructing Simone on how to accept her own peculiar position in the morphology of gender. It is only if she accepts "good splitting" that she can be a proper subject. This imposition of textuality relates her to the archive of psychoanalysis as a normal subject. However, it also denies her an *alpha-function of her own*, a principle of psychic creativity that genuinely belongs to her. Partially, this may be a shortcoming of a clinical modality that emphasizes interpretation of the here-and-now of the transference over a more sustained, freely-associative approach. The loss of polymorphous being, and even non-being, is particularly painful. I am saying this while being mindful that this change grants Simone some safety. In her I recognize a particular trans experience, that of the trans child, battered and abandoned, that moves out of the shadows, asking with the greatest of trepidation, "may I be here too?"

What are we to make of this yearning for arrival? Of being able to move between forms, even refuse them, but also cling to them? Quinodoz does welcome this child, she does not pathologize her, but she also assigns her a seat – that of heterogeneity. She buries Simone's own expressive function of psychic materiality under clinical teachings. The teachings that she dispenses hem in Simone's jouissance and limit her rather than enable her to confront the system of morphological assignation that she has faced so many times. Can there be a cure for this kind of imposition? Perhaps that of a deeper emptiness?

In his late work, Bion proposes the following: "Inability to tolerate empty space limits the amount of space available." (2014b, p. 292) This undated note from 1969 recasts an earlier formulation from 1967, in which Bion asserted, in a structural sense, that the "inability to tolerate frustration can obstruct the development of thoughts and a capacity to think" (2014a, p. 156). We find here our eternal struggle with the formless infinite out of which we create morphemes we can present to others. This struggle also animates Simone's journey. She yearns for a capacity to think, and Quinodoz is eager to supply her with the handed-down notions of psychoanalysis. What thus recedes into the background is the ability to forget such concepts – why not tolerate empty space and leave it empty, at least for a little while? This emptiness may be the cure for a psychoanalysis that operates by way of teaching its own archive over and over again. From this emptiness flows the awareness that repeating the archive's wisdom is its own compulsion. Quinodoz remains a teacher at heart, even though she is willing to abandon many of the strictures of her discipline, noting right from the outset that one must be somewhat mad to practice analysis nowadays (Quinodoz, 2003, p. 1). Her commitment to teaching is a result of fear over madness. We cannot overcome our mad or psychotic parts, because they belong to us. As fragments, they may lend themselves to creative sublimation. However, what can we do with the rest of our madness? The parts that are not merely suitable material for art, individuation, and becoming?

Before concluding, I want to emphasize once more the eminently political dimension of Simone's situation, something that Quinodoz does her best to occlude. Simone enters Quinodoz's consulting room as a person, who has grown up with the fetishization and objectification of the trans feminine body (as we all have). If she is alive today, she still has to contend with the near-constant oppression of trans feminine expressivity, which various institutions and social actors pathologize, ridicule, and belittle. Quinodoz's teachings participate in this reductive discourse by insisting that she be identifiably feminine socially, transsexual existentially, and a secret biologically. This model, though it gives trans feminine subjects wiggle room in the clinic, still confines them to this space, and their ability to find solace depends on them accepting this wiggle room as the sole acceptable locality of their becoming.

Simone enters the clinic and she becomes a Kleinian, and I am criticizing her therapist for this development – such may be a brief summary of my argument so far. One may argue that I, myself, merely seek to replace the Kleinian references with Bionian or Laplanchian references, and that all these "bad educations" are still very learned ones. I must readily concede that I have no solution for our near constant entanglement with the past. I want to suggest, however, that we can accomplish something by acknowledging the fact of a dark precursor, a hidden figure that inaugurates the constellation of questions we then examine. This dark precursor, Deleuze writes, "makes the different communicate, and makes it communicate with difference as such" (Deleuze, 1968, p. 189). Far from being "a friend," the dark precursor operates as an intensive force that gathers different notions and ideas within semiotic rubrics, without ever granting them full sovereignty. The dark precursor withdraws from our full understanding. In the case of Quinodoz's work, this dark precursor is not Klein herself. Her theories, which Quinodoz amply mobilizes, are the response to the various non-morphological disruptions Simone carries into the clinic. What precedes both her and Klein is the larger context of the constant diminishment of trans femininity, and of how this non-morphological force disrupts the possibility of touch itself. This presents a problem to Quinodoz, because her work rests on the implicit valorization of linguistic and affective touch.

My concern, then, does not lie with Kleinianism itself. I do not intend to juxtapose it with Bionian or Laplanchian thought to suggest that Kleinianism is inadequate. My critique is not about clinical efficiency or technique. One could equally argue that the modality of free association can be an interminable treatment that yields no change. My concern lies rather with the imposition of archival textuality, and the carceral landscapes this act of imposition generates. This landscape has its own play field, with rules and references, and it tames the unfettered thoughts of trans femininity.

Here, I want to introduce a distinction between concepts: faith and belief. In my view, belief represents an archaic investment in a certain notion or psychic disposition. Belief is blind to critique, and seeks to immunize itself from it. Oedipality is above all an archaic belief-system that guides our lives, and psychoanalysis is a method to problematize our own unconscious beliefs and phantasies. Faith, on the other hand, is about trust, and to a certain degree, the willingness to let go of an inhibition and instead give oneself permission to rely on something. To have faith in, for example, Oedipality is quite different from believing in it. The former suggests a trust in Oedipality's structuring force and its axiological importance. Belief connotes a more deep-seated investment in this structure, though this investment lies beyond symbolization. Belief is the fantasy that the super-ego's demands are fundamentally good ones.

The notion of "faith" has received great attention in psychoanalytic discourse, with, for example, Michael Eigen proposing the existence of an "area of faith" in Bion, Lacan, and Winnicott (Eigen, 1981). The area of faith, as per Eigen's reading of Winnicott, concerns transitional experiencing and object usage (Eigen, 1981, p. 413), both of which are aspects that matter greatly to Simone. Winnicott proposes that we must make room for the paradox that transitional objects come out of nowhere, falling neither into the realm of dreams or object-usage. The factors that underlie Simone's transition require their own particular function. Can one conceive of an alpha-function that grants the various factors of queerness and trans femininity their own meaning and space that are not reducible to inherited discourse? Factors such as the repudiation of reproduction, the sly play with secrecy, and the saccharine warmth of indeterminable femininity. Quinodoz's answer is to teach her patient about psychic bisexuality. However, psychic bisexuality is a level one theory, to borrow a concept from Laplanche. While a level two theory is generalizable and "properly" metapsychological, such as the distinction between ego, id, and super-ego, a level one theory belongs to a particular group of patients, such as the castration complex (Laplanche, 1996, p. 12). To engage in teaching this level one theory is to impose inherited textuality on another patient, and thus sabotage the possibility of genuinely novel and apposite alpha-function. Of course, the distinction between level one and two theories is somewhat specious. Can we at all speak of generalizable psychic structures? For now, I merely wish to emphasize that what protrudes transferentially are a series of factors that belong to functions that call for a different approach to structure. Established theory responds by proposing new imprisonments. As Donald Meltzer suggests, psychic carceral formations, which he terms "the claustrum," emerge because a person – an analyst – struggles or is unwilling to integrate foreign objects (Meltzer, 1992, p. 59); objects such as the trans feminine other. This is a problem of great urgency because the common societal response to trans femininity has been imprisonment.

The attempt at resituating trans being within the concept of psychic bisexuality means trapping trans being within someone else's anxious projective identifications. Meltzer utilizes the concept of the mental geography of the body to argue that such projective identifications utterly confound our relationship to our own body (Meltzer, 2000, p. 61). Given that Quinodoz's stated goal is to generate "words that touch," a particular psychic training is necessary to prepare her analysand for receiving touch – to make her a subject that can receive desiring touch is to make her properly morphological within the schema of psychic bisexuality. What Simone exhibits is certainly a *polymorphia*, owing to her shifting identifications, but also a suspension of morphological holding altogether. This suspension I would call "non-morphological," and its effects are forceful: it discombobulates intersubjectively shared views of the body, and the various mental geographies we have created of it. Simone's being thus invites us to reflect differently on the possibility of bodily being altogether. Her own statement about being a "lovable alien" directly speaks to her complicated relationship with morphology. The alien (or monster) is a common figure in queer literature. However, Quinodoz denies this alien its radical political force by projectively identifying it into her own model of carceral heterogeneity that goes by the name of psychic bisexuality.

Conclusion

My protracted reading of Quinodoz's vignette shows the various aspects that remain repressed throughout her treatment. To what extent these would have had meaning to Simone herself is impossible to tell, and not central to my argument. I am engaging neither in clinical admonishment nor in anti-ideological scolding.

Instead, it was a study of some of the disciplinary effects of (clinical) psychoanalysis, and of how these impose received notions of gender upon a person. Central to this is the consequence of heritage. The invocation of heritage offers a minoritized subject psychosocial stability. Simone has undergone a conversion and is now a properly sexuated person according to Freudo-Kleinian standards. This propriety renders her social and thus acceptable to be touched. This shift is significant, and alleviates her suffering; it also makes her internalize the clinic as a holding environment. However, it also traps her in other people's phantasies of what is right and wrong. She has thus re-experienced a foundational violence of trans feminine childhood, namely the prohibition to "merely be" according to the illegible workings of her own distinct and paradoxical creativity. She loses her own alpha-function again, and instead reformulates her incipient longings – her factors – according to functions of psychic conversion that belong to others, such as Freud, Klein and ultimately, Fließ.

Should trans feminine subjects reject or embrace the clinic? Perhaps the word "embrace" itself is decisive here. The physicality of the embrace, of allowing oneself to be held and protected, means to concede certain morphological norms. The words of the analyst can only reach the analysand if she concedes her psychic bisexuality as necessary fate – at least in the case of Quinodoz's treatment plan. Of course, other embodiments could find space in the clinic as well, but this requires that the invitation to polymorphia and suspension of morphology be embraced clinically.

It remains frustrating to me that my responses to Freudo-Kleinian limitations nevertheless make recourse to other hegemonic psychoanalytic figures, such as Bion or Laplanche. Something lurks behind all of this maneuvering: my desire to turn trans femininity into something that the establishment can recognize. I thus ultimately regress behind the very criticality I was insisting on in my reading of Quinodoz's work. It is as though I am pleading with the powers that be that they finally accept the trans feminine as psychoanalytically proper and reputable. After all, other great names of the discipline – Bion and Laplanche – offer us such fine theories to explain these confounding realities. The safety that thus follows, however, is its own prison. The masters have granted us the right to our existence, we may say. Such a gesture is Oedipal to the core, and while it is evidently productive and helpful, it is another attempt to deny the autonomy of trans feminine creativity. It seems to me that almost a hundred years after Radcylffe Hall's *The Well of Loneliness* queer people still live out as condemnation the very act that concludes Hall's novel, with its protagonist pleading, "'God,' she gasped, 'we believe; we have told You we believe... We have not denied You, then rise up and defend us. Acknowledge us, oh God, before the whole world. Give us also the right to our existence!'" (Hall, 2015, p. 510).

Any of my theoretical sleights of hand, which cast Bion or Laplanche as standard-bearers of liberation, preserve this very yearning. From this follows a question, which, albeit central to trans femininity, holds universal force: how do we *approach* the (trans feminine) other *without recourse to the established name*? And perhaps we ought to add: how may this other approach us? What would it mean to step entirely behind the world of morphological certainty? It is a world devoid of maps; perhaps it is not even a world, but a force of disarticulation. This force unties psychic bindings and confounds conceptual clarity. If it is a space, then it is one without name or structure. This space is empty, it deletes signification, and it is far-removed from the accumulation of psychosocial wealth and the promise of infinite growth.

Although it is empty, it not is not without potentiality. One may move in and out of this transitional space. Gender transition plunges someone into this space, and what begins to suffuse the worn-out body is playfulness over the completely contingent arrangement of objective belonging. This space is queer because it entails the refusal of a definite binding to society. While society continues to weave its infinite network of associations, queerness demands desubjectification. The cathexis of the world's entanglements brings joy, but due to their contingency, they are without captivity. The world rushes onward, creating again artworks, with their beauty, though evident to the trans feminine spectator, never moving into the realm of absoluteness. Instead, it all falls back again into the indelible darkness of muddled memory.

The world, then, proceeds by staying busy in all the usual ways, with the trans feminine subject staring rather bemusedly at the various contortions of the cisgender mind and body. If she wishes to join them, she has to accept the captivity of gendered morphology, and yet she can remain in the eternally suspended abeyance of a remark by the late Taubes, "I can imagine as an apocalyptic: let it [the world] go down. I have no spiritual investment in the world as it is" (Taubes, 2003, p. 103).

With belief in the world and its various defensive articulations – the law, theology, the clinic – receding, there emerges the possibility of a deeper faith; that the overcoming of inheritance and tradition may be the sole way toward a psyche floating freely and uncontrollably. Instead housing oneself in the prison of queer and trans feminine shame, which are necessary protections against the potential violence that corpsing could produce, the still emaciated body shakes off the imposition of unfreedom. The extent to which psychoanalysis can formulate and deepen these forces is the extent to which it is queer and trans feminine.

Bibliography

Barratt, B. (2017). "Opening to the Otherwise: The Discipline of Listening and the Necessity of Free-Association for Psychoanalytic Praxis." In: *The International Journal of Psychoanalysis,* 98.1, pp. 39–53.

Bion, W.R. (2014a). "A Theory of Thinking." In: *The Complete Works of W.R. Bion. Volume VI/ Second Thoughts.* Ed. by Chris Mawson & Francesca Bion. London: Karnac Books, pp. 153–161.

Bion, W.R. (2014b). "Cogitations." In: *The Complete Works of W.R. Bion. Volume XI.* Ed. by Chris Mawson. London and New York: Routledge, pp. 1–350.

Deleuze, G. (1968). *Différence et répétition.* Paris: Presses Universitaires de France.

Deleuze, G. (2013). "Controle et devenir." In: *Pourparlers. 1972–1990*. Paris: Les Éditions de Minuit, pp. 229–239.

Edelman, L. (2023). *Bad Education. Why Queer Theory Teaches us Nothing*. Durham: Duke University Press.

Eigen, M. (1981). "The Area of Faith in Winnicott, Lacan and Bion." In: *International Journal of Psycho-Analysis,* 62, pp. 413–433.

Freud, S. (1961). *Gesammelte Werke II/III. Die Traumdeutung. Über den Traum*. Ed. by Anna Freud, Edward Bibring, & Ernst Kris. Frankfurt: S. Fischer Verlag.

Gherovici, P. (2017). *Transgender Psychoanalysis: A Lacanian Psychoanalysis*. New York: Routledge.

Hall, R. (2015). *The Well of Loneliness*. London: Penguin Books.

Hansbury, G. (2017). "Unthinkable Anxieties. Reading Transphobic Countertransferences in a Century of Psychoanalytic Writing." In: *Transgender Studies Quarterly,* 4.3–4, pp. 384–404.

Heyam, K. (2023). *Before We Were Trans: A New History of Gender*. New York: Basic Books.

Klein, M. (1975). *Love, Guilt and Reparation and Other Works (1921–1945)*. Introduction by R.E. Money-Kyrle. New York: The Free Press.

Laplanche, J. (1996). "Psychoanalysis as Anti-Hermeneutics." In: *Radical Philosophy,* 79, pp. 7–12.

Laplanche, J. (2007). "Gender, Sex, and the Sexual." Trans. by Susan Fairfield. In: *Studies in Gender and Sexuality,* 8.2, pp. 201–219.

Meltzer, D. (1992). *The Claustrum*. London: Karnac Books.

Meltzer, D. (2000). "A Review of My Writings." In: *Exploring the Work of Donald Meltzer. A Festschrift*. Ed. by Margaret Cohen & Alberto Hahn. London and New York: Karnac Books. pp. 1–11.

Quinodoz, D. (2003). *Words That Touch. A Psychoanalyst Learns to Speak*. Trans. by Philip Slotkin. Foreword by Janine Chasseguet-Smirgel. London: Karnac Books.

Saketopoulou, A. & Pellegrini, A. (2023). *Gender without Identity*. New York: The Unconscious in Translation.

Taubes, J. (2003). *The Political Theology of Paul*. Trans. by Dana Hollander. Stanford: Stanford University Press.

Winnicott, D.W. (1985). "The Development of the Capacity for Concern." In: *Maturational Processes and the Facilitating Environment: Studies in the Theory of Emotional Development*. New York: International Universities Press.

Chapter 4

Tiresias, The Patron Saint of Psychoanalysis

On the Integral Mutations of Psychoanalysis

Simone A. Medina Polo

From the Symptom...

There is a pervasive restlessness at the heart of psychoanalysis. For an outsider, psychoanalysis comes across as sexist, homophobic, racist, transphobic, and Eurocentric – these have been historical resistances to psychoanalysis from feminism, queer theory, post-colonialism, and critical race theory, which argue that there is an irreducible excess that psychoanalysis fails to comprehend that is most evident in awkward attempts at universalizing psychoanalysis.[1] Even if at times psychoanalysis is caricaturized in these claims, these general insights contain an element of truth regarding psychoanalysis: these tensions cannot solely equate to a mere external impasse, but rather constitute an internal and constitutive impasse.

The tension at the heart of psychoanalysis is what we call the symptom of psychoanalysis. This chapter focuses on the mythical figure of Tiresias, who articulates this symptom in order to formulate psychoanalysis' integral capacity to mutate and change the bases from which it models its subjects and objects. Tiresias not only accomplishes this but can also help us model a *sinthome* of psychoanalysis as the patron saint of psychoanalysis. This is a creative strategy for the dislocative reinvigoration of psychoanalysis that comes to terms with this restlessness by treating it as an invitation for psychoanalysis to lose itself in such a truth and re-embody itself around this.

This chapter focuses on references to Tiresias throughout the work of Jacques Lacan, as well as in the contemporary work of Bracha L. Ettinger, Sheila L. Cavanagh, Patricia Gherovici, and Geneviève Morel, who lean on Tiresias and his significance in post-Lacanian psychoanalysis. We find that Lacan's references to Tiresias are ambivalent since Tiresias is seen as an impossible transsexual figure located outside of sex, while also being regarded as a figure close to Lacan's conceptualization of feminine non-all (2014). Gherovici appeals to Tiresias as a figure that articulates the oscillations between masculine and feminine sexuation, as well as life and death, as this is pertinent to what transgender cases teach us about psychoanalysis and sexuality (2017). Morel turns to the *sinthome* and Tiresias as a possibility for referring to sex without the phallic signifier (2006). Lastly, Ettinger and Cavanagh lean on Tiresias to transgressively articulate the matrixial borderspace besides the phallic signifier – as a model of individuated, sexuated subjectivity that

DOI: 10.4324/9781032624129-5

renders Tiresias impossible and the difference he breaches unknowable (Ettinger, 2020; Cavanagh 2023). Where Lacan sees a fundamental failure that constitutes the sexual non-relation and the unknowability of feminine sexuality by reinforcing the phallic signifying cut, Ettinger and Cavanagh highlight an impossibility of non-sharing and of not-knowing the feminine instead.

The Myth of Tiresias

Stories about Tiresias have different features, emphases, and versions with some basic elements remaining, including his birth from Everes, the shepherd, and Chariclo, the nymph, as well as his capacities for shape-shifting and prophecy. In "Tiresias and the Other Sexual Difference," Cavanagh surveys these different mythological and literary accounts of Tiresias including Homer's *The Odyssey*, Callimachus' poem "The Bathing of Pallas," Ovid's *Metamorphoses*, Sophocles' Theban plays, Guillaume Apollinaire's *Les Mamelles de Tiresias*, and T.S. Eliot's *The Waste Land* (Cavanagh, 2023).

In Ovid's *Metamorphoses*, Tiresias becomes a woman for seven years after disturbing two large snakes mating (1975). Zeus and Hera consult Tiresias on the question of whether women or men have the most pleasure – and further onwards, Tiresias' predictions play a role in the myth of Narcissus. In Callimachus' "The Bathing of Pallas," Tiresias is blinded after gazing upon a naked Athena – a significant encounter with the goddess of wisdom due to its symbolic weight with respect to Athena's association with virginity, shape-shifting, crossdressing, as well as multiple births (Callimachus et al, 1921). For Eliot, Tiresias' perspective grasps the stakes of the poem with all its figments of modern disjointedness (2001). For Apollinaire, Tiresias' breasts act as the bursting of a bubble of fantasy when Therese breaks the feminine masquerade for her husband and adopts the name Tiresias (1918). In Sophocles' plays, Tiresias counsels Oedipus and Creon regarding their respective tragedies (2008a, 2008b, 2015). And in *The Odyssey*, Tiresias continues to bear his gifts of prophecy even in the underworld (Homer, 2003).

Here are some interpretative threads with regards to the importance of Tiresias. Tiresias represents a vantage point to the partialities of sexuality, as Tiresias is portrayed as having an intimate knowledge of feminine and masculine sexual pleasure. In his blindness, Tiresias' knowledge and his capacity for prophecy are tied to a transgressive act – as in both Tiresias and *Oedipus at Colonus,* a grasp of a fundamental truth takes hold of these characters when they lose their sight (Sophocles, 2015). Not only does Tiresias transgressively oscillate between two sexual positions, but he also oscillates between life and death. Lastly, Tiresias embodies and fleshes out a difference in the instance of the lure of Tiresias' breasts. These are not exhaustive points to highlight from within Tiresias' myth by any means. However, they suffice for our understanding of the type of modeling that the Tiresian myth can offer for psychoanalysis.

We are not detouring through myth to exemplify psychoanalysis or the other way around. The deployment of myth in psychoanalysis offers a modeling of the psychoanalytic orientation as well as the structuring of the subjects and objects therein (Fink, 1997, p. 196; Felman, 1987, p. 103). As Lacan notes: "When we get on the trail of the unconscious, what we encounter are structured, organized, complex situations" (Lacan, 1991a, p. 65). The appeal to myth offers a symbolic and structural articulation of a model rather than a mere image, since what is at stake is the capacity to account for these formal situations of the unconscious according to clinical and practical efficacy (Lacan, 2006a, p. 718; Felman, 1987, pp. 104, 109, 122–123). We explore how Tiresias acts as a threshold for Lacanian psychoanalysis, as well as a herald of the mutations that characterize the future of psychoanalysis.

Phallic Impossibilities

The myth of Oedipus plays a central role in both Freud's and Lacan's deployment of myth. For Freud, Oedipus articulates an incestual and a patricidal set of thoughts that, even if they are detested in our most immediate and natural consciousness of them, speak to some fundamental drive of which we can only learn about through sources such as mythology, folklore, symbols, jokes, and other sublated formations of the unconscious (Freud, 1989, pp. 195, 212, 416–417).

Freud often points us to yonic and phallic symbolisms that articulate a certain sexual situation. From the feminine side, Freud refers to rescues from water, the fertility of landscapes in imageries of Mother Earth, oceanic mystical feelings, and uncanny womb fantasies sketching out a matrixial complex left untouched (Freud, 1989, pp. 195, 200; Freud, 1991, pp. 251–252; Freud, 2007, pp. 527–528; Ettinger, 2006, pp. 47–48). From the masculine side, there are well-known phallic symbolisms and the castration complex (Freud, 1989, pp. 203, 257–258; Freud, 2007, pp. 220, 230). Although we are dealing with implicative articulations of sexuality, feminine sexuality and sexuality itself remain a riddle in the final analysis, while the phallic remains a commonplace obviousness which is just as riddling – these are complexes that we grasp through myth and narrative even if we do not understand them (Felman, 1987, p. 150).

For Lacan, myth is a symbolic articulation of the drive and the libido – this is the contradiction that is the truth in the meaning of the myth (Dunand, 1996, p. 106). Besides his references to myths, Lacan makes his own like *l'hommelette* and the lamella (Lacan, 2006a, pp. 717–718). Thus, while Lacan is known for his transformative return to Freud formalizing mythemes into mathemes, Lacan insists on the deployment of myths as an act of modeling the antimonic psychic relations that we encounter in analysis (Lacan, 1992, p. 143; Lacan, 1991b, p. 227).

In the 1956–1957 seminar, myth is discussed through Lacan's commentary on Melanie Klein's treatment of Little Hans. Lacan treats myth as if it were a primary fact and activity akin to a narrative fiction and structure that maintains a singular relation to a truth because truth is structured like a fiction (Lacan, 2020, pp. 245–246). Thus, myth is what gives us "an idea of the weight, the presence, and the instance of the signifier as such, its specific impact" (Lacan, 2020, p. 248).

The signifier marks the beginning and the end of the Lacanian unconscious and its field. The signifier and its symbolic articulation as the Oedipus complex concern "the entire field of human relations... where the assumption of sex is decided" (Lacan, 1991a, p. 67). In "The Signification of the Phallus," the signifier is a contingent yet necessary disturbance of human sexuality around which the assumption of sex undertakes idiosyncratic and antimonic strategies articulating the disturbance – this is the irreducible crux of sexuation (Lacan, 2006b, p. 574). While in Freud, the distinction between the penis as the biological organ and the phallus as the symbol is not clear, for Lacan, the phallus has nothing to do with the anatomical distinction between the sexes: it is strictly a signifier which cuts on the imaginary and real registers of the subject as it introduces the symbolic.

The signifier has contradictory effects in the constitution of sexuated subjects as masculine and as feminine, no longer an unrecognizable and undifferentiated sexuality. Instead of the indistinguishable plenitude of the lamella as an indestructible organ of sexuality that spills everywhere, the cut of the signifier reveals the paradoxical space localizing two lacks: alienation as the constitutive failure in the subject and separation as the constitutive failure in the Other (Lacan 2006a, pp. 712–716). The unconscious is the short-circuit between the two failures, and the unconscious is sexual insofar as it is fundamentally skewed on the basis of the sexuated strategy around which both subject and Other are structured.

In "Position of the Unconscious" and *The Four Fundamental Concepts of Psychoanalysis*, Lacan breaks down the analytic situation as a retroactive operation beginning from the forced choice, which characterizes the *vel* of alienation, and ending the operation with a self-engendering attribution of this choice to oneself in the *velle* of separation. This movement from alienation to separation is nonetheless a return to alienation, as Lacan notes: "The *vel* returns in the form of a *velle*" (Lacan, 2006a, pp. 715–716; Lacan, 1998, pp. 209–215). This remark is suggestive and indicative of the oscillation between beginnings and endings around two superimposed lacks.

The *vel* to the *velle* is the movement from masculine and feminine expressions of the same term. This expression is symptomatic of the terminal point of the Lacanian unconscious and the Lacanian field on two accounts: (1) the phallic signifier as the operative impasse of the Lacanian field, and (2) the *sinthome* as an articulation of non-phallic psychic phenomena in the later Lacan. We can begin to refer to the myth of Tiresias as the articulation of a threshold in the Lacanian field as anchored by the phallic signifier here.

Before the introduction of the *sinthome*, Lacan's 1953–1954 seminar alludes to the limits of the Oedipal myth as a model for psychoanalysis. As Lacan notes, Freud offers us the first model of the complex situations of the unconscious through the Oedipus complex – and indeed it has become its standard (Lacan, 1991a, p. 65). Lacan addresses the privileged status of this complex:

That is what, in the life of the individual, resonates with the register of the law, as one discovers in the neuroses. [The Oedipus complex] is the most uniform point of intersection, the minimum requirement. That is not to say that it is the only one… The fact that the structure of the Oedipus complex is an ubiquitous requirement does not exempt us, for all that, from perceiving that other structures belonging to the same level, to the plane of the law, can, in a given case, play just as decisive a role (Lacan, 1991a, p. 198).

In the 1962–1963 seminar, Lacan comments that the signifying cut may not provoke the knotting of lack in woman like it does necessarily in man (Lacan, 2014, p. 183). While Tiresias is unequivocally referred to as the patron saint of psychoanalysis, Lacan's references to Tiresias tend to be ambiguous with respect to the feminine and transsexuality. Their fate remains tied up to each other through an impossibility inaugurated by the signifier, since sexual difference is structured around this same logical function which bars any knowledge of the Woman, the possibility of bypassing the phallic signifier through transsexuality, and a primary articulation of the Tiresian model of psychoanalysis besides the Oedipal complex (Lacan, 2006c, pp. 613, 619; Lacan, 2018a, pp. 9, 88).

In the 1971–1972 seminar, Lacan refers to Apollinaire's Tiresias at two instances where feminine sexuality and transsexuality are in question. With transsexuality, Lacan describes the transsexual as suffering a commonplace error that conflates the signifier and the organ (Lacan, 2018a, p. 9). Contrary to some accounts of this, such as Catherine Millot's (1990, p. 141), the transsexual struggles with an error that takes itself for a certainty not because they are confusing the signifier and the organ into a denial of the real sex, but because others have. However, what Lacan describes as the folly of the transsexual rests in the impossibility of being no longer signified by the phallus in sexual discourse and in the attempt to force this surgically as a passage to the real. Rather than denying the body and the real sex, one could say that the transsexual is passionately concerned with it. And Lacan adds that this is something that he has said in reference to feminine homosexuality in "Guiding Remarks for a Convention on Feminine Sexuality", claiming that a woman can only find jouissance in a symbolic break which excludes her from psychoanalytic discourse (Lacan, 2006c, p. 619; Lacan, 2018a, p. 9).

Lacan discusses feminine jouissance as the other jouissance that does not depend on phallic jouissance – this does not keep her from participating in phallic jouissance. This is precisely the meaning of the not-all: woman partakes in the symbolic through a masquerade without any masculine pretext that its relations are essential, unlike the masculine obsessions that convince themselves of the phallic necessity. As Lacan describes:

… she only participates in the phallic function by wanting it, either by stealing it from the man or, good heavens, by ordering him to serve it to her, so that in the… *or worse* of cases – mark my words – she may serve it back to him (Lacan, 2018a, p. 88).

Lacan refers to Apollinaire's Theresa dispelling the lure of her breasts for her husband as she shows herself to be Tiresias, thereby acting as the *objet a* appearing as lack lost in signification, which resists the function of the signifier (Lacan, 2014, p. 174). Or worse, this is precisely the crux of Oedipus gouging his eyes and of Creon's tragic turn upon encountering the *objet a* after disparaging the blind prophet Tiresias no less (Sophocles, 2008a, pp. 59–61).

Lacan comments on Hera's and Zeus' consultation of Tiresias' knowledge of sexual difference. Each of them was assuming that the opposite sex was having more pleasure. Though Zeus and Hera had not agreed upon the metric for the assessment, Tiresias answers that women enjoy nine times out of ten whereas men enjoy one out of ten (Apollodorus, 1921, p. 367). In her anger, Hera blinded Tiresias, while Zeus gifted the power of prophecy to Tiresias. Tiresias' answer is necessarily unsatisfying if we presume the measure of its truth beforehand. Tiresias' answers are often provoked by anger or provoke anger. Tiresian answers spoil Lacanian *jouissance* whether it be masculine (by spoiling the confidence of the phallic signifier) or feminine (by spoiling the masquerade) through transgression of the masculine-feminine and life-death. This much is remarked by Tiresias when the incestuous and patricidal truth of Oedipus, as well as the tragic transgression of life and death by Creon, are revealed to them.

> … when, with his eyesight turned to blindness,
> His wealth to beggary…
> … his children with him; and he will be known
> Himself to be their father and their brother,
> The husband of the mother who gave him birth,
> Supplanter of his father, and his slayer.

(Sophocles, 2008a, p. 63)

> Sickness has come upon us, and the cause
> Is you: our altars and our sacred hearths
> Are all polluted by the dogs and birds
> That have been gorging on the fallen body
> Of Polyneices…
> Because you have thrust down within the earth
> One who should walk upon it, and have lodged
> A living soul dishonourably in a tomb;
> And impiously have kept upon the earth
> Unburied and unblest one who belongs
> Neither to you nor to the upper gods
> But to the gods below, who are despoiled
> By you.

(Sophocles, 2008b, pp. 35, 37)

The Tiresian truth disorients all orientable relations, from sexual certainties to sexual ambiguities and from life to death, which we are compelled to address in some form. Tiresias remarks to Creon that:

> No man alive is free from error, but the wise and prudent man... does not persist, but tries to find amendment... It is the stubborn man who is the fool.
>
> (Sophocles, 2008b, p. 35)

We can think of *Oedipus at Colonus* as a portrayal of Oedipus precisely finding some amendment and letting go of his stubborn folly while Creon adopts his own. The major tension in *Oedipus at Colonus* concerns the location where Oedipus will die and be buried since this will give divine benefit to the city that is near the burial. Because of this and the on-going battle between Oedipus' sons about Thebes' throne, Thebes is seeking Oedipus after he was exiled for his blood-guilt, since it was prophesied that Oedipus would be the key to their security regardless of whether he was found dead or alive. Creon seeks Oedipus to keep him close enough to Thebes but not in Thebes (to keep themselves unpolluted by Oedipus' blood-guilt), tolerating Oedipus without internalizing him and appreciating his value. Nonetheless, Oedipus and Antigone find themselves welcomed in Colonus by their leader Theseus. Theseus sees himself in the alienness of Oedipus, and thus Oedipus gives himself away to Colonus over Thebes because the people of Colonus recognize the importance of Oedipus (Sophocles, 2015, pp. 240, 246). This point is driven home when Polynices seeks to finally acknowledge Oedipus' significance. Oedipus condemns his sons' ruthless despotism while his daughters tend to him in his exile – he holds love only for them:

> My children, on this day your father is no more.
> My life is wholly finished now,
> and you no longer need to bear
> the weary task of looking after me.
> It has been harsh, I know, my girls,
> but there is one small word
> redeems these many sufferings:
> You never could have had a *love*
> More full than from this heart of mine.
> But now henceforth you'll live a life devoid of me.
>
> (Sophocles, 2015, pp. 273–279 and 285)

Therefore, the Oedipus that we find at Colonus is much closer to Tiresias in the queer wisdom around his blind resoluteness to death and the feminine. However, when it comes to placing Lacan and psychoanalysis at Colonus, Lacan insists that the fate of the Tiresian myth remains undecided – in the end, the *velle* returns to the *vel*.

Joycean Heresies and Transgender Transgressions

It is opportune for us to turn to Patricia Gherovici's *Transgender Psychoanalysis* and Geneviève Morel's "The Sexual Sinthome," which bring together the impasses of the phallic signifier and the *sinthome* as an articulation of the non-phallic psychic phenomena such as that of queer and transgender subjects (Gherovici, 2017a). While we are departing from Lacanian orthodoxy, Lacan's 1975–1976 seminar on the *sinthome* can offer a groundwork for contemporary reformulations of sexual difference and psychoanalysis.

The *sinthome* can be thought of as a "but not that," as in "anything but not that," which characterizes the feminine not-all. The sinthome rolls with things, to put it idiomatically, in that it goes along with the current through the assumption of its own home rules [*sint' home rule*]. The *sinthome* is explored through reading the work of James Joyce and its significance can be grasped by an earlier presentation by Lacan, "Joyce the Symptom" (2018b). Joyce is a peculiar writer since his use of language appropriates its structuring of narrative with portmanteaus and stream of consciousness, as well as oscillating interior and exterior narratives described by one and the same sentence while breaking any linearity. Another significant aspect of Joyce's writing is the attempt at joining the spiritual liberation of Ireland under British colonialism, an intra-linguistic resistance within the language of the oppressor to the point of being met with censorship by British authorities condemning Joyce's language as obscene.

Lacan regards Joyce as embodying the symptom in himself to elude death – specifically through a posterity of keeping academics busy (Lacan, 2018b, pp. 143, 147). Joyce's elusiveness constitutes both his saintliness and his heresy. His saintliness in that Joyce embodies a pure symptom concerning the relationship to language as *lalangue*, a language oriented around *jouissance* rather than communication – here, Joyce uplifts the symptom to a power of language without concern for its being analyzable (Lacan, 2018b, pp. 142, 146). Joyce's heretical move stems from the very thing that captivates his saintliness insofar as English is appropriated for the aims of *jouissance* rather than communication. Joyce dislodges the English language, disrupting the sensibilities of the Anglophone settled into their monolingualism much like the feminine masquerade spoiling phallic masculine *jouissance*. In a sense, Joyce recalls Derrida's proclamation that "I have one language and it is not mine" (Derrida, 1998, p. 5). However, whereas for Derrida this unleashes a proliferation of undecidable difference, the Joycean difference entails a decision unlike the decisive cut of the phallic signifier which remains phallogocentrist. According to Lacan, Joyce sets a limit, but the ambiguity is what we are to understand by it (2018b, p. 147).

Lacan argues that Joyce avoided psychosis through the productive limitation of the symptom as *sinthome* without restricting himself to the Name-of-the-Father and the phallic signifier. Lacan argues that the *sinthome* is a decision of singular "home rule" in the manner that it knots the subjective registers of the symbolic (language and speech), the imaginary (the body, the senses, and images), and the real (jouissance) in taking on its limit. Usually, we understand Lacanian psychosis as the undoing of a delusional metaphor that holds a loose knot over these subjective registers to prevent a conflation of the imaginary and the real through the symbolic which regulates how *jouissance* may be inscribed. While normally the Name-of-the-Father manages this attachment of the knot in Lacanian perversions and neuroses, the *sinthome* offers an alternative that knots the unconscious with what is singular to the individual, while captivating the universality of structural modeling around them. In this sense, the *sinthome* is heresy done just the right way and that captivates the truth, as in "it just hits the spot" (Lacan, 2018b, p. 7).

There are unequivocal cases of the Freudian man and the Lacanian woman insofar as they inscribe their *jouissance* in familiar paradigms (Morel, 2006, pp. 65–66). However, as Morel notes, when we pose a Turing-esque experiment on whether by listening alone we can determine our analysands' sexuation, things become troubling when they do not fit these paradigms as we take them case by case. This is an invitation to come up with a different concept of sexual difference and to test out our capacity to model them. For example, Morel's case study of Ilse helps address this question with the creation of "the Parent" as a sinthome that helped Ilse bypass the sexual ambiguities surrounding the phallic forced choice through a choice of her own at the point where she did not want to play the role of "second mother" nor the role of "father" in her relationship to Marie and their child (Morel, 2006, p. 79).

In *Transgender Psychoanalysis*, Patricia Gherovici takes up the *sinthome* at work in transgender cases by highlighting the embodiment of the symptom as an attempt to get a body to get a hold of itself – this runs explicitly counter to Millot's claim that transsexualism aims for being outside-sex [*Horsexe*] as a sign of its psychosis which delusively denies the real of sex and the body (Gherovici, 2017a, pp. 143–144, 146; Millot, 1990, p. 15). Instead, the transgender sinthome takes the body seriously as its artwork, an embodiment that is a work in progress concerning the consistency of its form as its knot (Gherovici, 2017b, pp. 378–380). Not only that, but the transgender sinthome attempts to establish a sexual difference rather than being outside-sex. Furthermore, Gherovici highlights an element that even she overlooked in *Please Select Your Gender*: while we often focus on the sex and gender question in transgender cases, there is also a dimension of it that concerns boundaries of life and death (Gherovici, 2017a, p. 166). While Tiresias represents a transgression of sexual difference that some may treat as if it were outside-sex, Tiresias concerns a truth beyond life and death. This is where trans aesthetics and the contentious notion of passing become relevant to us: not only does passing concern how we own up to our body, but also how that assumption of the body is perceived as realness in the social world by its own right (Gherovici, 2017a, pp. 82, 103–104). Trans analysands are still concerned with the body, the drive, and sexuality – but what ties these things together is the *sinthome* of transition as a creative reclamation of life as livable (Gherovici, 2017a, pp. 164–167).

Through these reorientations of psychoanalysis, Gherovici and Morel agree that the myth of Tiresias offers us an opportunity to model these cases that hit a threshold in Lacanian psychoanalysis. There is an invitation that we are met with akin to Odysseus' consultation of Tiresias in *The Odyssey*. In *The Odyssey*, Odysseus performs rites and blood-offerings so that Tiresias can tell Odysseus the way home (Homer, 2003). Gherovici's interpretation articulates the stakes concerning Tiresias, as she points out that in speaking with ghosts, we are offering our living substance to make our journey worthwhile (Gherovici, 2017a, pp. 169–170). What we need to add is that Odysseus is warned about the difficulties ahead and his future re-enacting of a circle of vengeful violence which would mark his death – and in the end, Odysseus makes a difference concerning the nature of his death in finding peace through the divine intervention of Athena to stop Odysseus' perpetual struggle (Homer, 2003, pp. 322–324). With regards to interpreting this aspect of Tiresias' prophecy, we can turn to Simon Critchley's reading of the act of blood-offering to the ancients as he notes that when we offer our living substance to the ancients, they do not speak to us about themselves but about us, as we are invited into a "we" that is articulated creatively through a mutual dependence and vulnerability that provokes thought (Critchley, 2020, pp. 7–8).

Matrixial Openings

Another appropriation of the Tiresian myth by Bracha L. Ettinger and Sheila L. Cavanaugh articulates this mutual dependence and vulnerability as the matrixial borderspace: a trans-subjective edge besides personalized experiences as an axis of sexual difference that stands beside that of the phallus. In the matrixial borderspace, we can articulate what is experienced as a missed encounter and as a constitutive impossibility for individualized subjectivity that emerges through the phallic cut since the matrixial facilitates subtle transmissions, links, and acts of witnessing between anyone interwoven in its fabric (Ettinger 2006, pp. 42, 72–73). Ettinger's crucial intervention in psychoanalysis is that we can articulate the phallic while also giving structural support for the expression of transgenerational and trans-subjective trauma even if it is by means other than the Name-of-the-Father.

Ettinger does not challenge Lacan's position as this would be beside the point for her since the matrixial and the phallic operate concurrently even if the matrixial predates the phallus and the emerging subject is cut from the matrixial by the phallic signifier – a separation-in-jointness. What Ettinger problematizes with respect to Freud and Lacan is the terms under which they formulate feminine sexuality as impossible, unknowable, and regressive through figurations such as Freud's oceanic feeling and Lacan's transitivism that reduce the m/Other as potentially psychotic and inaccessible in-itself (Ettinger 2020a, p. 361). Where the phallic signifier sees that there is no sexual relation and there is no knowledge about the feminine, the matrixial borderspace articulates a space where there is a sexual relation and it is impossible not to share – the *objet a* turns on itself into a *link a* in the same way that we find ourselves implicitly connected to something other than ourselves when we ponder the emptiness of our navel that opens up a metaphysical speculation about our origin (Ettinger 2020a, pp. 355, 369).

The matrixial borderspace shares through metramorphosis, which Ettinger defines as "a co-poietic activity in a web" composed by the encounter that engendered *jouissance*, traumas, and affects. Their affected traces avow a partnership-in-difference between partial subjects and partial objects (Ettinger 2020a, pp. 360–361; Cavanagh 2023, p. 211). Thus, the womb operates as a modeling complex apparatus rather than an organ, by articulating the matrixial through figurations such as intrauterine relations between the becoming-mother and the becoming-subject as com-passion clusters that *com-pass* between oneself and inside others and outside. Matrixial encounters are transgressive events of one's own personal handling, yet one knows them without knowing whose trauma it is.

Ettinger articulates this as knowledge of *co-naissance* (being-born-together) corresponding with the matrixial alliances that bind the partialities of the feminine cluster into a unique sort of unity. Ettinger's matrixial space recalls the invitation into the "we" in the force of tragic theater insofar as a foundational vulnerability and dependence is revealed in the Oedipal drama when Oedipus unravels a matrixial web – specifically, after Tiresias tells him the truth and the fact that Antigone and Ismene were tending to him at Colonus. The impossibility of non-sharing is transformative and fragilizing for Oedipus in wit(h)nessing a trauma that has spanned and will span generations (Ettinger 2020b, pp. 338–339). The Thing that compels us about Oedipus has bonded a generational transmission. Ettinger's notion of *metramorphosis* is the aesthetic process of this matrixial transformation not contained to dramatic theater since Ettinger articulates it through visual art. The stage and the surface of the artwork share an aesthetic potential for facilitating a spasm of co-emergence of subjectivity-as-encounter.

This comes with ethical implications because the artwork borderlinks us by the outreaching experience of wit(h)nessing across time and space; and the therapeutic approach has to be faithful to its ethical significance. One can grasp the ethics of psychoanalysis around the matrixial aesthetic through Ettinger's Demeter-Persephone complex and the figure of Sylvia Plath as articulations of motherhood and primordial love. In myth, Demeter turns Heaven and Earth on its head upon losing Persephone, who has been dragged to the Underworld for a marriage with Hades. When Persephone is met by Orpheus in his quest to retrieve Eurydice from Hades, Persephone is touched by his song evoking the name of love which reminded her of Demeter through an erotic shock of maternality. For Ettinger, the Demeter-Persephone complex is the articulation of the unconscious complexity of this primordial love and sharing besides the phallic poles of love-hate around Oedipus and the signifier – this is a matrixial love held by resonances and inspirations, rather than identifications that otherwise treat this love as incestuous and psychotic according to phallometrics. The stakes of the matrixial ethics become apparent when one denies the possibility of the Demeter-Persephone complex as in the case of Sylvia Plath's poetry, where the alternative is abjection that reduces the womb to a suicidal tomb ("Ariel") and hatred for the mother by her children since there is nothing in between them ("Medusa") (Ettinger, 2014, pp. 123–124, 135–137). The ethics of psychoanalysis amount to nothing more than empathy without compassion here, an empty empathy unable to overcome the projective semblances of transference and countertransference with nothing in between the analyst and the analysand (Ettinger, 2014, p. 127). Counter to the well-known tendency to sacrifice something to enter into the analytic situation, the matrixial cannot be clean cut and separated from. Therefore, the analytic responsibility, care, respect, and compassion of the matrixial extends beyond transference and countertransference by accounting for the trans-subjective in asking: What impact do these interventions have on future helpless others?

... To the Sinthome: On the Integral Mutations of Psychoanalysis

This chapter continues an argument from another piece on psychoanalysis' capacities to change in response to Gabriel Tupinambá's *The Desire of Psychoanalysis*.[2] What we are trying to articulate is the possibility of a genericity inherent to psychoanalytic thinking otherwise obscured by the logic of the signifier and Oedipus. These structures are contingent operative limits for the procedures of psychoanalysis in Freudian, Lacanian, and object-relations, among other orientations of psychoanalysis. The problem is their quasi-transcendentalization of its contingency through a retroactive illusion presuming the necessity of its model.

While generic psychoanalysis makes great strides opening up the psychoanalytic field, we can still value and appreciate these orientations within their own operational limitations, such as the Oedipus complex and the logic of the signifier. As Morel argues in "The Sexual Sinthome:"

[The sinthome as a separation and as transgenerational transmission] turns the sinthome into a concept which theoretically "fills in for" the Name-of-the-Father, to the degree that the latter... loses its central position in his theory... the Name-of-the-Father retains a clinical interest: it is no more than a particular modality of the sinthome... The phallus... becomes a contingent signifier of jouissance... This is not to say these structures are useless or that we have to replace the "old" paradigm of the Name-of-the-Father by the "new" paradigm of the sinthome, because these structures are still valid in relation to the classical signs, the Name-of-the-Father and the phallus, which remain important in a number of cases (Morel, 2006, p. 70).

At most, one could say that the *sinthome* relativizes the privileged modalities of the *sinthome*. Thus, generic and impure psychoanalysis are the difference between analysis terminable and interminable, between the finite and the infinite in psychoanalysis – between psychoanalysis and psychoanalysis as a short-circuit of theory and practice, which the figure of myth is able to articulate (Felman, 1987, p. 155; Lacan, 1991b, p. 227). As Tupinambá argues: "Psychoanalytic thinking is generic because it is terminable and interminable, a set of finite processes that stitch together an infinite procedure" (Tupinambá, 2021, p. 117). The myth of Tiresias, the Persephone-Demeter complex, Ilse's "the parent," and many others show us this. With every mythotopological structure, psychoanalysis is not what it used to be – and perhaps never was!

There are changing tides regarding what psychoanalysis is at any one point. From Freud's turn from his early pastorialism to the death drive as the core negativity; from the early splits to Lacan's return to Freud; from the Lacanian teaching to the Millerianisms, Badiouianisms, Zizekianisms, and Ettingerianisms of "Lacanian" psychoanalysis, psychoanalysis is in a constant retrieval of itself through psycho-analysts (Felman, 1987, p. 11). Psychoanalysis is not a *sinthome*, however, the psychoanalyst is a *sinthome* (Lacan, 2018c, pp. 115–116). Psychoanalysis forgets itself in productive ways unconscious to it. Psychoanalysts are the mutant results of this forgetful activity which forgets that it has nothing but an ignorance of the *sexualle* unconscious – except that we are recollecting something from it, about it, and that we can realize this knowledge through the very plasticization with which it short-circuits.

This knowledge of psychoanalysis is the transformation of psychoanalysis itself. This minimal insight opens the field of psychoanalysis so that Oedipus is a frag-ment of a broader myth. Psychoanalysis models unconscious formations through myths that captivate "its apparent fixities and ostensible flexibilities", whilst psy-choanalysis is the transformation of its own self-consciousness in what it means to be psychoanalysis (Nobus, 2017, p. 355). It is not that psychoanalysis has to be-come a mutant psychoanalysis with a new epistemology of sex, gender, and sexual difference (Preciado, 2021, pp. 97–98). Rather, psychoanalysis is itself a mutant psychoanalysis, and it is just realizing that it cannot help but impurify itself through operative limits to process a complex situation.

Notes

1 For another treatment on this problem, see the forthcoming "Guerrilla Psychoanalysis: On Generic and Impure Psychoanalysis" (Medina Polo, S., 2023).
2 See the forthcoming "Guerrilla Psychoanalysis: On Generic and Impure Psychoanaly-sis" (Medina Polo, S., 2023).

Bibliography

Apollinaire, G. (1918). *Les Mamalles de Tiresias: Drama Surrealiste en Deux Acts et un Prologue*. Paris: Editions Sic.
Apollodorus. (1921). *The Library, Volume I*. Trans. J.G. Frazer. London: William Heinemann.
Callimachus, Lycophron, Aratus. (1921). *Hymns and Epigrams. Lycophron: Alexandra. Aratus: Phaenomena*. Trans. A.W. Mair and G.R. Mair. [Loeb Classical Library 129.] Cambridge, MA: Harvard University Press.
Cavanagh, S.L. (2023). "Tiresias and the Other sexual difference: Jacques Lacan and Bracha L. Ettinger." In P. Gherovici and M. Steinkoler (Eds.) *Psychoanalysis, Gender, and Sexu-alities: From Feminism to Trans**. London: Routledge. pp. 197–211.
Critchley, S. (2020). *Tragedy, the Greeks, and Us*. London: Profile Books.
Derrida, J. (1998). *Monolingualism of the Other: Or, the Prosthesis of Origin*. Trans. P. Mensah. Stanford: Stanford University Press.
Dunand, A. (1996). "Lacan and Lévi-Strauss." In R. Feldstein, B. Fink, and M. Jaanus (Eds.) *Reading Seminars I and II: Lacan's Return to Freud*. Albany: State University of New York. pp. 98–108.

Eliot, T.S. (2001). *The Waste Land: Authoritative Texts, Contexts, Criticism*. Ed. M. North. New York: W.W. Norton & Company.

Ettinger, B.L. (2006). "The matrixial gaze." In B. Massumi (Ed.) *The Matrixial Borderspace*. Minneapolis: The University of Minnesota Press. pp. 40–90.

Ettinger, B.L. (2014). "Demeter-Persephone complex, entangled aerials of the psyche, and Sylvia Plath." *ESC: English studies in Canada*, 40(1): pp. 123–154.

Ettinger, B.L. (2020a). "Transgressing with-in-to the feminine." In G. Pollock (Ed.) *Matrixial Subjectivity, Aesthetics, Ethics: Volume I, 1990–2000*. London: Palgrave Macmillan. pp. 347–374. (Original work published in 1997.)

Ettinger, B.L. (2020b). "Art as the transport-station of trauma." In G. Pollock (Ed.) *Matrixial Subjectivity, Aesthetics, Ethics: Volume I, 1990–2000*. London: Palgrave Macmillan. pp. 325–345. (Original work published in 1999.)

Felman, S. (1987). *Jacques Lacan and the Adventure of Insight: Psychoanalysis in Contemporary Culture*. Cambridge: Harvard University Press.

Fink, B. (1997). *A Clinical Introduction to Lacanian Psychoanalysis: Theory and Technique*. Cambridge: Harvard University Press.

Freud, S. (1989). *Introductory Lectures on Psychoanalysis*. Trans. and Ed. J. Strachey. New York: W.W. Norton & Company.

Freud, S. (1991). "Civilization and its discontents." Trans. J. Strachey. In A. Dickson (Ed.) *Volume 12, Civilization, Society, and Religion: Group Psychology, Civilization and its Discontents and Other Works*. New York: Penguin Books. pp. 251–340. (Original work published in 1929.)

Freud, S. (2007). "The 'uncanny.'" In D.H. Richter (Ed.) *The Critical Tradition: Classical Texts and Contemporary Trends, Third Edition*. Trans. J. Strachey. New York: Bedford/ St. Martin's. pp. 514–532.

Gherovici, P. (2017a). *Transgender Psychoanalysis: A Lacanian Perspective on Sexual Difference*. New York: Routledge.

Gherovici, P. (2017b). "Sexual difference: From symptom to sinthome." In N. Giffney and E. Watson (Eds.) *Clinical Encounters in Sexuality: Psychoanalytic Practice and Queer Theory*. Goleta, CA: Punctum Books. pp. 369–381.

Homer (2003). *The Odyssey*. Trans. E.V. Rieu and D.C.H. Rieu. New York: Penguin Books.

Lacan, J. (1991a). *The Seminar of Jacques Lacan, Book I: Freud's Paper on Technique, 1953–1954*. Ed. J-A. Miller. Trans. J. Forrester. New York: W.W. Norton & Company, Inc.

Lacan, J. (1991b). *The Seminar of Jacques Lacan, Book II: The Ego in Freud's Theory and in the Technique of Psychoanalysis, 1954–1955*. Ed. J-A. Miller. Trans. J. Forrester. New York: W.W. Norton & Company, Inc.

Lacan, J. (1992). *The Seminar of Jacques Lacan, Book VII: The Ethics of Psychoanalysis, 1959–1960*. Ed. J-A. Miller. Trans. D. Porter. New York: W.W. Norton & Company, Inc.

Lacan, J. (1998). *The Seminar of Jacques Lacan, Book XI: The Four Fundamental Concepts of Psychoanalysis*. Ed. J-A. Miller. Trans. A. Sheridan. New York: W.W. Norton & Company, Inc.

Lacan, J. (2006a). "Position of the unconscious." In Écrits. Trans. B. Fink. New York: W.W. Norton & Company, Inc. pp. 703–721.

Lacan, J. (2006b). "The signification of the phallus." In Écrits. Trans. B. Fink. New York: W.W. Norton & Company, Inc. pp. 575–584.

Lacan, J. (2006c). "Guiding remarks for a convention on feminine sexuality." In Écrits. Trans. B. Fink. New York: W.W. Norton & Company, Inc. pp. 610–620.

Lacan, J. (2014). *The Seminar of Jacques Lacan, Book X: Anxiety*. Ed. J-A. Miller. Trans. A.R. Prince. London: Polity.

Lacan, J. (2018a). *The Seminar of Jacques Lacan, Book XIX: ... or worse*. Ed. J-A. Miller. Trans. A.R. Price. London: Polity.

Lacan, J. (2018b). "Joyce the symptom." In J-A. Miller (Ed.). *The Seminar of Jacques Lacan, Book XXIII: The Sinthome*. Trans. A.R. Price. London: Polity. pp. 141–148.

Lacan, J. (2018c). *The Seminar of Jacques Lacan, Book XXIII: The Sinthome*. Ed. J-A. Miller. Trans. A.R. Price. London: Polity.

Lacan, J. (2020). *The Seminar of Jacques Lacan, Book IV: The Object Relation*. Ed. J-A. Miller. Trans. A.R. Price. London: Polity.

Medina Polo, S. (2006). "The sexual sinthome." Trans. R. Végső. In *Umbr(a): Incurable*, (1), 65–83.

Medina Polo, S. (2023). "Guerilla psychoanalysis: On generic and impure psychoanalysis." In N.A. Barria-Asenjo and S. Žižek S. (Eds.) *Revista de Humanidades de Valparaíso: An International Journal of Philosophy*, (23), 163–178.

Millot, C. (1990). *Horsexe: Essay on Transsexuality*. Trans. K. Hilton. New York: Autonomedia.

Morel, G. (2006). "The sexual sinthome." Trans. R. Végső. In *Umbr(a): Incurable*, (1), 65–83.

Nobus, D. (2017). "Undoing psychoanalysis: Towards a clinical and conceptual metistopia." In N. Giffney and E. Watson (Eds.) *Clinical Encounters in Sexuality: Psychoanalytic Practice and Queer Theory*. Goleta, CA: Punctum Books. pp. 343–356.

Ovid (1975). *Metamorphosis*. Trans. M.M. Innes. Great Britain: Penguin Books.

Preciado, P.B. (2021). *Can the Monster Speak? Report to an Academy of Psychoanalysts*. Trans. F, Wynne. Cambridge, MA: semiotext(e).

Sophocles (2008a). "Oedipus the king." In *Antigone, Oedipus the King and Electra*. Trans. H.D.F. Kitto. Oxford: Oxford University Press.

Sophocles (2008b). "Antigone". In *Antigone, Oedipus the King and Electra*. Trans. H.D.F. Kitto. Oxford: Oxford University Press.

Sophocles (2015). "Oedipus at Colonus." In *Oedipus the King and Other Tragedies*. Trans. O. Taplin. Oxford: Oxford University Press.

Tupinambá, G. (2021). *The Desire of Psychoanalysis: Exercises in Lacanian Thinking*. Evanston, IL: Northwestern University Press.

Chapter 5

H.D. and Bryher

Psychoanalysis, Mysticism, and Gender

Elisabeth Punzi

H.D. and Bryher were two queer writers, poets, and lovers, whose work and lives were profoundly marked by their interest in mysticism and psychoanalysis. They were important figures in the modernist literary movement. They also made significant contributions to art cinema, both as editors of the cineaste magazine *Close-up* between 1927 and 1933 together with Kenneth Macpherson, and through the films they created – films that, according to them, expressed psychoanalytic processes. Bryher became a spokesperson for psychoanalysis, encouraging friends, family, and colleagues to attend psychoanalysis. He also rescued psychoanalysts from Nazi prosecution, was an early subscriber to the *International Psychoanalytic Journal*, and was a patron of the International Psychoanalytic Press (Souhami, 2020, p. 175). H.D. also had a serious interest in psychoanalysis and attended psychoanalysis with Sigmund Freud during 1933 and 1934. She wrote about her analysis in the volume *Tribute to Freud* (H.D., 1956).

In this chapter, I will present H.D. and Bryher and their encounters with psychoanalysis. I will specifically focus on how their queerness and life choices – including non-normative gender identifications and presentations, and relationships – were acknowledged as valid and not pathologized by the psychoanalysts they encountered. I will also reflect on the queerness of Pallas Athena, since a Pallas Athena statue from Freud's collection of antiquities was important in H.D.'s presentation of her own psychoanalysis.

H.D. and Bryher

H.D.'s full name was Hilda Doolittle. She was born in Bethlehem, Pennsylvania, USA, in 1886. Her family belonged to the Moravian Church, a part of Protestantism in which mystical experiences and spirituality were important. Her father was a professor of astronomy, and she grew up in a privileged environment (H.D., 1982). Even as a child, she was drawn to poetry and mystical experiences. As a teenager, her interest in poetry was strengthened and she was engaged to another modernist poet, Ezra Pound. Their engagement was short, but their friendship lasted a lifetime, as described in *End to Torment. A Memoir of Ezra Pound* (H.D., 1979). It was Pound who suggested the pen name H.D., which she adopted. Early in life, H.D.

DOI: 10.4324/9781032624129-6

acknowledged her desire for both men and women. In 1911, together with her then partner, Frances Josepha Gregg and Gregg's mother, she traveled to Europe where she stayed lived the rest of her life, occasionally visiting America. From 1913 until 1938 she was married to Richard Adlington.

H.D. published her first book, *Sea Garden*, in 1916. Her poems repeatedly involved mystical and mythological themes, not least symbols and tales from Egypt and from Greek mythology (see, for example, H.D., 1973), and she translated Greek dramas into English. She was considered a prominent writer, and in 1960 she was awarded an American Academy of Arts and Letters medal (Hollenberg, 2022).

Throughout her life, she experienced a series of traumas, crises, and shocks, including the sudden and traumatic death of family members, serious somatic illnesses, and a miscarriage. She also struggled with serious mental health issues, including short and prolonged episodes of extreme mental states – in medical terminology called psychosis, profound states of derealization, paranoia, and breakdowns – and during these episodes Bryher provided emotional, practical, and financial support (McCabe, 2021a, pp. 99–100, 259). The last years of her life, she mostly lived in a mental health institution in Switzerland, arranged and paid for by Bryher (McGabe, 2021b).

H.D. was ambivalent about her so-called occult experiences and her tendencies for derealization. She perceived them as benevolent and as a form of spiritual realism, although simultaneously she and her close ones perceived them as distressing, to the extent that Bryher provided sedatives and analgesics (McCabe 2021a, pp. 106, 247). Her distress contributed to her wish to start analysis. Another reason for starting analysis was that she experienced writer's block. During analysis, Freud supported her to overcome her writer's block, (Friedman, 2002, p. 392).

It is difficult to draw a line between spiritual experiences and mysticism on the one hand, and extreme mental states that impact a person's wellbeing and capacity to live a satisfying life on the other. During the days when H.D, and Bryher engaged in mysticism, occultism and seances, this was part of the Zeitgeist (McCabe, 2021a, p. 233). Freud also had an interest in mystical and occult phenomena, specifically the possibility of telepathy (Rottenberg, 2017, pp. 310–18). It should be noted that a person may experience severe distress and altered mental states and have difficulties in handling life for shorter or longer periods of time, and still have capabilities, a satisfying life, and mutual relationships (see, for example, Bentall, 2004). It should also be noted that H.D.'s and Bryher's non-normative gender expressions and identifications exposed them not only to ridicule and prejudice, but also meant that they often had to hide who they were and how they lived – circumstances that in themselves may trigger mental health issues, due to chronic trauma and stress. Both H.D. and Bryher had their difficulties, and both supported each other (McCabe, 2021a, pp. 114–15).

Bryher was born Annie Winifred Ellerman, in 1894, into an exceptionally wealthy family. Sir John Ellerman, Bryher's father, was a shipowner and considered the richest man in England. Since Bryher was born a girl, a major part of the wealth was dedicated to the younger brother. Social and financial injustices due to gender assigned at birth, were ever-present. As a child, Bryher identified as a boy and was concerned by the dresses and ruffles Bryher had to wear. Later in life, Bryher preferred clothes that were coded as masculine, and, in personal correspondence, H.D. often referred to Bryher as he or him. In prior and current literature, Bryher is often referred to as a woman and a lesbian – a term that at the time was often used, not only in the way the word is used today, but also for women who had a non-normative gender identity or expression or non-normative sexual orientation (Souhami, 2020, pp. 3–4). McCabe (2021b) underlines the couple's queerness and Bryher's desire to be approached as male. It is difficult and risky to use contemporary terminology in hindsight. Terms such as trans or non-binary were not used in Bryher's and H.D.'s lifetime. I would, however, like to acknowledge that, since childhood, Bryher identified as male, and therefore I will refer to Bryher as he or him.

Halperin (2003) writes that the terms queer and queerness are disruptive and invite reflections, possibilities, and acknowledgment of multiple differences. By using the terms queer and queerness in relation to past times, history can be understood in new ways (Halperin, 2003, p. 341). Therefore, I will use the terms queerness and queer identifications, expressions, and desires. The possibility to understand history could also be connected to Rohy's term *straight time* and her reflections on *anachronism*. Rohy (2009) describes straight time as not simply heterosexual, but as an idealization of regularity, linearity, and progress. These simplified forms of temporality are challenged, however, since we live our lives in circumstances of anachronism. In psychoanalysis, memories, the acknowledgment that personal past, present, and future exist simultaneously, as well as the metaphor of psychoanalysis as an archeological excavation, demonstrate that straight time is not in focus. Likewise in mysticism, as well as in the poetry of H.D., time is nonlinear. Memories, dreams, past, present, and future overlap each other. Time is simultaneously ever-present and challenged. Such temporality is queer, it resists linear progression and normative constructions of time.

Early in life, Bryher wanted to write and had a serious interest in archeology, history, and literature. He read H.D.'s debut *Sea Garden* and learned the poems by heart. In the summer of 1918, Bryher visited H.D., who by then was staying in Cornwall together with her lover Cecil Gray (Souhami, 2020, p. 124). Their love story began immediately, and when H.D.'s daughter Perdita was born in 1919, Bryher took care of the seriously ill H.D. and the child, as well as practical and financial issues. Meanwhile the biological father, Cecil Gray, and Adlington withdrew from H.D. and Perdita.

H.D.'s and Bryher's relationship did not exclude others, and they were involved in what today could be described as polyamorous relationships. H.D. had many lovers of various genders and gender orientations. Bryher was married twice, to Robert McAlmond from 1921 to 1927 and to Kenneth Macpherson from 1927 to 1947. These marriages increased Bryher's financial inheritance and created a normative façade, which suited his family. Macpherson and Bryher adopted Perdita. When

H.D. became pregnant with Macpherson's child, she had an abortion. McCabe (2021a, p. 176) describes that Bryher and H.D.'s relationships involved jealousy and strivings to create emotional effects in each other and in their partners – for example, through love affairs or flirtations with others. For long periods Bryher and H.D. did not see each other. Nevertheless, their relationship was solid, and they were life companions.

Psychoanalytic Encounters

By the time of H.D. and Bryher's encounter and evolving love story, psychoanalysis was in the air. Psychoanalysis as clinical treatment developed and became increasingly diverse. Interventions for children, people with psychotic experiences, and soldiers with war neuroses were explored and established. The poverty among people in Europe after the end of World War One was extreme. Freud took the initiative to establish free clinics for those who could not afford treatment or counseling – a psychotherapy for the people – establishing sex education for teenagers and adults, as well as ambulatory clinics (Danto, 2007). Simultaneously, the connections between psychoanalysis and the humanities and the artistic domain became increasingly important, as exemplified by the journal *Imago*, established in 1912 and devoted to psychoanalysis's intersection with the arts, humanities, and social sciences. Freud sensed that psychoanalysts needed thorough knowledge of religion, mythology, history, and literature in order to understand their patients. Art and literature were important to him, and he cherished writers such as Goethe and Schnitzler for their capacity to understand and present the depths and conflicts of the human soul.

Analysts explored connections between psychoanalysis and the arts; and writers, visual artists, and film makers incorporated psychoanalytic thinking in their works. In Berlin, the connections between the arts and psychoanalysis became clearly pronounced. Alexander Döblin integrated literature and psychoanalytic thinking in his groundbreaking book *Berlin Alexanderplatz* (Fuechtner, 2011, pp. 18–64). The 1926 silent movie *Secrets of a Soul* (in German *Geheimnisse einer Seele*), directed by Pabst, strived to show psychoanalytic processes through images and processes (whether it succeeded is a question I will not try to answer here). The analyst Hanns Sachs, who had established himself in Berlin, was important for making the movie come into being, representing the wish to popularize psychoanalysis and go beyond treatment of patients (Fuechtner, 2011, p. 11).

Bryher frequently stayed in Berlin. In 1927, he met Hanns Sachs, and in 1928 became Sachs's analysand (McCabe, 2021a, pp. 134–9). Their relationship went beyond patient and analyst. When Bryher, H.D., and Macpherson published *Close Up*, Sachs wrote for the magazine. Bryher had met Freud in 1927, and, in 1934, Sachs encouraged Bryher to write to Freud and ask him to accept H.D. as an analysand, since H.D. was increasingly distressed and behaved erratically. Within a week Freud responded to Bryher's letter, writing that he remembered their meeting and addressed Bryher as "Sir" (McCabe, 2021a, p. 158).

H.D.'s analysis started in March 1933, and, after a break, it was resumed in 1934. Before they met, Freud read H.D.'s poetry, and during their first meeting he showed her the consulting room with its mythological statues and archeological artefacts (Friedman, 2002, p. 34). These forms of heritage became central in H.D.'s presentation of the analysis in *Tribute to Freud* (H.D., 1956). The book is no straightforward presentation of the analytic process but, rather, it is dreamlike, nonlinear, associative, and anachronistic. Thereby, it resembles the psychoanalytic process itself. H.D. describes how the analysis involves reflections on religion, mythology, mysticism, and creative expressions, and how dreams, objects, memories, and mystical experiences are approached with openness (Punzi, 2022). Also questions of gender and gender identity were approached with openness. While in analysis, H.D. wrote to Bryher and told him that she had showed Freud (whom she in personal letters called Papa) a photo of Bryher, taken by Man Ray. "Papa made a most brilliant remark," she wrote, and added, "He turned to me and said, 'but she is ONLY a boy.' I think that rather wonderful" (Friedman, 2002, p. 112). Moreover, McCabe (2021a, p. 163) describes that, after Freud had encountered the couple, he understood that girls do not always transfer their emotions from the mother to the father – something that McCabe perceives as "huge." Considering that this was a time when homophobia was ever-present and atypical identities and desires were oppressed, I agree that this is "huge." Freud's acknowledgment of Bryher as a boy, and of girls not necessarily transferring their emotions to their father, can also be seen as a return to his statements that both hetero- and homosexual tendencies are present in everyone, and that the physical gender, the perceived gender, and the object choice, are varying and come in many forms (Freud, 1920, pp. 146–8). This reveals that despite the many oppressive and pathologizing psychoanalytic interventions and theories that were developed during the 20th century, psychoanalysis holds a queer heritage, a core that acknowledges queerness as an issue that concerns us all.

Bryher's identification as a boy, sensed already in childhood and presented in fictional form in the short novels *Development* (published 1920) and *Two Selves* (published 1923) (Bryher, 2000), was acknowledged by Freud and Sachs. Bryher was on the Executive Committee of the psychoanalytic publishing house, *Verlag*, and took part in international psychoanalytical congresses during the 1930s (McCabe, 2021a, pp. 157, 177, 197, 205). Freud and Sachs supported Bryher's wish to become a lay analyst. They suggested to him that he could train in France or Switzerland since the institutes there were more "liberal" and open to lay analysts. Freud and Sachs offered support and recommendations, but due to the political climate of Europe and the subsequent war, Bryher was unable to proceed with these plans (McCabe, 2021a, p. 169).

I would like to call attention to the fact that if Freud and Sachs had disdained queer identifications, sexualities, desires, or relationships, or had considered them pathological, they would not have supported Bryher to become a psychoanalyst. In *Close Up*, Sachs wrote about how witch hunts served to demonize women who were not docile and who escaped their roles as subservient housewives. He also told Bryher that psychoanalysis had no conventional morals (Souhami, 2020, p. 170–2). Nowhere do H.D., Bryher, or Freud himself, describe Freud as discouraging Bryher and H.D.'s queer identities, expressions, and desires, or their life choices. Rather, he supported them. In a personal letter, H.D. writes to Bryher that during analysis, she and Freud discussed that she has "a sort of perfect bi-sexual attitude" and that while she previously had strived to be man or woman, she now realizes that she has to be both (Friedman, 2002, p. 503). She added that Freud said that she had "two things to hide," that she was a girl and that she was a boy. According to McCabe (2021a, p. 181), this thrilled H.D., and I must admit that it thrills me, too. It means that Freud approached the idea of non-binary identifications and expressions.

This implies that Freud acknowledged, and in this case even supported, queer identifications and expressions. This nuances the prevalent idea that Freud and psychoanalysis are skeptical of women and femininity, and neglectful or even dismissive of what we today would call queer identifications, expressions, desires, and lives. There have certainly been misogynist, homophobic, and condescending perceptions and treatments of queer people within psychoanalysis. There have also, however, been recognition and support, as exemplified by H.D.'s encounter with Freud. I perceive this as a psychoanalytic cultural heritage that should be cherished and appreciated. Cultural heritage includes objects and sites, as well as narratives and practices, that are inherited from previous generations, in this case from previous generations of psychoanalysts. Practices and narratives that are remembered and used become part of our shared material and immaterial heritage. Heritage is about how the past is connected to the present and the future, which means that some parts are continuous while others change (Harrison, 2013). In this way, heritage can be seen as a connection to our collective memory (Engström & Punzi, 2022). If we explore the traces of how queer lives were acknowledged in psychoanalysis, we can contribute to the recognition of queer lives in the present and in the future. We can also contribute to amending oppressive and pathologizing practices, within as well as outside of psychoanalysis. We may also discover that we have a lot to learn from those who came before us, not only when it comes to gender and queer lives but also when it comes to the acknowledgment of mysticism, and the intersection of queerness and mystical themes.

Mystical themes

H.D. and Freud both grew up in milieus in which mystical themes were ever-present, and these mystical themes could also be intermingled with sexual themes. In the Moravian Church, which H.D. and her family belonged to, the idea that both the individual believer and the church community were in a mystical marriage with the divine was central and had implications for the sexual lives of the members. The sexual act between a married couple (and it perhaps goes without saying that this was a husband and a wife) was, for example, perceived as a liturgical ritual (Bauer, 2018, p. 71; Peucker, 2006, p. 31). Moreover, single men saw their mystical union with Christ as a sexual unity. In this union religious feelings were expressed in homoerotic terms. The male biological sex was perceived as neutralized through the mystical union with Christ, and in this process everyone in the Moravian community became brides (Bauer, 2018, p. 76; Peucker, 2006, p. 32). This meant that H.D. grew up in a milieu that was paradoxically both heteronormative and open to mysticism and gender fluidity (even though they obviously did not use this term).

The same holds true for Freud, who grew up in a milieu characterized by Jewish mystical traditions that influenced him and his thinking, even though he characterized himself as "a Godless Jew" (Bakan, 1958; Berke, 2015). For a Jewish person, religiousness is not required for identifying as a Jew. This holds true for Freud, who was an atheist and simultaneously had a profound Jewish identification. I submit that to understand the dialogue between H.D. and Freud, the Jewish heritage of psychoanalysis and its founder needs to be acknowledged. In the mystical tradition Freud grew up in, there is a name, *Shekhinah*, for the feminine aspect of God, since it is assumed that God incorporates male as well as female elements (Bakan, 1958). Moreover, human beings incorporate both feminine and masculine aspects, since all human beings incorporate all aspects of creation (Bakan, 1958; Berke & Schneider, 2006). This means that it was not alien to Freud to perceive feminine and masculine elements to be intermingled. Throughout *Tribute to Freud* (H.D., 1956), mystical themes are explored. In their discussions, H.D. and Freud often related mysticism to questions of gender. Perhaps the roots both Freud and H.D. had in mystical traditions that did not perceive gender as strictly binary primed an openness in them to acknowledge queer gender identifications, expressions, and desires.

I have previously (Johansson & Punzi, 2019) explored "The Princess Dream," a dream H.D. and Freud discussed during H.D.'s psychoanalysis (H.D. 1956). In the dream, an Egyptian princess walks down a marble staircase, toward a watercourse. H.D. herself is positioned at the foot of the steps, having a feeling of concern. In the water, there is a basket with a child in it. It does not take much experience in dream interpretation to understand that the dream portrayed Moses and the Pharaoh's daughter. According to H.D., the dream resembled an illustration in the Doré bible. H.D. and Freud discussed this illustration and attempted to understand the position of H.D. in the dream, including with whom she identified. Freud asked if she identified with the baby in the basket – in other words with Moses. He also asked if H.D. remembered another child in the illustration, Miriam, the sister of Moses, who hides in the bushes. Freud thereby emphasized the role of Miriam, a woman of utmost importance in Jewish tradition, not only because she contributed to saving Moses but also to saving the people. Because of Miriam, a well of water miraculously followed the people during the 40 years in the desert (Rosenfeld, 2010). Miriam is a prophetess and a leader, and she signifies female power. I have previously argued that when Freud introduced Miriam, when he and H.D. reflected on "The Princess Dream," he likely intended to acknowledge female power and the importance of women throughout history, and strived to support H.D. in trusting her own capacity as a writer and as a woman (Johansson & Punzi, 2019). Prior explorations of the encounter between H.D. and Freud were most often performed from a feminist perspective, assuming that H.D. had to challenge and fight Freud and his supposed misogynistic thinking (e.g., Buck, 1991; Friedman, 1981; Kennedy, 2012). This is of course important, since Freud certainly made some questionable statements about women and femininity. It is also important to recognize female writers, since they tend to become invisible (Friedman, 1981). H.D. has, for example, become somewhat forgotten despite her importance as a modernist poet, whereas her male counterparts have been, and continuously are, cherished and canonized.

Moving Beyond Binary Thinking

It is, however, important to move beyond various forms of binary thinking, even my own thinking, when I understood H.D. and Freud's discussions of "The Princess Dream" as an acknowledgment of female power. If we move beyond binary thinking, the encounters between H.D., Bryher, and Freud can be explored in ways that acknowledge the fact that H.D. and Bryher embraced queer identifications and expressions. It should, for example, be noted that in a letter to Bryher and Macpherson, H.D. related that, during her analysis, she explored how she had tried to be either man or woman but needed to be both (McCabe, 2021a, pp. 10, 182). Moreover, Freud acknowledged that love could be directed toward someone who is both masculine and maternal, referring to H.D.'s love for Bryher (McCabe, 2021a, p. 166).

If we perceive the encounter between H.D. and Freud not only as a gendered one, to use Kennedy's (2012) terminology, but also as a queered one, a more complex and thought-provoking image evolves. In this image, queerness and queer identifications and expressions, as well as racialized stereotypes, come forth. This permits explorations of the queer heritage of psychoanalysis, as well as the queer heritage of Freud. Perceiving the encounters as queered also illuminates how psychoanalysis, during the first decades of the 20th century, was not inherently gender stereotypical or pathologizing of non-normative gender identifications and expressions; the queer heritage of psychoanalysis comes forth.

It is open to debate whether mystical traditions have contributed to an openness to gender and various gender identifications. As previously discussed, my interest in mystical traditions – specifically in Moravian and Jewish contexts and how gender was and is perceived in these contexts – has shaped my readings and understandings. Acknowledgment of mystical traditions is however relevant for understanding the encounters between H.D., Bryher, and Freud, beyond a specific interest in mysticism. When H.D. and Bryher established themselves as writers, and when psychoanalysis was established, mysticism was not considered awkward, but rather part of the Zeitgeist – a fact that is sometimes neglected. One example is that the Bauhaus movement, which has been perceived as representing rational modernism, also included mystical themes as well as explorations of gender fluidity and queer identifications (Otto, 2019). Bryher indeed appreciated the Bauhaus movement and established a Bauhaus Villa, Kenwin, in Switzerland

(Souhami, 2020, p. 180). Freud had an interest in mystical and occult phenomena, specifically the possibility of telepathy (Rottenberg, 2017, pp. 310–18), as well as kabbalistic traditions, including numerology (Bakan, 1958). Sachs (1941, p. 359), who collaborated with H.D. and Bryher in *Close Up* and was Bryher's psychoanalyst, wrote that all forms of psychotherapy are close to the magical origin of medicine, which makes it difficult for patients to have modest hopes and expectations, and which in turn may make them disappointed with the results of the analysis.

I would like to underline that acknowledgment of mysticism does not provide the "true understanding" of H.D., Bryher, Freud, or psychoanalysis, or how they perceived gender and queerness. There is no final understanding of H.D., Bryher or Freud – or of anyone, or anything, for that matter. I, however, submit that through recognizing mystical traditions, queerness, and non-binary identifications, the risks of being caught in stereotypes and prejudices are reduced. One risk is to perceive persons who lived non-normative, non-binary lives – as H.D. and Bryher did – according to ideas of binary genders, as many researchers, including myself, have done. Another risk is to perceive psychoanalysis in stereotypical ways, including seeing Freud as a privileged, white, man. Freud lived during a time when antisemitism was ever-present. Jews were considered representatives of the "dark-skinned races," with the "dark-skinned races" seen as inferior, and "blacks" and Jews were assumed to have similar negative characteristics (Gilman, 1994, pp. 12, 122). Moreover, Jewish men were considered overly sexual and effeminate, as half-women even, and negative stereotypes of women (for example, being overly talkative, neurotic, sexually inferior, and unreliable) were attributed to Jewish men (Gilman, 1995; Salberg, 2007). Such ideas often came from the medical discipline, a discipline to which Freud himself belonged. It should also be considered that Freud came from an impoverished background. For him, as for many other Jews, academic achievement was an opportunity to counteract marginalization, escape poverty, and become part of society (Beller, 1989; Richards, 2014).

This means that Freud knew well what it meant to be "other"-ed, seen as inferior and sexually deviant. At the same time, he valued his outsider position. In a letter to the Jewish organization B'nai Brith on his seventieth birthday, he expressed that, as a Jew, he was placed in opposition. This gave him a certain position with regard to understanding prejudice and being able to see what those who belonged to the majority did not see. Boyarin argued that Freud's racial difference made him sensitive to the nuances of sexual differentiation, and that he accepted the perception of male Jews as female (2003, p. 172). Moreover, it has been argued that there is a queerness to Jewishness itself, since both queerness and Jewishness transgress the expected and challenge normative, gendered ways of life (Boyarin, Itzkovitz, & Pellegrini, 2023).

Neither Freud, nor H.D. and Bryher conformed to norms or expectations, not those of the society they lived in, nor those of their own families, religions, or communities. Freud challenged religion and Jewish religious practices, just as he challenged prevailing ideas of the human mind as unitary and rational, and just as he challenged the medical discipline. Bryher and H.D. challenged gender

identifications and expressions, their respective families' expectations, and normative ideas of how one should live one's life, establish relationships, spend one's
money, and write poetry. In their own ways, and in their own contexts, the three
of them struggled against prejudice and discrimination in creative and courageous
ways, making unique cultural contributions. They also shared an interest in mysticism, mythology, literature, history, and archeology. As a young person, Bryher
wanted to study archeology but was not permitted to do so by his parents (Bryher,
1962). Bryher had wanderlust all his life. Together with H.D. he traveled to Greece,
Italy, and Egypt, among many other places (Hollenberg, 2022). H.D. and Freud
knew ancient Greek, and H.D. even translated ancient Greek dramas into English
(McCabe, 2021a, p. 191).

Throughout *Tribute to Freud*, mythology – not least Greek mythology – was a
medium through which H.D.'s experiences and conflicts were explored and understood. In this process, a Pallas Athena statue became important. Of all the statues
and artefacts in Freud's collection, this was his favorite (H.D., 1956, pp. 67–70).
According to H.D., Freud handed the object to her. She took it in her hands, and
Freud said, "She is perfect, only she has lost her spear." Through making the statue
the focus of attention, Freud and H.D. could explore the missing spear, and what it
symbolized. Thereby, they could approach H.D.'s perfection as a phallic bisexual
woman, with the lost spear symbolizing her writer's block, which was one reason
for seeking out psychoanalysis; and it was indeed overcome (Martin, 2008).

Freud's comment about the lost spear has been interpreted as derogatory view of
femininity, since the spear has been seen as a phallic symbol and by focusing on the
lost spear, it has been assumed that Freud made lack the center of femininity (Buck,
1991; DuPlessis & Friedman, 1981). I have previously (Johansson & Punzi, 2019)
reflected on the possibility that Freud viewed femininity as perfect in itself, and his
comment on the perfection of Pallas Athena, was intended to encourage H.D. to
abandon her non-productive self-doubt.

Pallas Athena was goddess of wisdom and war. She was also a goddess with
attributes that are normatively characterized as masculine, and her persona is
non-binary. One example of such an attribute is the plate armor she is wearing, and
it should be noted that she is the only goddess presented with plate armor. Other
examples are the shield she holds in her hand and the spear. Pallas Athena was far
from portraying normative femininity; she was rather a goddess with non-binary
characteristics. Freud and H.D. knew ancient Greek and Greek mythology well.
Of course they understood that the Pallas Athena statue embodied attributes that
are normatively coded as masculine as well as feminine. Thereby Pallas Athena
eluded binary gender classifications. Martin (2008) describes that, for Freud, symbols and objects (for example, the Pallas Athena statue or the children in "The
Princess Dream") should not be understood as a wish for a particular object or a
particular relation but as a representation of a wish. In my interpretation, this means
that beyond the specific statue, the lost spear and the perfection of the goddess, is
a representation of a wish to be both man and woman (McCabe, 2021a, pp. 10,
182). This wish is embodied by Pallas Athena, and integrating her into the analytic

work opens a possibility to explore these themes, so that H.D. recognizes her own strength, her queer gender identifications and relationships, and herself as a writer.

Final reflections

I have described instances of how queer identifications, expressions, and desires were explored by H.D. and Freud during psychoanalysis. I have also provided examples of how Freud did not pathologize queer identifications and gender expressions – on the contrary, he validated them – and I have given examples from H.D.'s psychoanalytic process, such as Freud's recognition of H.D.'s love for Bryher and the importance of the queer goddess Pallas Athena. Other examples are how Freud approached Bryher as "Dear Sir" and supported him to become a psychoanalyst, which Freud would not have done if he had considered Bryher's gender identification and expression as pathological.

I have also reflected on how mystical themes and religious backgrounds must be recognized when striving to understand the encounter between H.D., Bryher, and Freud, and how psychoanalysis and queer identifications, expressions,and desires became intermingled during the time when the three of them met. For Bryher, psychoanalysis served as a medium to break the limits of literature and cinema, and psychoanalysis supported self-understanding; it was a method for peeling away layers of repressive childhood experiences in order to find liberation and truth. Not being true to oneself was, according Bryher, the hardest to bear.

If we contrast straight time with ideas of linear progress (Rohy, 2009), and add some mysticism, the courageous and truth-seeking struggles of H.D., Bryher, and the psychoanalysts, not least Freud and Sachs, who recognized queer identifications, expressions, and desires, come forth also in our time. Thereby, they not only nuance our understandings of history, but they also give strength to contemporary struggles.

Bibliography

Bakan, D. (1958). *Sigmund Freud and the Jewish Mystical Tradition.* Princeton: D. Van Nostrand.

Bauer, B. (2018). "Bridal mysticism, virtual marriage, and masculinity in the Moravian hymnbook Kleines Brüdergesangbuch." *Journal for Religion, Film and Media*, 4(2), 67–79.

Beller, S. (1989). *Vienna and the Jews 1867–1938: A Cultural History.* Cambridge: Cambridge University Press.

Bentall, R. (2004). *Madness Explained: Psychosis and Human Nature*. London: Penguin.

Berke, J.H. (2015). *The Hidden Freud. His Hassidic Roots.* London: Karnac.

Berke, J.H., & Schneider, S. (2006). "The self and the soul." *Mental Health, Religion & Culture*, 9(4), 333–54.

Boyarin, D. (2003). "Homophobia and the postcoloniality of the Jewish Science." In D. Boyarin, D. Itzkovitz and A. Pellegrini (Eds.) *Queer Theory and the Jewish Question.* New York: Columbia University Press, pp. 166–198.

Boyarin, D., Itzkovitz, D., & Pellegrini, A. (2003). "Strange Bedfellows: An Introduction." In D. Boyarin, D. Itzkovitz and A. Pellegrini (Eds.) *Queer Theory and the Jewish Question*. New York: Columbia University Press, pp. 1–18.

Bryher. (1962). *The Heart to Artemis. A Writer's Memoirs*. Melbourne: Hassell Street Press.

Bryher. (2000). *Two Novels. Development and Two Selves*. Ed. by Joanne Winning. Madison: University of Wisconsin Press.

Buck, C. (1991). *H.D. and Freud. Bisexuality and a Feminine Discourse*. New York: Harvester Wheatsheaf.

Danto, E.A. (2007). *Freud's Free Clinics. Psychoanalysis and Social Justice, 1918–1938*. New York: Columbia University Press.

DuPlessi, R.B. & Friedman, S.S. (1981) "Woman is perfect: H.D.'s debate with Freud." *Feminist Studies, 7*, 417–430.

Engström, A., & Punzi, E. (Eds.) (2022). *Mad studies, kulturarv & konst*." [Mad studies, cultural heritage & arts]. Vimmerby, Sweden: Trapart Books.

Freud, S. (1920). "The psychogenesis of a case of female homosexuality." *The International Journal of Psycho-Analysis*, 1, 125–49.

Friedman, S.S. (1981). *Psyche Reborn: The Emergence of H.D.* Bloomington: Indiana University Press.

Friedman, S.S. (Ed.) (2002). *Analyzing Freud. Letters of H.D., Bryher, and Their Circle*. New York: New Directions.

Fuechtner, V. (2011). *Berlin Psychoanalytic. Psychoanalysis and Culture in Weimar Republic Germany and Beyond*. Oakland: University of California Press.

Gilman, S. (1994). *The Case of Sigmund Freud. Medicine and Identity at the Fin de Siècle*. London: Johns Hopkins University Press.

Gilman, S. (1995). *Freud, Race and Gender*. Princeton: Princeton University Press.

H.D. (1956). *Tribute to Freud*. New York: New Directions.

H.D. (1973). *Trilogy*. Cheshire: Carcanet Press.

H.D. (1979). *End to Torment. A Memoir of Ezra Pound*. New York: New Directions.

H.D. (1982). *The Gift*. New York: New Directions.

Halperin, D. (2003). "The normalization of queer theory." *Journal of Homosexuality*, 45(2–4), 339–43.

Harrison, R. (2013). *Heritage. Critical Approaches*. London: Routledge.

Hollenberg, D.K. (2022). *Winged Words. The Life and Work of the Poet H.D.* Ann Arbor: University of Michigan Press.

Johansson, P.-M. & Punzi, E. (2019). "She is perfect – Nuancing Freud's view of femininity through reading 'Tribute to Freud' with respect to mystical and religious themes." In V. Sinclair (Ed.), *Rendering Unconscious: Psychoanalytic Perspectives*. Vimmerby, Sweden: Trapart Books, pp. 283–96.

Kennedy, M. (2012). "Modernist autobiography, hysterical narrative, and the unnavigable river: The case of Freud and H.D." *Literature and Medicine*, 30(2), 241–75.

Martin, T. (2008). "From cabinet to couch: Freud's clinical use of sculpture." *British Journal of Psychotherapy*, 24(2), 184–96.

McCabe, S. (2021a). *H.D. & Bryher. An Untold Love Story of Modernism*. Oxford: Oxford University Press.

McCabe, S. (2021b). "Writing H.D. & Bryher in double dimensions – an invitation to H.D. & Bryher: An untold modernist love story." *Feminist Modernist Studies*, 4(1), 22–35.

Otto, E. (2019). *Haunted Bauhaus. Occult Spirituality, Gender Fluidity, Queer Identities, and Radical Politics.* Cambridge: The MIT Press.

Peucker, P. (2006). "Inspired by flames of love: Homosexuality, mysticism and Moravian brothers around 1750." *Journal of the History of Sexuality*, 15(1), 30–64.

Punzi, E. (2022). "Reflections on the integration of poetry therapy and psychodynamic practice based on an analysis of the book *Tribute to Freud* by the poet H.D." *Journal of Poetry Therapy*, 35(3), 186–97.

Richards, A.D. (2014). "Freud's Jewish identity and psychoanalysis as a science." *Journal of the American Psychoanalytic Association*, 62(6), 987–1003.

Rohy, V. (2009). *Anachronism and its Others. Sexuality, Race, Temporality*. Albany: State University of New York Press.

Rosenfeld, Y. (2010). "Skin deep: Scratching the surface of Miriam in Numbers 12". *Women in Judaism*, 7(2), published online, ISSN 1209–9392.

Rottenberg, E. (2017). "What are the chances? Psychoanalysis, telepathy, and the accident." *Paragraph*, 40(3), 310–28.

Sachs, H. (1941). "Psychotherapy and the pursuit of happiness." *American Imago*, 2(4), 356–64.

Salberg, J. (2007). "Hidden in plain sight: Freud's Jewish identity revisited." *Psychoanalytic Dialogues: The International Journal of Relational Perspectives*, 17(2), 197–217.

Souhami, D. (2020). *No Modernism Without Lesbians*. London: Head of Zeus.

Chapter 6

Trans Childhoods and the Family Romance

M.E. O'Brien

Introduction: Belonging Among Aliens

Until her unexpected death in February 2024, Cecilia Gentili lived as a well-respected trans activist, consultant, and performer in New York City. Growing up as a child in Gálvez, Argentina in the 1970s, Cecilia tried to reconcile how she fit into the social world around her. Following a childhood confrontation with authority figures who insisted upon her assigned gender, she developed a fantasy that she did not originate from her parents. She recounts this story in both an oral history interview and in her published memoir: She would frequently be taken by her family to visit her grandmother in the rural countryside. The area was well-known for UFO (unidentified flying object) activity. On one such drive when she was about five years old, her brother told her they were passing the area where their family first found Cecilia as a baby, abandoned and naked.[1] She recounts the scene in an oral history interview that I conducted with her:

> During the rest of the trip to my grandma's house, I put two and two together and I thought, this is an area with a lot of UFO activities. I am a girl with a fucking dick. And I was found there? I know what happened here. I was left by mistake by a UFO, and I thought that somewhere there would be a planet where all girls could have penises like me. And for me it was kind of—I think I always found magical ways to deal with reality (NYC TOHP, 002, p. 6).[2]

The story is one of many traces of questions of origins, adoption, and not belonging in her family throughout her published memoir. Her imagining that she belonged among aliens is an example in psychoanalytic theory of *the family romance*: a child's fantasy that they do not belong to their parents, but instead with some other, true family elsewhere. In his 1909 essay, "Family Romances," Freud describes common forms of this fantasy, and uses his explanation of its basis to make sense of children's changing understanding of sexual difference, biological origins, and the child's relationship to their parents.

Various forms of family romances are common among trans children, appearing frequently in first-person accounts, oral histories, memoirs, clinical work, and on

DOI: 10.4324/9781032624129-7

social media. These fantasies share common themes: that there is somewhere the trans child belongs, someone who could understand and make sense of them, and some future time when they will find acceptance. Gentili's memoir, along with other references to the family romance gathered from the New York City Trans Oral History Project (NYC TOHP), can help illuminate how trans children grapple with the gendered demands of caregivers and the broader social order. (The NYC TOHP is a collection of nearly two hundred oral history interviews with trans and gender non-conforming New Yorkers, available as an online public archive. The author previously worked as a coordinator for the project.)

The family romance, for Freud and in the trans accounts here, is the child's response to a confrontation with what Jacques Lacan terms *the symbolic*. Through the symbolic, Lacan theorizes a set of interconnected problematics: the subject's relationship to and constitution through language and signifiers, paternal lineage and kinship, one's place in a broader social order, sexual difference and castration, and much else. Through the family romance, Freud identifies and theorizes elements of the symbolic register as confronted by a child.

The family romance offers trans children a means of preserving gendered desire in the face of sexual difference as a social order. It constitutes an imaginary fantasy space through which they attempt to respond to confrontations with gender, both in relation and in opposition to the desires of others. Trans children often face difficult questions about sexual difference, lack of recognition from their parents and other authority figures, and a fraught relationship with the dictates of a gendered social order. Trans children may turn to the family romance as a fantasy to stage these conflicting desires and to defend against social expectations. The family romance offers us an opportunity to think with trans children, and to theorize along with them in the way that they make sense of the impossible contradictions and fraught demands of the gendered world. Through the taking up of the family romance by trans children, we can begin to trace the vicissitudes of the subject's iterative encounters and their incomplete psychic reconciliation with the symbolic order.

Trans Childhood Fantasies

Cecilia Gentili shares with many trans children her practice of often turning to versions of the family romance. In trans narratives, a few characteristics of the family romance circulate, sometimes together, sometimes in separation: a belief that one's own parents must be in some way false relations, a desire to escape from one's family and life conditions, a sense that there is somewhere else to go where one's experience would be more tolerable, and the belief that there are other kinship and familial ties or an alternative social order where one may better belong. As with Cecilia's account, these fantasies all share a desire to escape some of the demands of this order.

Traces of the family romance frequently appear across first-person accounts by trans adults describing their childhoods and imaginative lives. Many of my trans patients report that they imagined themselves as children within their favorite video game, television world, or fictional universe from childhood books, sometimes through the fantasy sub-genre of portal fiction where one is magically transported elsewhere. There a child imagines that they may find some adventure or intrigue, but more often a desired form of recognition and belonging. Others describe being magically linked to other children, families, or places elsewhere in the world, suggesting this other place was where they belonged. Popular depictions of trans childhoods include versions of family romance fantasy, such as the 1997 French-Belgian film *Ma Vie in Rose* (Berliner), where the film's protagonist constructs elaborate fantasy worlds to cope with parental and social opposition to her gender identification.

In the NYC TOHP archive, several versions of family romance fantasies appear:

One version is the same as Gentili's: identifying as an alien from another world. Nogga Schwartz said that beginning in first grade, when asked "Are you a boy or a girl?," Nogga would respond: "I'm an alien from another planet. I've come here to observe your race. You're failing miserably" (099, p. 5). Hazel Katz said: "Everything is so weird and it doesn't make sense and it feels like you're an alien. Or, I feel like I'm an alien half the time" (134, p. 9). Many other interviews mention childhood identification with non-human characters in popular culture.

NYC TOHP narrators often reported experiences of not belonging in their families of origin, sometimes coupled with the desire to escape, hide, disappear, or to be without family ties. Jay Toole was often raped by their father and brother and began to hide on a grassy hill across the street from their home where they imagined "nobody could see me" (003, p. 3). Their first memory was sitting in a tree, realizing "no one was going to take care of me and I had to do it myself" (003, p. 4). Genevieve Tatum always felt she was "different," that "no matter how close I got to other people, there was always that sense of detachment" (011, p. 19). Renee Imperato, like some other narrators, saw changing her family name as a way of disowning her family and her experience of abuse and violence committed by her father (009).

These fantasies of leaving one's family can include imagining a place that might be more supportive. Many narrators reported childhood fantasies of escaping their family and place of origin through establishing other ties. For Dean Spade, this took the form of what he later calls the "romance myth," the fantasy that a romantic relationship would enable him to flee the violence, alcoholism, and lack of emotional support in both his birth and foster families. He wanted "to leave, and go far away" (001, p. 8). As a child, Bianey Garcia saw cinematic depictions of the city and imagined New York would be a place they could "become a trans woman," unlike Mexico (004, p. 6). Shannon Harrington similarly felt deeply limited by growing up in Arizona and was "itching to break out. To go somewhere else to live a life" (022, p. 3). Spade's interview was one of the few where questions of social status – a central component of Freud's formulation – figured in childhood family romance fantasies. For Spade, it took the specific form of "social climbing," making a concerted effort at school to obscure the poverty of his family from classmates. Spade followed their mother's aspirations that he marry into wealth.

In adolescence he abandoned this plan, but still "wanted to get out of Virginia and like, leave this world" (001, p. 7).

Narrators also report seeking out fictional fantasy worlds as children as providing a way into reimagining sexual and gender difference. Naomi Clark frequented a bookstore where she would read science fiction and fantasy novels for hours. At eleven years old, Clark moved to Japan and encountered the "mind-blowing" extensive themes of magical sex changes in Japanese comics, "a fucking gender swap fantasia" (013, p. 6). Image Object "loved books," and "read a lot of fantasy and fiction and dabbled in writing" (079, p. 4). Pauline Park said she would "bury myself in books" (012, p. 10). Son Kit developed an adolescent love of "fandom gay erotica" that provided Kit's introduction to "queer anything" (113, p. 10). JD Davids was a "voracious reader" because JD was "a pretty lonely kid" (019, p. 3). Yanyi found life unable to sustain their interest; he "read a lot of like, fantasy novels," imagining the fantasy book he would write (042, p. 15). Zephyr D Merkur Herrera "discovered fantasy as a genre," and was particularly enamored with a novel describing the copasetic relationship between the protagonist's father and his father's dragon companion (096, p. 10). Lauren Simkin Burke describes the importance of reading for them as a response to the lack of agency for children:

> [Reading] was a way to experience more than you could experience in your day to day reality... I think that childhood is challenging. You have no power. Everyone is telling you what to do... I was like, biding my time until I was able to have a little more agency in my life (066, p. 11).

Many extended their love of fantasy fiction into creating their own fantasy worlds. Federico Jalwa would make up "imaginary stories of escaping... mimicking fantasy tales" (058, p. 5). Evan would "delve into into my own fantasy world" amidst his family's "turmoil and some trauma" (067, p. 2). El Roy Red "really created a world for myself," later leading to Red's work as a writer (021, p. 4).

Other narrators describe the moment of meeting others that they identified with, forming chosen family, or discovering a supportive queer- or trans-affirming community for the first time. Although these are not childhood fantasies, they are fulfillments of a form of the family romance, articulated as desires to find positive alternative kinship relations. Paris Milane described a friend she lived with after leaving her family as her "real sister" (010, p. 5). Genevieve Tatum found in a queer neighborhood that "you're just one big, happy family" (011, p. 4). These new relations, however, often fell short of the desired fantasy. J Soto referred to his "chosen family," but said that they were never a "replacement for blood relatives" (017, p. 8). In describing the extensive mutual aid relations of New York's Kiki ballroom scene, Gia Love said, "it's like the family aspect. You know? I'm providing people with a space" because "some people don't have family... New York is the escape" (116, p. 17). In the ballroom scene Love describes in depth, trans and queer youth of color identify their relationships with each other with familial titles: house mother, house father, house sister. Love's interview emphasizes that these chosen families can become fraught sites of conflict, as participants repeat their childhood traumas.

For some narrators, the family romance is wrapped up in the actual reality of being adopted, living in the foster care system, or otherwise under the family policing system. Trans children are disproportionately overrepresented in the foster care system (Prince, et al. 2022). For NYC TOHP narrators, actual separation from their families of origin intensified and complicated family romance desires. Dean Spade connected his desire to flee the world to the violence of both his birth family and multiple foster parents. For him to leave Virginia depended on and was complicated by the survivor's benefits available to him through lacking a legal guardian. Pauline Park was born in Korea but was adopted by a white American family. She spoke of the challenges of her group of all-non-white siblings growing up in an "all-white Southside of Milwaukee" to a "Christian fundamentalist family" (012, p. 6). Knowing that she was adopted and being racially out of place became tied up in a complex way to Park's cross-gender identification.

These interviews from NYC TOHP include narrators with widely varying experiences of trans childhoods. Some, like Cecilia, share an experience often over-documented in writing about trans children: identifying strongly with their chosen gender from an early age, sharing that gender identification with caregivers and facing considerable opposition, and eventually moving to find a more supportive queer and trans community. However, elements of the family romance are also articulated by trans narrators who did not have any defined clarity on their gender as children and instead came to understand themselves in their chosen gender much later in life. Some elements of the family romance are also articulated by narrators with comparatively supportive parents, or those who had the chance to encounter queer or trans people relatively early in life.

Shannon Fawkes reported that similar family romance stories were widespread among the trans youth they work with. Fawkes is a Midwest radical trans activist who ran a support group for trans and gender nonconforming youth for twelve years in Northwest Ohio. In an interview I conducted with Fawkes on the topic, they reported that trans youth frequently believed themselves to be one of a broad range of non-human creatures: fairies, mutants, aliens, and human/animal hybrids (Fawkes, 2023). The youth drew from popular culture for their fantasies, and varied from apparently sincerely believing these fantasies to seeing them as only a fictional identity for gaming and role-playing. In the queer youth group that Fawkes ran, these children could find peers who joined in their fantasies of belonging elsewhere and of having non-human traits in their bodies and souls. Fawkes described that as the youth found more social acceptance and support from peers, parents, and authority figures for their gender identity, they would often move away from their fantasies of non-human belonging. The fantasies served as a transitional support when belonging was not easy to find.

Trans people imagining that they belong among non-humans is not limited to childhood. Trans studies scholar Abram J. Lewis has documented extensive references to alien kinship by trans activists in the gay liberation era of the early 1970s, themes reappearing frequently in the later work of trans artists (2014, 2017a, 2017b). Angela Keyes Douglas, founder of the Transsexual Action Organization (TAO) in 1970, frequently referred to UFOs and extraterrestrials. She said TAO would "welcome extraterrestrials as liberators," and practically "protect and assist extraterrestrials" upon their arrival (Quoted in Lewis, 2017b, p. 65). Douglas began to be interested in UFOs as an adolescent. She wrote in her memoir: "Sex and UFOs came into my life about the same time. My feelings about sex were ones of shock and disbelief" (Quoted in Lewis, 2014, p. 23). Douglas was deeply moved to discover that one of her closest friends was a "reptilian, transsexual ET," and was confident that otherworldly forces were operating to aid the cause of trans rights (Quoted in Lewis, 2017a, p. 210). Trans philanthropist and activist Eric Erickson actively funded research to communicate with dolphins, and declared his pet leopard as a life partner. While often dismissed (not without warrant) as psychosis or eccentricity, Lewis argued that these other-worldly experiences are a major component of the archive of trans history and require expansively rethinking approaches to the historiography of trans activism.

Throughout these accounts, trans children yearn for an alternative to their families of origin, often in the form of escaping from humanity and human society altogether. To really understand the subtle logic of these fantasies – how they link questions of sexual difference, social authority, violent transphobia, paternal lineage, and language – requires a close reading of Freud's essay.

Freud's "Family Romances"

In 1909, Freud contributed a section to Otto Rank's volume *Der Mythus von der Geburt des Helden*. Only with its second German printing was Freud's essay given a title – "Der Familenroman der Neurotiker," literally "The Family Romance of Neurotics." Rank's collection, with Freud's essay, was translated into English four years later as *Myth of the Birth of the Hero*. Freud's contribution found its way into English as "Family Romances" (Rank, 1909a/1914). The shifts in the essay's translated title touch on unacknowledged ambiguities between the specific and the general which are already present in Freud's essay: the category of neurotic as both a psychopathology and a means of theorizing human psychic life generally; and the family romance as both a particular trope and as broadly relevant to childhood daydreams. At just under fifteen-hundred words – four-and-a-half pages in the *Standard Edition* – the essay is quite succinct (1909a/1959).

Freud had previously referred to "family romance" in his letters to Fliess. In the "Draft M" letter on May 31, 1897, he cites the "romance of alienation (cf. paranoia)… as a means of illegitimizing the relatives in question" as an example, followed by a dense account of the construction of unconscious fantasy (1985, p. 248). In a letter from October 15 of that year, he comes upon "the invention of parentage in paranoia" in the self-analysis of his own dream, which helps to illuminate a link between Freud's mother and a nurse that abruptly disappeared from his life (1985, p. 272). In a letter dated June 20, 1898, he writes that the "so-called" family romance is universal to neurotics. Here, Freud identifies the family romance as both a means of "self-aggrandizement" and a "defense against incest." He contends that the (presumably bourgeois) neurotic draws the trope of illegitimate children from the "lower social circles of servant girls," particularly in cases of seduction by a servant (1985, p. 317). The family romance appears twice according to Freud, both as a "fantasy about the mother" and as a "real memory of the maid" (1985, p. 317). In this early formulation, encounters with class difference in the form of sexual seduction are essential to the constitution of the family romance. In these early letters, the violent rivalry with the father and sexual desire for the mother is already at play in the family romance of the unconscious landscape of neurotics.

The 1909 essay offers both a clear exposition of a particular psychic phenomena and a subtle set of theoretical pivots and leaps. Freud's focus in the essay is a particular conscious fantasy among children, as reported by his adult neurotic patients when recounting their early lives. Having come to a "low opinion" of their parents, the child imagines that they must be adopted (Freud, 1909a/1959, p. 238). They replace their parents with others in a fantasy, imagining their true parents are of "higher social standing." Freud's examples are taken from the remnants of feudal society which were still present at the time in Central Europe: a "Lord of the Manor," or a "member of the aristocracy" (Freud, 1909a/1959, p. 239).

Freud opens the essay with "the liberation of the individual" from parental authority as both "most necessary" and "most painful" (Freud, 1909a/1959, p. 237). Neurotics are those who have failed to adequately accomplish this generational separation. Already in the first paragraph, Freud has established several key coordinates which the rest of the essay grapples with: the problem of social authority and the social order as incarnated in the parents, the fraught difficulty for subjects needing to come to terms with their relationship to this order, and the broader social and psychic stakes in the problem of lineage.

Freud then moves to the problem of gender identification. The child identifies with "the parent of his own sex" (Freud, 1909a/1959, p. 237). Freud specifies that at this early inception of the family romance, "the child is still in ignorance of the sexual determinants of procreation" (Freud, 1909a/1959, p. 239). Although no semantic distinction between sex and gender was available to Freud, sexual differences in the absence of an understanding of procreation points to *gender* as an appropriate concept to understand this moment of Freud's theorizing of the child's early and "momentous wish" to be like their parents (Freud, 1909a/1959, p. 237).[3] Paired with the nearly contemporaneous essay "On the Sexual Theories of Children," the children at this previous phase of gender identification may not even be aware of anatomical sexual difference (1908/1959). For Freud, the child initially enjoys a total imaginary, gendered identification with their parents. This identification is expressed through a wish to become like them and to share in their characteristics.

The rupture from this gendered identification with the parent occurs when the child discovers "the category to which his parents belong" (1909a/1959, p. 237). Here, Freud locates the neurotic's family romance at the moment in which the child intuits a feature of the symbolic order: the placing of individuals within categories – in this case, the treating of their specific parents as among a class of parents. This then allows the child to engage in comparison with other parents, recognizing for the first time their inadequacies, and allowing the child's growing sense of slights at a perceived non-reciprocation of his affection. The disappointments made possible through the parents' placement within a symbolic category give rise to the fantasy of the family romance. The rupture quickly takes on a gendered cast. The child primarily directs their hostility towards the parent of their own gender. With his not infrequent passing misogyny, Freud suggests that girls have weaker imaginations and are less in the grip of parental rivalry.

The family romance emerges as a wish fulfillment in the face of these mounting disappointments and new knowledge. The family romance's initial asexual ambitious motivation is expressed by the child imagining themselves as belonging to a higher social status. As the child begins to understand the basics of procreation and "sexual processes," the fantasy shifts in contradictory directions. The child can no longer question their maternal origin, but their paternal lineage is still in doubt. As the child understands the role of sexual difference in procreation, patrilineal descent remains as a preoccupation. At this phase, the family romance serves the child's desire for erotic intimacy with their mother through imagining her in a variety of illicit affairs. The family romance proves versatile, serving a diverse range of psychic wishes.

In a concluding twist, Freud reads the stated hostility toward one's parents in the family romance as an expression of devotion. The child's imagined regal parental figures bear the attributes of their earlier exalted esteem of their own parents. The child's family romance links their earlier idealization of their mother and father with their later disappointments. The fantasy, Freud argues, persists in even normal adults, through the appearance of the parental figures in dreams in the form of "the Emperor and Empress." Freud's short essay offers a peculiar and complex theorization of the relationship between sex and gender, and imaginary identification and symbolic location.

Rank puts Freud's argument to use in his analysis of mythology (1909). He draws attention to the family romance trope in a cross-cultural survey of mythology, including in the fable of Oedipus, in the biblical story of Moses, in the Hindu Mahabharata, and in the epic of Gilgamesh. Freud returned to his family romance essay 30 years later in *Moses and Monotheism* (1939). He used the difference between Moses's story and his original account of the typical family romance – namely, that although Moses's family of origin is humble, his adopted family is of exalted royalty – as a key pivot in the book's argument that Moses was an Egyptian who adopted the Jewish people to advance his discredited Egyptian monotheistic sect.

Uses and Abuses of the Family Romance

"Family Romances" was never particularly central to the canonization of psychoanalysis. There is a scattering of literature that addresses the essay. Here, I briefly summarize the major trends in this literature, focusing more on essays of particular relevance to this argument.

Like my attention to Gentili's memoir, one current of psychoanalytic writing on family romance focuses on popular-cultural and literary analysis.[4] Phyllis Greenacre (1958) extensively develops one theme, namely, how the family romance in children can serve to cultivate an inner fantasy life and, later, to foster creativity and artistic expression in adulthood. This inner space for the child's fantasy is recognized by Johanna K. Tabin as maintaining a defensive protection against social expectations: "The family romance serves so well because it is a personal secret of a fantasy that one can keep in mind, thus feeling free to conform to outer reality" (1998, p. 291).

Another body of literature addresses the relationship between family romance fantasies and actual adoption, both historically and in an adopted child's "genealogical bewilderment."[5] In their 1991 essay, Thomas M. Horner and Elinor B. Rosenberg ground the family romance in the extensive reality of actually existing adoption, foster parenting systems, child selling, and other practices through which children were raised by those other than their birth parents. They see the prevalence of family romance variations in the folklore of Medieval Europe as a reflection of the reality of mothers dying during childbirth, of wet-nursing, and of foster care. Children face dilemmas of uncertainty with respect to "their personal origins, their kin, and the nature of social bonds," which "although far from being uniformly patterned, are universally present" (Horner & Rosenberg, 1991, p. 142).

This use of the family romance by trans children finds parallels in Ken Corbett's exploration of the "nontraditional family romance," where children from queer and other nontraditional families develop novel and creative means of making sense of the question of biological origins and kinship. Drawing from Judith Butler, Corbett argues: "No one develops outside a system of norms, but no one develops as a simple mechanical reiteration of such norms" (2001, p. 602–603). Corbett locates the family romance as the site where the child begins to understand new facts about parental sexuality, their own conception, sexual difference, and generational change. Corbett shares this attention to new knowledge as the motivation for the family romance with Freud and a subset of literature on the family romance, most notably Klein (1920).

Most psychoanalytic writing on the subject treats the family romance as an elaboration and specification of the Oedipus complex. In this literature, the family romance is treated as a stage in a normative trajectory of development, one whose persistence is pathological. This is most clearly argued in Anna Freud's 1949 essay "On Certain Difficulties in the Preadolescent's Relation to His Parents," where she locates the family romance as a key developmental stage emerging shortly after the breakdown of the Oedipus complex, leading to a "more ruthless disillusionment" in preadolescence (1968). Similarly, Helene Deutsch proposes that the family romance is a means of compensating for feelings of inferiority brought on by the Oedipus complex (1936). Here, status anxiety and status fantasies provide an antidote to the fraught parental relationship following the passing of the Oedipus complex. Philip R. Lehrman correlates various iterations of the family romance to different developmental trajectories (1927). Linda Kaplan identifies several variants of the family romance across multiple developmental stages (1974). Though her argument is distinct, it shares with Anna Freud's a normative framework of development. For Kaplan, there is a pre-Oedipal version of the romance (initiated by the loss of infantile omnipotence) delaying the advent of Oedipal guilt. In the Oedipal phase, the child has full awareness of their parents as sexual beings and fears retaliation for incestuous wishes.

Herman Westerink and Philippe Van Haute challenge this reading of "Family Romances" as fully integrated with Freud's later theories of the Oedipus complex (2020). In their close reading of the essay, they note that the Oedipus complex is not mentioned in Freud's essay, nor does the essay start by focusing on a conflicted relationship with a controlling father. Instead, they locate the 1909 essay at a pivotal cusp of Freud's thought, written concurrently with "On the Sexual Theories of Children" (1908) and just before "Analysis of a Phobia in a Five Year Old Boy" (1909b). In the 1905 edition of *Three Essays on Sexuality*, Freud argues that there is no inherent, natural relationship between the sexual drive and its objects. Infants experience sexual drive, but in an autoerotic form without an object. It is not until puberty that sexual life is normatively organized, requiring the overcoming of many obstacles and detours. Westerink and Van Haute note that "Family Romances" shares this divide between infantile and adolescent sexuality. Unlike his writing from only a few years later, the child does not yet fully sexualize their relationship with their parents. When writing "Family Romances," Freud still held that the adolescent sexualization of parents depends upon "the knowledge of sexual difference, reproduction and descent (*Abkunft*) – a knowledge first established in puberty" (Westerink and Van Haute, 2020, p. 182). But Freud rethought this point; in the study of Little Hans written within a year of completing the manuscript of "Family Romances," he argues that children are capable of clear object choice (1909b).

Westerink and Van Haute argue Freud's essay is on the cusp between two contrasting accounts of the child's sexuality: the first depends primarily upon sexual knowledge and self-preservation; the second, upon the Oedipus complex and childhood sexual object choice. The letters to Fliess make it clear that Freud was not fully consistent on these points. When writing "Family Romances," Freud was grappling with questions of childhood sexuality and considering multiple conflicting answers. This transitional moment in Freud's changing theorization strangely parallels another cusp described within the essay itself, one that is faced by the child of the family romance: between an early objectless sexuality that soon includes a non-sexualized gender identification, and an adolescent sexuality that depends on acquiring new knowledge of sexual difference and the social order. This point in Freud's work is helpful for understanding the fraught questions facing trans children. For trans children, discovering the sexual organization of society as articulated within and through the familial order can be devastating. The family romance provides a means of enduring this fraught moment of unwelcome knowledge and the symbolic order it articulates.

Questioning Developmentalism

Stage-based developmental frameworks such as those that dominate psychoanalytic writing on the family romance have been particularly insidious for trans analysands and for the psychoanalytic theorizing of trans life. Such frameworks often imply a normative trajectory against which a patient's experience is contrasted as pathological. When taken up in this way, developmental frameworks have often been used as part of the very process of gender discipline against which a trans child may first turn to the family romance. When psychoanalytic theory and practice treats transgender people as deviations from a proper developmental course, the field acts in the service of the most violent and regressive logics that objectify the patient into a symbolic order.

Although he does not write about the family romance directly, Lacan offers a counterpoint to the preponderance of normative Oedipal developmental frameworks in writing on the family romance. Insofar as the family romance has something to do with the child's encounter with the symbolic order, "the category to which his parents belong," Lacan cautions against treating the symbolic as historically arising at a particular stage of development. Side-stepping a developmental framework that seeks out a genetic origin of the symbolic to the Oedipus complex or a stage in psychosexual development, Lacan treats the symbolic dimension as always-already engulfing the subject and constituting the subject's pre-history, even prior to birth. In his seminar on January 11, 1956, Lacan challenges us to not be overly fascinated with the first entry into language:

> The young child whom you see playing at making an object disappear and reappear, who is thereby working at apprehending the symbol, will, if you let yourselves be fascinated by him, mask the fact that the symbol is already there, that it is enormous and englobes him from all sides—that language exists, fills libraries to the point of overflowing, and surrounds, guides, and rouses all your actions—the fact that you are engaged, that it can require you to move at any moment and take you somewhere—all this you forget before the child being introduced into the symbolic dimension. So let us place ourselves at the level of existence of the symbol as such, insofar as we are immersed in it (Lacan, 1981, p. 81).

Regardless of a patient's ability to symbolize (as understood by various psychoanalytic schools), the symbolic has already played a fundamental constituting role in positioning a child in the social world of their family, society, and language. This caution against assuming a developmental and temporal trajectory is essential in the argument that follows, and I return to it towards the essay's end.

Cecilia Gentili's *Faltas*

Gentili's memoir, paired with her interview with the NYC TOHP, provides an extensive exploration of family romance fantasies for a trans child. At 17 years old she was a sex worker and entered into a social network of other trans women in her Argentine city of Rosario. Eventually, Gentili moved to the US, where she continued sex work in Miami, San Francisco, and New York, during which she struggled with drug addiction. After a residential drug treatment program, Gentili became an outreach worker at a HIV/AIDS health clinic. Despite her relative lack of both education and English literacy, Gentili proved capable, and moved up through various non-profit positions. She eventually became the Director of Policy at Gay Men's Health Crisis (GMHC), one of New York City's largest HIV service organizations. It was during her time at GMHC, in 2017, that I met Gentili and interviewed her for NYC TOHP. After she left GMHC, she became a non-profit consultant, further developed her practice as a stage performer, and played a leading role in a campaign to decriminalize sex work in New York State. Gentili's death was a devastating event for New York City's trans communities, and for activists across multiple movements.

Her 2023 memoir, *Faltas: Letters to Everyone in my Hometown Who Isn't My Rapist,* offers an in-depth account of her childhood relationships, told through a series of letters. The family romance is woven throughout the book, appearing in multiple forms. The most explicit example of the family romance is the one recounted at the opening of this chapter: the belief that she had been left by aliens. She describes the scene again in the novel, with minor variations from her oral history interview. On the drive when she was about five years old, her brother pointed out railroad tracks as they passed, whispering: "That is where we found you" (2023, p. 29). He described her as found alone and naked. "You are not my brother," her brother said to Cecilia. In response, Gentili writes: "If he was telling the truth, this explained so much. I had always felt like I was not part of this family" (2023, p. 30). She wondered if she was "some kind of new Moses," recognizing the parallels between her fantasy and other family romance myths previously identified by Freud (2023, p. 30).

On arrival, she told her loving grandmother about her newfound realization:

> I am an extraterrestrial. Do you see all the spaceships being spotted in the sky around us? They are looking for me, Grandma. Claudio told me I was found by the railway, and I just found out in school that what I have makes me a boy, and I just couldn't tell them I am not. They would not understand because they are not like me! But I am from a planet where girls like me have peepees! The lady called it *penis* (2023, p. 31, emphasis in original).

That evening, her grandmother helped her pack a bag, and they went out to spend the night in the desert, waiting for aliens to return to pick Cecilia up and take her to where she belonged. The aliens did not come, her brother's story did not fit with their mother's frequent account of Cecilia's difficult childbirth, and Cecilia returned to the world where girls with penises do not easily find their way.

Condensed into this passage are multiple threads of the family romance. The fantasy's immediate use here is clear, and relevant for many examples of trans children turning to the fantasy: Gentili was not being accepted or supported by her family, who largely rejected her self-understanding as a girl. As a means of holding fast to her sense of her gender and of preserving her gendered desire, she found a fantasy that explained her physical differences from other girls. This fantasy also allowed her to imagine that there is a place where she belongs, providing a supportive and necessary distance from parental authority. This use of the family romance does not necessarily depend on Gentili's particular experience of having an early and well-defined identification with her chosen gender. For a child that will only later identify with a non-assigned gender, a similar use of the family romance could emerge out of inchoate or partial gender dysphoria, including a vague sense of not quite fitting.

Using Freud's essay and Lacan's seminar, *Faltas* offers us even more for understanding the use of the family romance beyond this logic of belonging. Here, I use Gentili's memoir to focus on five facets of the family romance: the family romance (1) as the product of a conflictual encounter with the social organization of sexual difference; (2) as a means of reconciling and defending against knowledge of biological origins and their social meanings; (3) as both the rupture and preservation of an idealizing identification with a parental figure; (4) in relation to the limits of belonging, here specifically through childhood sexual violence; and (5) in relation to death and social violence.

Confrontation With the Order of Sexual Difference: "The Lady Called it Penis"

In both her memoir and interview, Gentili tells another story immediately prior to recounting the trip to her grandmothers. A couple of weeks after beginning school, the young Cecilia was confronted with a forceful education in the gendered order. She was called into the principal's office, where her teacher, a psychologist, and her mother were also gathered. She writes:

> Mama was there. My first thought was she was giving me up to another family. I felt relief and sadness at the same time. I loved her, but I already knew at that age we were not a good match. I hoped they would send me to a rich family. I didn't care if they were bad people, just as long as they were rich! (2023, p. 23)

After this initial iteration of a family romance fantasy, Cecilia then briefly considered that the meeting may be the result of the army taking over the government, with the intention of explaining to her that they now lived in a different province. Instead, the assembled authority figures presented Cecilia with a schematic drawing of sexual genitalia. Gentili writes of the diagrams:

> They were weird; I didn't understand them at all. As an adult, now, I see them clearly, and I know what they were intended to schematize. But at the time I was only five or six. I had no idea what I was supposed to be seeing. (2023, p. 24)

The diagrams offered a new form of sexual knowledge, one articulated by institutional authority. The psychologist explained that she herself had a vagina, and asked Cecilia to identify which drawing corresponded to her own genitals. Cecilia was not sure, asking herself, "What *did* I have?" (2023, p. 25). She tentatively chose the penis, saying she could be wrong. Her mother quietly cried throughout the scene. The psychologist then explained that because she had a penis, she was a boy and had to use the boy's bathroom.

Here is a moment of collective institutional violence, seeking to discipline young Cecilia's gender identity and expression. By this point in her life, Cecilia's gender identification was already established, though it is less clear whether she declared it to others or would have articulated it to others in the terms that she did in adulthood. But at five years old, she is already regularly using the girl's bathroom, styling her school uniform to be as feminine as possible, and seeking out relationships and activities where her femininity is partially acknowledged by others. Where much psychoanalytic literature focuses on the process of gender formation and identification – an important theoretical and clinical question – in this case, like in Freud's essay, the family romance emerges after the initial establishment of her gender identity. The fantasy here comes into its fullest fruition when authority figures reject and attempt to forcefully correct her gender. Her mother, Gentili explains elsewhere, does not particularly understand or support her childhood gender expression, but appears relatively powerless in this scene in the face of an outside authority, represented by the principal, psychologist, and a teacher.

Cecilia turns to the family romance in response to her confrontation with the order of sexual difference. This is not instigated by an encounter with corporeal reality in the form of seeing her own genitals or those of a family member, as Freud identifies elsewhere, but specifically as insisted on by institutional authority. It is not anatomical difference itself that constitutes a primary problem for Cecilia, or what Lacan calls the *real*. For Cecilia the problem is *the social organization* of sexual difference, as enforced and imposed upon her: a dimension of the symbolic. The problem for her is not that she discovers that she has a penis, it is that "the lady called it a penis," with imposed social meanings and implications. Even prior to genital diagrams, Cecilia's first thought in seeing the authority figures in the meeting represents a partial family romance – that her mother was giving her up for a rich family, because they "were not a good match" – recognizing both their authority over her family and the class stratification and poverty of her household. It is the structural character of sexual difference as constituted and enforced by social authority that leads Cecilia to turn to the family romance fantasy.

This distinction between gender identification and sexual difference as a social order, already subtly present in Freud's essay, is of broad significance for trans children and likely for gender as a general phenomena. One significant moment is when the child first has an imaginary identification with a parent that includes a gendered dimension – "the child's most intense and momentous wish" to be like "the parent of his own sex." This first moment cannot primarily be about sex as an anatomical category, because the child does not yet understand procreation or possibly even anatomical difference at all. But the family romance does not emerge until a second moment, when the child, according to Freud, recognizes their parents as belonging to "the category to which his parents belong," as positioned within a symbolic order beyond them. It is here that gender as parental identification gives way to sex as a social category in which one is placed, willingly or unwillingly. The family romance for Freud enables the child to bridge this earlier identification and the symbolic moment of the category; the family romance is a response to an encounter with the symbolic and the social organization of sexual difference.

Biological Origins: "Confusion and Strife Around the Question of Who the Fathers Might Be"

Cecilia faced multiple forms of parental absence. Her father disappeared for an extended period and when he returned he remained completely psychically unavailable. Though she no longer doubted that her mother gave birth to her, she remained doubtful throughout her life that her mother was at all maternal, that she fulfilled the role of a mother:

> Whenever I write about Mami it seems like my words carry the feeling that she was a bad person. Do I need to say that she wasn't? Though I am sure we can both agree that… I was going to say, 'We can both agree that she was not a good mother,' but I think it's closer to say she was just not a mother. She had the love and empathy of a good soul, but she was never motherly. I wonder where that absence came from? (2023, p. 137, ellipsis in original).

The relative absences of both her father and mother were likely among the disappointments that led Cecilia to imagine she belonged among aliens. After that fantasy passed, their psychic absences remained unresolved problems.

In Freud's essay, the question of biological origins is central to the child's turn to the family romance. The family romance is a dimension of the evolving sexual theories of children through which they try to explain their own origin. The problem of origins, in Freud's framework, is a challenging one for children, and the family romance serves as an intermediary way of theorizing what he will later describe as the primal scene. Specifically, the family romance takes a different form before and after the child begins to understand the biology of procreation. As the child understands the basics of biological procreation, they come to no longer have doubts about their mother, but maintain uncertainty about their father. This enables the child to begin to explore various sexual fantasies about their mother.

Following the structure of Freud's essay, Gentili's memoir similarly marks a difference between the initial fantasy of believing that she was left by aliens and a later reflection on the uncertainty of paternal relations. She writes in a letter to her deceased grandmother: "I am not questioning the legitimacy of your motherhood here. That you were the mother was always clear, despite all the confusion and strife around the question of who the fathers might be" (2023, p. 138). The confusion about fathers is multiple, both doubts about Cecilia's father and more substantiated doubts about the fatherhood of her grandmother's children. These doubts later preoccupy Cecilia and her cousins, one of whom receives ongoing support from the greengrocer, whom she and many others suspect to be her true grandfather.

The problem of doubt about fatherhood includes both the imaginary experience of paternal absence, and a symbolic dimension which puts into doubt one's place in social life. Intergenerational symbolic inheritance, embodied in part by the paternal name and paternal lineage, is a psychic problem in the constitution of neurosis. In Lacan's essay, "The Neurotic's Individual Myth," he understands the Rat Man's neurosis to be rooted in an inherited mythology of his own origins. The Rat Man's father's story of conflicted interests in a poor girl and a rich girl structure the Rat Man's compulsive and apparently nonsensical behaviors (1953). In one Lacanian clinical technique, an analyst asks the patient for their associations with their names (Luepnitz, 2009). The subject confronts the problems of patrilineal descent, generational debts, and biological origins as a mode of what I term *encountering the symbolic*.

Trans people face these problems in particular and challenging ways. My trans female patients contend with the multiple meanings of rejecting both their assigned position in a lineage of patrilineal descent and the expectations and obligations that their parents placed on them through it. To declare oneself as not male is often to reject one's place in a line of fathers and male ancestors. Trans men, by contrast, may wish to enter into a familial relation of patrilineal descent, but they are often not welcome to do so. Even to change the name given by one's parents can be to complicate and reject familial expectations, including symbolic debts and expectations. The complexity of these symbolic questions can manifest in fraught and conflictual relations with actual fathers and grandfathers.

Idealization and Identification: "They are Looking for Me."

For Freud, prior to the family romance is an earlier moment of strong gendered identification with the parent. In his essay, this moment is not explored directly as it is not remembered or reported by the child. Instead, it is reconstructed from the traces that this moment leaves in the family romance itself, through providing the idealizing material which is later incorporated into the family romance fantasy. For Freud, this primarily takes the form of the aristocratic, high-status, and wealthy character of the imagined other family. This earlier idealization expresses itself in the family romance in gendered terms: "when his father seemed to him the noblest and strongest of men and his mother the dearest and loveliest of women" (1909a, p. 241).

Freud's analysis is helpful for identifying how an earlier idealizing identification may shape Cecilia's fantasy. Like Freud's account, Gentili does not clearly mark this earlier moment of idealizing gender identification. A few hints suggest earlier, more positive identifications with her family members. Her father returns after a lengthy disappearance; Gentili says little about him before his absence, but after she suggests that he is changed by becoming "no more than a body that slept and ate with us," implying that he had possibly once been something more to her. Her grandmother was consistently loving and supportive; though not calling her a girl she allowed Cecilia to act femininely. When she first reports her alien realization to her grandmother, her response is one of understanding: "I love you," her grandmother replied. "That makes so much sense. I just don't know how to help you. Do you want us to wait for them tonight?" Cecilia "felt such relief": "Yes, Grandma. I knew you would get it" (2023, p. 32).

Later Cecilia discovers her grandmother had a close friend who was secretly intersex, with both a vagina and a penis. Gentili also positively references her mother's femininity, and was able to later establish a positive relationship with her mother once Cecilia moved away from the area. Cecilia even makes associative links between the aliens and her closest female relatives: when her mother was not depressed, they would sit outside trying to identify UFOs; Cecilia confided her alien fantasy to her grandmother.

These traces also appear in her fantasy. She initially hopes that the family she may be given up for is rich. She tells her grandmother that the aliens spotted in the sky are "looking for me," that they desire her return, and are seeking her out. Among these aliens, her anatomy would not distinguish her from other girls; she would belong and would be accepted as a girl without the imposition of a mismatched gendered order. By imagining other kin relations, Gentili identifies the characteristics that stand in for ones that she may have felt in an earlier, more devoted moment to parental objects. Unfortunately, Cecilia does encounter a surrogate parent who offers many of these characteristics, at great cost.

The Limits of Belonging: "He Saw Me as I Was"

The subtitle of Gentili's memoir identifies the figure whose absence as an address haunts her epistolary work: her rapist. Her rapist was a father in her neighborhood who established a multi-year sexual relationship with Cecilia. Cecilia clearly identifies the relationship as extremely harmful, coercive, and non-consensual. But she also explores her childhood investment in the relationship, and the reasons that motivated her to enter into and stay in the relationship beyond the force of coercion.

In the book's opening letter, addressed to the rapist's daughter, Cecilia describes what she encountered when first entering their home: the signifiers of familial stability, with its class, gendered, and sexual logics:

> I envied your TV. I envied everything. That house looked like the house a family lived in. There was furniture and it indicated: *family*. I think I fell into some kind of reverie, thinking of how my life would be if I lived in this home, if your parents were my parents. I would be happy, watching TV in your dad's lap, wearing a cute pink dress while your mom smiled at us from the kitchen, where she was preparing dinner (2023, p. 37, emphasis in original).

It was at this moment that Cecilia's rapist first touched her. Her rapist was the first person and, for years, the only person, who unambiguously affirmed her as a girl:

> And there was one other thing he knew: I was a girl. He understood my femininity as normal, and used that, too. I remember the first time he laid eyes on me: I saw it, I saw he would give me that thing everyone else was denying me. He saw me as I was, and I didn't have to explain how I felt inside because for him it was visible. He saw I was Cecilia. He saved my life and ruined it forever. (2023, p. 37)

She felt completed, experiencing an idealized unity:

> He called me his "little girl"! You know when you put that last Lego in whatever shape you are making? Or add the last piece to a puzzle? That kind of satisfaction I had never had, and that is how I felt. Something completed me. Something was just perfect (2023, p. 19).

He framed their sexual activity in familial terms: as appropriate between fathers and daughters, but something that Cecilia's father shamefully would not provider her. The novel includes a great deal on their relationship, how Cecilia made sense of it as a child and later as an adolescent, and how it shaped her subsequent romantic relationships.

Gentili's account challenges the centrality of belonging as an idealized endpoint of many conventional trans narratives. Not supported by one's parents or immediate social context, it is often imagined that the trans child eventually encounters a supportive community, one where their gender is affirmed and embraced by others. They fulfill the wish of the family romance as shared by many trans children: they will find a place that they belong. For many, including Cecilia, this dream is partially realized later in their lives, with much benefit. Adult trans people often have much more opportunity to pursue lives where they are in relation to other trans people and to cultivate trans-affirming community, resulting in improvement for their mental health and wellbeing. But belonging and recognition can also be means of harm. Cecilia's rapist uses her desire and need for gendered belonging to establish and maintain a relationship of child sexual abuse, with negative consequences for Cecilia's life. It is not simply a false belonging; her rapist desires her as a girl, recognizes her as Cecilia, and sincerely affirms her femininity, alongside and inseparable from the violent sexual abuse. This is a necessary corrective to the predominance of simplified and idealized accounts common in representations of trans life.

It is also a brutal, concrete example of a more subtle and general problem of the family romance. Belonging is also always a question of the desire of the other. The family romance is taken up by trans children as a fantasy of belonging, of a different world where they may experience social acceptance. For trans children, the social organization of sexual difference may be particularly violent and harmful, and a better, more trans-affirming social world may be possible and desirable. Yet the family romance also marks or covers over a fundamental alienation of the desire of the other, the impossibility of a fantasy of full self-congruence. The family romance attempts and fails to resolve forms of alienation that operate in both imaginary and symbolic registers. To encounter the world as a system of social categories that exceed oneself is to be subject to social authority, alienated through a language that is never one's own. But the fantasy of escaping this symbolic alienation – a longing for full belonging and recognition which amounts to a false repetition of an idealized relationship with an imagined pre-symbolic parental object, often depicted in the family romance as a return to one's true exalted parents – is equally an experience of subjugation and self-alienation, with potentially horrific consequences. The very act of belonging is also always a moment of self-alienation, of constitution through the desire of the other, as made possible through an impersonal order of language.

Social Violence: "Those Children Were Sold"

As with Horner and Rosenberg's (1991) recognition that the family romance bridges psychic life amidst prevalent social violence, Gentili's interview and memoir locate her family romance in a broader context of a counter-insurgent war. When Cecilia first enters the meeting with her principal, psychologist, teacher, and mother, she thinks that it may be somehow related to changing provincial boundaries resulting from a recent military seizure of the Argentine state. In her oral history interview, immediately after her story of awaiting her return to the aliens, I ask Cecilia about the political context in Argentina at the time. In her description of Argentina's "Dirty War" and her family's complex relationship to the political context, she quickly cites a specific feature of the war:

> People were being kidnapped and killed and that pregnant people were being kidnapped and their children were stolen from them and then they were killed, and those children were sold, and everything that was not totally in line with the dictators and dictatorship that was going on was simply eliminated (NYC TOHP, 002, p. 6–7).

Among the many egregious human rights violations of the Dirty War and its varying facets of political terror, here Cecilia refers to one closely related to the family romance: the practice of murdering left activists, stealing their children, and then giving their children as adoptees to military families and those friendly to the regime (Lazzaro, 2013). Cecilia's childhood fantasy is, at least in her adult recounting, deeply tied up with the broader context of the child theft as mass terror that was happening around her.

Violent, involuntary separation of parents and children has been a central feature of racial capitalism for centuries.[6] Black feminist scholars like Saidiya Hartman (1997), Angela Davis (1972), Tiffany Lethabo King (2018), and others consider the practice of separating enslaved mothers and children as central to the racial and gender order of plantation slavery, with lasting implications for US racial politics of the family. Separation of families and children was central to the system of boarding schools for indigenous children established through the US and Canada, resulting in the mass death of many children and many others being allocated to white families as domestic workers (Glenn, 2010). Recent organizing and scholarship have focused their critique on the "family policing system," recognizing the anti-Black violence of the child welfare policies (Roberts, 2022). Trans children are disproportionately subject to the family policing system, and face high levels of abuse by both parents and institutional caregivers (Prince et al., 2022). As the interview with Shannon Fawkes details, among the trans youth that they worked with, family romance fantasies often overlapped with actual separation from their parents and living in foster arrangements with extended relatives or relative strangers. Many of these children had faced extensive trauma and violence throughout their lives.

The family romance both reflects and attempts to cover over this violent social order. Children, even when their understanding is fragmented and partial, turn to the family romance to both incorporate and defend against a society of racial capitalism where the murder of parents, the separation of children and parents, and the use of mass violence to police family life is widespread.

The violent social context of Gentili's life and the world of racial capitalism may appear for the subject through questions of death and mortality. In Lacanian theory, sexual difference is constituted by differing relationships with an absolute limit necessary to language and subjectivity (see, for example, Lacan, 1999). Generally, this limit is understood in terms of castration, sharing with Freud a recognition that differing attempts to respond to the problem of castration constitute the split of sexual difference. This limit that constitutes sexual difference could also potentially be theorized as death. The symbolic poses but cannot answer the question of death. The signifier represents something in its absence; our names represent us after our death; through the family name the dead continue to structure the lives of the living. The absolute limit of death that haunts the symbolic may also be constitutive of sexual difference. In an evocative passage from his seminar on May 30, 1956, Lacan suggests the symbolic constitution of sexual difference is also the position from which we view our mortality:

> The two sides, male and female, of sexuality are not given data, are nothing that could be deduced from experience. How could the individual situate himself within sexuality if he didn't already possess the system of signifiers, insofar as it institutes the space that enables him to see, at a distance, as an enigmatic object, the thing that is the most difficult of access, namely his own death? (Lacan, 1981, p. 248–249).[7]

Retheorizing the Family Romance[8]

The family romance is a means through which trans children attempt to use a fantasy to reconcile and defend against new knowledge. This new knowledge arrives in the form of the desire of the other; it is articulated through a social order which places the children in categories of sexual difference. The family romance is used by the trans child to create and maintain an inner space for the preservation of the child's desire.

Like many of the family romance fantasies of trans children that I have found, and in contrast to the claims of Freud's essay, Cecilia does not primarily frame the family romance in terms of other parents as specific imagined people. Though she has a brief wish to be adopted into a wealthy family, social status and wealth do not figure as centrally for trans children's accounts as they do in Freud. Cecilia's main fantasy, that she belongs among aliens, is common for trans children, yet does not follow the specific logic that Freud details. Where for Freud the mark of the social order in the family romance manifests through the (cis) child's understanding of feudal remnants of social status hierarchies, for trans children it often takes the form of being a member of a species where their gender incongruities no longer mark a distance between their sense of themselves, social expectations, and social acceptance.

What accounts for this difference? There are obvious concrete and contingent factors: Freud's social context was dominated by concerns with class position and the tumultuous historical clashing of multiple modes of production with their accompanying status hierarchies. Further, higher social classes would not likely provide trans children with greater opportunities for acceptance. But there is another, more challenging possibility: that the family romance is always a response to the violence of the social imposition of sexual difference, but cis children are able to repress this and substitute the problem of sexual difference for a phallic fantasy centered instead on social status. Freud's essay, with its multiple references to questions of sexual difference as confronted by the child, offers traces of this other potential interpretation. Freud repeatedly returned to the problem of how children respond to, cover over, and are transformed by the encounter with sexual difference and knowledge of biological reproduction. Written shortly before "Family Romances," his essay "On the Sexual Theories of Children" is centrally focused on the fantasized theories that children generate as a means of making up for and defending against knowledge of sexual difference.

Freud recognized in his developing theories of castration that sexual difference is experienced by the child – cis and trans alike – as a traumatic rupture. The cis child is able to more thoroughly cover over this rupture through fusing their imaginary gendered identification with the parent of their sex with their symbolic placement in a social order of sexual difference, through a partial and imagined congruence between their internal experience of gender and external expectations. Through this fusing of gender identification and placement within sexual difference, the cis child is then able to repress the problem of sexual difference altogether, replacing it with a phallic fantasy centered instead on social status in class society. The repressed problem of sexual difference, for the cis person, later reemerges in the neurotic symptom. This repression, perhaps, is less available for the trans child. The rupture of sexual difference persists, and the gap remains between imaginary gender identification and their socially assigned sex and its meanings. The trans child may then turn to a more drastic fantasized solution: alien kinship and an escape from human society altogether, with its accompanying codes of sexual difference. The trans child, for whom the problem of sexual difference may be much more intractable and persistent, can use the fantasy of alien kinship to maintain an internal distance between their own desire and the social expectations imposed upon them.

This use of the family romance by the trans child corresponds to elements of Lacan's understanding of fantasy. For Lacan, fantasy is always partially defensive (see, for example, Lacan, 1966). The structure of fantasy is a way of staging the subject as divided with respect to the Other, using the object cause of desire, the object a. Because the object a belongs neither to the subject nor the Other, it can serve as a separation. The trans child, too close to the social demands imposed by their parents, must produce an internal fantasy that opens up a gap in which the child's desire can survive. The family romance, perhaps, is always a fantasy constructed by the child to defend against sexual difference. For the trans child, this is more starkly apparent because it is less successful.

Returning to Lacan's emphasis on the symbolic as constituting the pre-history of the subject rather than as a solely developmental phase, trans children have to construct their gender and this fantasy space that preserves their desire using preexisting cultural forms. A child may come to experience something new about their gender at some developmental juncture, but that gender order proceeds them altogether, imposed consciously and unconsciously by all those around them from before birth and throughout their life. The trans child may reject gendered expectations from parental caregivers, but they do so using the very material of gender expression and identification. Trans people take up, rework, and constitute themselves through existing gendered signifiers.

The subject's encounter with the symbolic is iterative, repeated, and as a logical rather than developmental phase. On multiple occasions throughout the subject's life, they confront, learn, reject, or work with new knowledge about multiple interconnected questions that situate them into a symbolic order. These need not occur only at a specific phase of childhood. The family romance, in various guises, could similarly be taken up at any moment where the subject is confronted with a dimension of the symbolic order that disrupts and complicates previous identifications, that disappoints previous idealizations, or that poses in a new way the intractable questions of birth and death, origins and ends.

Like all subjects, the trans person must navigate their relationship with gender with respect to a sexual order that exceeds them. Sexual difference is a fundamental problem of human existence, impossible for anyone to fully resolve. It appears in neurotic and psychotic symptoms. It constitutes human psychic life. The trans child's family romance is one way to survive and evade the full force of this violence of sexual difference.

Conclusion: Listening for desire

This chapter is not meant to offer a definitive theory of gender, nor a full theory of the symbolic. Instead, it uses Freud at this theoretical conjuncture of his work to identify the particular uses that trans children make of the family romance. Like this moment in Freud's evolving theories, these children are at a cusp between different dimensions of sex and gender identification. At five years old, Cecilia already strongly identified with femininity and girlhood, but did not yet know how to relate to the figures of authority that dictated the meaning of sexual difference. Such moments between conflicting and partial accounts of sexual difference reappear, in various forms, throughout trans narratives. The family romance is a provisional fantasy that gives way to the subject finding other ways of relating to gender and sex, but it can also serve as a strategy for reconciling conflicting knowledge that the subject may repeatedly return to.

In these senses, there is a provisional and transitional character across three registers in this essay: in Freud's changing theories of childhood sexuality in 1909, for these children at a moment of developing sexual knowledge, and in this essay's effort to contribute to a fuller theory of sexual difference that could adequately speak to the experiences of trans lives.

Cecilia, like many trans children, used fantasy to survive a harsh and violent world. For her, fantasy was a powerful tool to postpone a capitulation to the social order of sexual difference, and its interwoven contexts of mass state terror, predatory sexual abuse, and profound social exclusion. Through her fantasies, she was able to preserve and cultivate something of her desire. Through this desire, Gentili was eventually able to play a powerful and far-reaching role in movements of trans people and sex workers in New York City, touching and transforming the lives of many thousands of trans people and others. Her memoir can be read as an attempt to bring the fierce wisdom of her adult life back into relation with her childhood, with the place of her origin, and with her family in which she could not belong. The child Cecilia called forth to aliens to rescue her; through her life in trans-liberation movements and through the creative act of her testimony, an adult Cecilia responded. Throughout her life in writing, organizing, performing, and speaking, Gentili claimed a radical subjectivity of her own desire, one that demanded and pursued fundamental changes in the social world.

Psychoanalysis, however violent and horrific its history in working with trans people, can also foster a space for articulating trans desire. In the gap between social expectations and private fantasy, between the symbolic order of sexual difference and the imaginary identification of gender idealization, between a normative developmental trajectory and a child's refusal to confirm, something of the subject's desire can emerge. By theorizing with and alongside trans life, psychoanalysis can challenge longstanding harms and biases in the field, and rediscover the radical kernel of the practice. In doing so, psychoanalysis can offer something back to trans narratives – returning speech in an inverted form and providing potential theorizations that can speak to the complexity and richness of trans life. Psychoanalysis is powerfully suited to listen carefully to trans desire, to foster and facilitate its unfolding, aiding the trans subject to speak and act toward the remaking of the world.

Acknowledgements

My thanks to those who read and provided extensive and thoughtful feedback on this essay, especially Loren Dent and Myriam Sauer. Thanks to Vanessa Sinclair for commissioning this piece, and Hannah Zeavin for proposing its publication in *Parapraxis*. I am grateful to all the narrators of the NYC Trans Oral History Project, who courageously and publicly shared the narratives of their lives, their brilliance, and their wisdom. I also thank Shannon Fawkes for agreeing to a research interview. My deepest gratitude, and to whom this essay is, of course, dedicated, goes to Cecilia Gentili. May you rest in power.

Notes

1 Throughout, I refer to Cecilia Gentili as Gentili when referring to her as an adult author and interview narrator, and as Cecilia when describing her in childhood, partially in keeping with her self-referencing herself as Cecilia at moments in the memoir.
2 Gentili's interview was through the New York City Trans Oral History Project (NYC TOHP), a project discussed further later. NYC TOHP interviews are cited using the three-digit number assigned to their interview in the project and page numbers from their posted transcripts. NYC TOHP interviews are posted under a Creative Commons license that permits essays like this. All interviews and transcripts can be found online at https://nyctransoralhistory.org.
3 The differential meanings of "gender" and "sex" have been extensively debated in the fields of feminist politics, queer theory, and sexology. In this essay, I inconsistently put the terms to provisional use to mark a particular distinction – between gender as identification and sex as a categorical place in the social order – without the intent to assert these as general definitions.
4 Backus, 1994; Lang, 1990; Meyer, 1964; Silverstein, 1977; Warner, 1993; Widzer, 1977.
5 Quote from Sants, 1964; see also Blum, 1983; Donoghue, 2017; Glassman, 2013; Wieder, 1977.
6 I review this literature in O'Brien, 2023.
7 This passage is one of a few in Lacan's work that can be read as compatible with an affirmation of trans experience. For others, see Gherovici (2011, 2017). Lacan is also widely read, not without reason, as condemnatory of trans identity, gender transitioning, and trans women. This essay is not meant to defend Freud and Lacan as necessarily in support of trans life, but to identify something in their projects that is of use in making sense of an aspect of trans experience.
8 A number of the ideas in this section were offered by Loren Dent in response to reading an early draft. Errors are of course my own.

Bibliography

Backus, M.G. (1994). "'Looking for that Dead Girl': Incest, Pornography and the Capitalist Family Romance in *Nightwood, The Years* and *Tar Baby,*" *American Imago*, 51(4), pp. 421–445.
Berliner, A. (1997). *Ma Vie en Rose*. Haut et Court, Blue Light Distribution.
Blum, H.P. (1983). "Adoptive Parents." *The Psychoanalytic Study of the Child*, 38(1), pp. 141–163.

Corbett, K. (2001). "Nontraditional Family Romance." *The Psychoanalytic Quarterly*, 70(3), pp. 599–624.

Davis, A. (1972). "Reflections on the Black Woman's Role in the Community of Slaves." *The Massachusetts Review* 13(1/2), pp. 81–100.

Deutsch, H. (1936). "On the Genesis of the Family Romance." *The Psychoanalytic Review*, 23, pp. 104–105.

Donoghue, O. (2017). "The 'Replacement Child': On Adoption, Haunting, and the Unlived Life." *Studies in Gender and Sexuality*, 18(4), pp. 313–317.

Fawkes, S. (August 17, 2023). Interview conducted by the author (online).

Freud, S (1956). "Analysis of a Phobia in a Five-Year-Old Boy." In J. Strachey (Ed.) *The Standard Edition of the Complete Psychological Works of Sigmund Freud (SE)*, Vol. X. London: Hogarth Press, pp. 3–152. (Original work published 1909b).

Freud, S. (1959). "Three Essays on the Theory of Sexuality." In J. Strachey (Ed.) *The Standard Edition of the Complete Psychological Works of Sigmund Freud (SE)*, Vol. VII. London: Hogarth Press. (Original work published 1905).

Freud, S. (1959). "On the Sexual Theories of Children." In J. Strachey (Ed.) *The Standard Edition of the Complete Psychological Works of Sigmund Freud (SE)*, Vol. IX. London: Hogarth Press, pp. 205–226. (Original work published 1908).

Freud, S. (1959). "Family romances." *The Standard Edition of the Complete Psychological Works of Sigmund Freud (SE)*, Vol. IX. London: Hogarth Press, pp. 235–241. (Original work published 1909a).

Freud, S. (1964). "Moses and Monotheism: Three Essays." In J. Strachey (Ed.) *The Standard Edition of the Complete Psychological Works of Sigmund Freud (SE)*, Vol. XXIII. London: Hogarth Press, pp. 1–140. (Original work published 1939).

Freud, A. (1968). "On Certain Difficulties in the Preadolescent's Relation to His Parents." In *The Writings of Anna Freud, Vol. 4*. New York: International Universities Press, pp. 95–106. (Original work published 1949).

Freud, S. (1985). *The Complete Letters of Sigmund Freud to Wilhelm Fliess 1887–1904*. Cambridge: Belknap Press of Harvard University Press.

Gentili, C. (2023). *Faltas: Letters to Everyone in my Hometown Who Isn't My Rapist*. New York: Littlepuss Press.

Gherovici, P. (2011). *Please Select Your Gender: From the Invention of Hysteria to the Democratizing of Transgenderism*. New York: Routledge.

Gherovici, P. (2017). *Transgender Psychoanalysis: A Lacanian Perspective on Sexual Difference*. New York: Routledge.

Glassman, N. (2013). "Narrative, Family Romance Fantasy, and the Adoption Triad." *Psychoanalytic Perspectives*, 10, pp. 116–119.

Glenn, E.N. (2010). *Forced to Care: Coercion and Caregiving in America*. Cambridge: Harvard University Press.

Greenacre, P. (1958). "The Family Romance of the Artist." *The Psychoanalytic Study of the Child*, 13(1), pp. 9–36.

Horner, T.M. and Rosenberg, E.B. (1991). "The Family Romance: A Developmental-Historical Perspective." *Psychoanalytic Psychology*, 8(2), pp. 131–148.

Kaplan, L.J. (1974). "The Concept of the Family Romance." *Psychoanalytic Review*, 61(2), pp. 169–202.

King, T.L. (2018). "Black 'Feminisms' and Pessimism: Abolishing Moynihan's Negro Family." *Theory & Event*, 21(2), pp. 68–87.

Klein, M. (1920). "The Psychic Life of the Child." Originally published in *Internationale Zeitschrift für Psychoanalyse*, 6(2), pp. 151–155. Trans. by S. Leighton, Melanie Klein Trust. https://melanie-klein-trust.org.uk/wp-content/uploads/2020/04/The-Psychic-Life-of-the-Child-by-Klein-1920.pdf.

Lacan, J. (1953). "The Neurotic's Individual Myth." *The Psychoanalytic Quarterly*, 48(3), pp. 405–425.

Lacan, J. (1981). *The Seminar of Jacques Lacan, Book III, 1955–1956, The Psychoses*. Trans. by R. Gregg. New York: W.W. Norton.

Lang, R. (1990). "Batman and Robin: A Family Romance." *American Imago*, 47(3–4), pp. 239–319.

Lazzara, M.J. (2013). "Kidnapped Memories: Argentina's Stolen Children Tell Their Stories." *Journal of Human Rights*, 12(3), pp. 319–332.

Lehrman, P. (1927). "The Fantasy of Not Belonging to One's Family." *Archives of Neurology & Psychiatry*, 18(6), pp. 1015–1023.

Lewis, A.J. (2014). "'I Am 64 and Paul McCartney Doesn't Care': The Haunting of the Transgender Archive and the Challenges of Queer History." *Radical History Review*, 2014(120), pp. 13–34.

Lewis, A.J. (2017a). "TRANS ANIMISMS." *Angelaki*, 22(2), pp. 203–215.

Lewis, A.J. (2017b). "Trans History in a Moment of Danger: Organizing Within and Beyond 'Visibility' in the 1970s." In R. Gossett, E.A. Stanley and J. Burton (Eds.) *Trap Door: Trans Cultural Production and the Politics of Visibility*. Cambridge: MIT Press, pp. 57–90.

Luepnitz, D.A. (2009). "Thinking in the Space Between Winnicott and Lacan." *International Journal of Psychoanalsis*, 90, p. 957–981.

Meyer, B.C. (1964). "Psychoanalytic Studies on Joseph Conrad: IV. The Flow and Ebb of Artistry." *Journal of the American Psychoanalytic Association*, 12(4), pp. 802–824.

New York City Trans Oral History Project (2024). *Interviews*. https://nyctransoralhistory. org/interviews.

O'Brien, M.E. (2023). *Family Abolition: Capitalism and the Communizing of Care*. London: Pluto.

Prince, D.M., Ray-Novak, M., Gillani, B. and Peterson, E. (2022). "Sexual and Gender Minority Youth in Foster Care: An Evidence-based Theoretical Conceptual Model of Disproportionality and Psychological Comorbidities." *Trauma, Violence, & Abuse*, 23(5), pp.1643–1657.

Rank, O. (1914). *Myth of the Birth of the Hero: A Psychological Interpretation of Mythology*. Trans. by F. Robbins and S.E. Jelliffe. New York: The Journal of Mental Disease and Nervous Disorders Publishing Company. (Original work published in 1909).

Roberts, D. (2022). *Torn Apart: How the Child Welfare System Destroys Black Families – and How Abolition Can Build a Safer World*. New York: Basic Books.

Saidiya, H. (1997). *Scenes of Subjection: Terror, Slavery, and Self-Making in Nineteenth-century America*. New York: Oxford University Press.

Sants, H.J. (1964). "Genealogical Bewilderment in Children with Substitute Parents." *British Journal of Medical Psychology*, 37(2), pp. 133–141.

Silverstein, H. (1977). "Norman Mailer: The Family Romance and the Oedipal Fantasy." *American Imago*, 34(3), pp. 277–286.

Tabin, J.K. (1998). "The Family Romance: Attention to the Unconscious Basis for a Conscious Fantasy." *Psychoanalytic Psychology*, 15(2), pp. 287–293.

Warner, L.L. (1993). "Family Romance Fantasy Resolution in George Eliot's Daniel Deronda." *The Psychoanalytic Study of the Child*, 48(1), pp. 379–397.

Wieder, H. (1977). "The Family Romance Fantasies of Adopted Children." *The Psychoanalytic Quarterly*, 46(2), pp. 185–200.

Widzer, M.E. (1977). "The Comic-Book Superhero." *The Psychoanalytic Study of the Child*, 32(1), pp. 565–603.

Westerink, H. and Van Haute, P. (2020) "'Family Romance' and the Oedipalization of Freudian Psychoanalysis." *Psychoanalysis and History*, 22(2), pp. 175–187.

Chapter 7

Transsexuality at the Origin of Desire

Or, Schreber's Satanic Handjob

Luce deLire

Introduction

What would a psychoanalytic approach to gender and desire look like that takes trans experiences as its point of departure? Trans and non-binary people, and trans women in particular, have been exploited and mistreated by the psychoanalytic community since the inception of this practice. Thus, McKenzie Wark's 2022 piece "Dear Cis Analysts" calls for psychoanalysts to pay us for our work, stop gate keeping, and set up a fund to help trans people with real expertise. I agree. If this provokes you in some way, consider this conversation started. Wark, however, also suggests: "It's time to ask what is wrong with the methods and concepts of psychoanalysis itself, rather than treating [the] horrors [committed against trans and non-binary people in the name of psychoanalysis] as mere deviations from 'best practice.'"[1] In this text, I want to pick up on this call. If you are a psychoanalyst, you might want to consider picking up on that same call from the other side. Reading this article and others in this volume is a great start. But paying your trans patients and other trans people for their work might make a tangible difference as well.[2]

What would a psychoanalytic approach to gender and desire look like that takes trans experiences as its point of departure? Instead of reforming some cis analysts' authority, I choose another path. "Maybe Schreber is a better theorist than either Freud or Lacan for our purposes."[3] What I find is that one is not born cis but rather becomes cis by virtue of an original displacement of the traumatic organization of the human psyche. In other words: what I call "the transsexual paradigm" privileges an allegedly given, actual body over and against a corporeal indeterminacy, a natural surplus in which a body points beyond itself. That surplus is denigrated and pathologized in the term "transsexuality" – and it is appropriated in trans, transgender, non-binary, and other forms of life. I argue that this transsexuality, understood as the violent displacement of a body that is *more than* one's actual body, is *not* a minority issue, but a *common* issue, shared by all subjects of patriarchal societies, – cis, non-binary, trans, and others alike. Real social change starts with an emancipation of such corporeal indeterminacy. Consequentially, an emancipatory psychoanalysis must center trans experience as it occurs in trans, cis, non-binary

DOI: 10.4324/9781032624129-8

and other people alike, rather than just including trans perspectives as yet other voices in the choir.

In the first part of this chapter, I read Freud's analysis of Daniel Paul Schreber, a German judge who experienced three distinct periods which might today be classified as psychosis (1884–1885, 1893–1902, and 1907–1911). Schreber captured some of these experiences, made in the period 1893 to 1902, in the book *Memoirs of My Nervous Illness* (German: *Denkwürdigkeiten eines Nervenkranken*).[4] The book extensively describes how and why God wants to turn Schreber into a woman but only partially succeeds for interference through other actors.

I focus on the degree of madness and contagion that Freud ascribes to Schreber. Citing Immanuel Kant as a saint of rationality, Freud likens Schreber's madness to a gay Satanic ritual that indulges excess pleasure and runs a danger of catching on, making other people crazy as well, notably Freud himself.

Yet, if anything, Schreber's "delusions" must be read as symptoms of a violent regime that I call "the transsexual paradigm," understood as the institutionalized reduction of gender diversity into medicalized transitions that involve body modifications.[5] I argue that Schreber existed within the vortex of the transsexual paradigm *avant la lettre,* and that as such, she was subject to maximized epistemic violence, understood as the complete lack of any resources for any political or libidinal self-understanding. So, in an act of extremely creative political resistance, from most sparse conceptual resources, Schreber generates a framework that is geared towards making her intelligible as a woman. Her *Memoirs of My Nervous Illness* scream for a heterogenous socio-political order that would allow her to exist in the first place.

Note that transsexuality as a medical condition and psychotic experiences (and related diagnoses) have been and still are deemed to be mutually exclusive. Sandy Stone reports as much for US medicine in the 20th century, and German regulations, for instance, are still very explicit about this.[6] You can either be trans or you can be crazy. "When the first academic gender dysphoria clinics were started on an experimental basis in the 1960s, the medical staff would not perform surgery on demand, because of the professional risks involved in performing experimental surgery on 'sociopaths'."[7] My reading of Schreber's memoir as creative resistance against epistemic violence also suggests that any distinction between trans identification and psychosis (and its relatives) may really function as an aspect of epistemic violence itself: it runs the risk of taking the psychotic response to an ultimately hostile world as the cause to deny appropriate treatment. Instead of providing care for disenfranchised trans people, making "sanity" a condition for trans affirmative care actually runs the risk of increasing the suffering.

But why Schreber today? In the third part, I argue that hers is a model of identity formation *in general*, not restricted to trans and non-binary people. In a reading of Judith Butler's *Gender Trouble* and Gilles Deleuze's *Difference and Repetition*, I argue that transsexuality should be understood as an original displacement of the traumatic organization of the human psyche. More concretely, Western cultures continuously call to repress corporeal indeterminacy, the natural surplus or *more than* that co-constitutes our actual physical existence. "Transsexuality" is a name that pathologizes the enjoyment of this surplus – and Schreber was an expert in such enjoyment. Yet all bodies have indeterminate aspects. Transsexuality is therefore *not* a minority issue, but a *common* issue, shared by all subjects of patriarchal societies.

I find this confirmed by Griffin Hansbury's work on "the transgender edge" in the psychic formations of some of his cis analysands. The libidinal organization of *all* bodies is rooted in a certain displacement of corporeal indeterminacy that I have suggested to call "transsexuality." This is *not* a minority issue. Freud himself faces his own transgender edge in his encounter with Schreber, or so I shall argue. Libidinal organization *for all people* entails the active *creation* of these bodies – be it by means of hormone therapy, regular work outs at the gym, dietary habits, implants, self-destructive behavior, particular sexual practices, or the most phantasmatic of all fantasies: the ideology of the "literal" biological body that we call "cis-gender." Our corporeal indeterminacy functions as engines that actively shape our actual bodies. In this sense, all people transition into their genders – cis, trans, non-binary, and other people alike. Consequentially, one is not born cis, but rather becomes cis. And transsexuality is disavowed enjoyment at the edge of each and every one of us.

A Diabolic Handjob

> The two main elements of Schreber's delusion, the transformation to the woman and the privileged relationship with God are linked in his system by the feminine attitude towards God. It becomes an unavoidable task for us to establish an essential genetic relationship between these two pieces. For otherwise our explanations of Schreber's delusion would assign us the ridiculous role described by Kant in the famous parable of the Critique of Pure Reason as that of the man who holds the sieve while another milks the he-goat.[8]

This is how Freud describes his project in the analysis of Schreber's memoir. The passage in Kant referenced here looks as follows:

> What is truth? [...] It is already a great and necessary proof of prudence or insight to know what one should reasonably ask. For if the question is in itself unrhymeful [*ungereimt*] and demands unnecessary answers, it has, besides embarrassing the person who raises it, sometimes the disadvantage of tempting the imprudent hearer to give unrhymeful [*ungereimte*] answers, and giving the laughable sight of one (as the ancients said) milking the he-goat and the other holding a sieve.[9]

In the following two sections, I read these two quotes. I argue that both Kant and Freud avoid asking tough questions about fundamental features of their respective systems. Kant derails from a problem inherent in the notion of truth, namely that a definition of truth cannot be verified nor falsified other than by dogmatic decree. Freud derails from the principle reversibility of both gender and desire that put basic features of his theoretical edifice and personal identity at risk. Both, gender and truth are inherently *indeterminate,* and as such they are subject to a surplus of desire or pleasure. Schreber experiences that surplus desire, and Freud exiles it into an allegedly absurd scenario of excess and moral depravity (milking the goat, etc.). But today, it backfires.

Kantian Excesses and the Abyss of Truth

Truth, Kant tells us, can only be reached if the question we ask makes sense. If it does not, our reasoning may appear sound but will nevertheless miss the mark. Bullshit questions yield bullshit answers.[10] So far, so uninteresting. What *is* interesting, however, is the image Kant draws for us in the event of asking bullshit questions. The purpose of this image is clearly to dissuade us from asking the wrong questions. It is meant to make the dramatic consequences of bullshitting affectively persuasive to us. Hence, he offers an image of absolute ridicule – and terror.

It is the image of a man "milking the he-goat and the other holding a sieve." Clearly, a male goat does not give milk. But he may well give a similar fluid: sperm. And really, the activity of milking, rubbing up-and-down an organ, is not unlike masturbation. Thus, although we cannot literally milk the he-goat, we may well give him a handjob. Yet there is more to the image: another man is holding a sieve. There are thus three male bodies involved: two humans and one goat. Kant is thus projecting a small gay orgy. Now, if one was to milk a cow one would probably want to catch the milk in some kind of vessel. Yet the Kantian handjob uses a vessel with holes – a sieve. Chances are that semen will go to waste. The goat literally dis-seminates.[11] The idea that unproductive sexuality was unnatural comes right out of the archives of religious morality: every signifier needs its signified and every semen needs its womb, or so bourgeois cis-het-sexuality wants us to think. Now, the two men in this image have sex with a male goat. Besides the zoophilia, the scene also touches on the quintessential Christian fantasy: sex with the devil. For the goat with his horns, hoofs, and hairy legs is a traditional symbol of Satan. With the history of Christian morality in mind, one might think that sex *is* the devil. In any case, the charge of sex with the devil as a form of witchcraft plays a particular role in the submission and oppression of women in Western society in particular. Because one *might* have (had) sex with the devil, female desire in particular could always cause suspicion of infernal influence. In order to avoid this suspicion, you better perform chastity. In this way, the fantasy of sex with the devil and its proximity to witchcraft were often used to discipline female desire.[12]

Back to the truth: according to Kant, those who do not know which question to ask risk having gay sex with the devil. Desire takes over. Libido gone wild drives people to cross all boundaries of morality (homosexuality), the species (zoophilia), and religion (sex with the devil). In other words: responding to wrong questions is too much fun. It is desire let loose, without anchoring in procreation, reproduction, the creation of new things (BABIES).

Kant uses the image of this animalistic handjob to discredit scholastic syllogisms, such as:

All humans are mortal.
Socrates is human.
Socrates is mortal

The argument may be sound – but is it really the case? Kant's worry is that the mere form of the logical progression cannot tell us whether the conclusion is true or not. Compare:

All humans are made of green cheese.
Socrates is human.
Socrates is made of green cheese.

This argument is sound, but it is not true. If you think it is funny, you are on track: the wrong may tickle our enjoyment by virtue of its sheer absurdity. Kant, however, tells us that adhering to the syllogistic form in abstraction from its content causes the namely effect: wrong question (is it formally correct?), wrong answer (Socrates is a cheesy boy). Kant squares this libidinal effect of wrongness, its humor, with sexual desire gone wild. Once we cross the boundaries of truth, he seems to say, we are overwhelmed by desire and will end up way off track – in a gay threesome with the devil, for example. Maybe the image transgresses its textual situatedness and makes you laugh or smile or frown. Kant at least indicates that the image should give off a "laughable sight." It should cause a physical response in its reader – in this case: you.[13] Consequentially, the passage is supposed to enact the libidinal surplus it simultaneously prohibits: cracking a joke about libidinal excess, Kant in turn intents to produce the namely excess, causing an affective reaction that we are simultaneously asked to discipline. The argumentative force of Kant's call for an analysis of truth procedures is thus anchored in an immediate, affective understanding: "sex with the devil... yeah that would be bad..." At the far end of the metaphor, it is witchcraft (sex with the devil) serving as the specter of an allegedly bad, desire-driven thinking – a figuration of "immaturity" (*Unmündigkeit*) as Kant calls it in his famous essay on Enlightenment.[14]

On the other side of the equation, Kant will present his own transcendental method. In this method, we already know at least some true judgments and we use them to reflect on their conditions of possibility so as to build a model of epistemological adequacy. Thus, for Kant, our mathematical judgments are undeniably true. Hence, we can use them to work our way up to the necessary presuppositions of rational thinking. We already know some truths – we just need to reflect on them and build a model. Likewise, we know what we do not want: unproductive, gay sex with an animal-devil. In this way, Kant brings his point across in an affective manner: we know which questions to ask and which not to ask. Procreative truth procedures = good. Excessive libidinal dis-semination = bad.

But what is wrong with fun and flimsy arguments? Sure, they are wrong – but the slippery slope to complete moral disintegration seems far-fetched. Yet the exaggeration has a purpose. Kant installs it here to deflect from a real philosophical problem: truth cannot have a concept. The problem is that once we ask the question, "What is Truth?", there is no real way to answer it. For once asked, there is no possible pre-established truth procedure that could back up any possible answer. Either we have already decided what truth is or we do not yet know what truth is. If we ask the question with a response in mind, then our question was mere rhetoric to begin with – it is not a real question and, hence, will not yield a real investigation nor a real answer. Inversely, if we commence our inquiry without any understanding of "truth" in mind, there is no guide, no template for a possible answer. For how would we know what kind of answer adequately responds to this question without a notion of truth that would back up that judgment? As long as we do not know what truth is, no answer to the question will stand any possible scrutiny. And once we know what truth is, we cannot seriously ask the question anymore. The question, "What is Truth?", hence, comes with a peculiar indeterminacy, a real undecidability. It sure is a relevant question. But every possible answer must reduce the question to some area of application, make a somewhat arbitrary decision. Truth, adequately understood, remains inherently problematic. The crucial question, "What is Truth?", cannot possibly produce a verifiable answer. The concept "truth" must thus remain indeterminate of sorts. Yet it cannot remain completely indeterminate either. For in order to understand my argument about the indeterminacy of truth, we need a brought agreement about certain features of truth already. If that was not the case, my argument might as well be mere gibberish, poetic writing, mental acrobatics. Yet once we try to spell out what those agreements are, they would have to be checked against a notion of truth which we do not yet have. Thus, *there is* truth. Yet it dissolves (disseminates?) into indeterminacy once we try to tackle the issue head on. It is as though there was a strange disorientation living at the heart of this basic concept: as long as we have some concept of 'truth' to back up our statements, we are fine. But as soon as we investigate the concept directly, it inevitably escapes us *while simultaneously* presupposing itself. Truth is strange – like the horizon: we can see that it is there. But once we move towards it, it recedes.

What to do? Kant chooses violence: he proclaims a witch hunt on the question, links the amazement of the question's indeterminacy to libidinal involvement with evil, and interpellates us to engage our intuitive knowledge of what is right (such as mathematics) and what is wrong (such as gay sex with animals). Thus, at the origin of Kantian reflection on the conditions of possibility of thought, we find deflection from the abyss of truth and its real metaphysical indeterminacy.

Freudian Entropy and the Indeterminacy of Gender

Let us return to Freud, who uses the same image in a different context. Here, the overwhelming, unproductive homo-handjob marks the limit of our engagement with Schreber. More particularly: God wants to transform Schreber into a woman, says Schreber. This happens by virtue of nerves that give off particularly feminine sensations of lust. The nerves were installed in Schreber's body by external forces.[15] Schreber is thus on the receiving, perceptive end of pleasure. One might think that Schreber was a trans woman whose emancipated body image (I am [becoming] a woman!) has a vitalizing, exciting and libidinally stimulating effect. In other words: Schreber has gender euphoria.[16]

But this is not Freud's interpretation. In fact, to Freud, the connection between the divine feminizing intervention into Schreber's body and Schreber's own feminine affects require us to provide an explanation of their "genetic relationship."[17] Freud thus inscribes the necessity for a *reproductive* connection ("genetic") between the two most prominent aspects of Schreber's delusion: feminizing divine intervention and the experience of feminine desire. In a sense, one of them must be the BABY of the other ("genetic"). *Lest* we end up back in Kantian excess desire, involving hand jobs, animals, wasted semen (dissemination), and allusions to Satanic practices – of which we get a taste in the "ridiculous" image and its physiological counterpart in our own reaction to it. The relation to unhinged libidinal excess is of particular interest in this context because it matches Schreber's own experience: the feminine nerves implanted by divine intervention do in fact produce whole body pleasure and inspire Schreber to become a connoisseur of the practices of lust and desire – whereas before the divine intervention, Schreber's sexuality had been a rather mellow affair. If we do not find the BABY in Schreber's pleasure palace, we effectively side with Schreber's delusion – says Freud. Note that by quoting the Kantian scenario of excessive desire, Freud also proclaims that he himself has skin in the game, "For otherwise *our explanations* [meaning: Freud's explanations] […] would assign *us* the ridiculous role described by Kant […] as that of the man who holds the sieve […]."[18]

If we side with Schreber, *we ourselves* join in on the Satanic threesome. Now, the "we" in this case is, or at least entails, Freud himself. Consequentially, what is at issue in Freud's treatment of Schreber is Freud's own sanity. Apparently, then, Freud feels somehow challenged by Schreber's memoir – so much so that he must write an imposing treatise, hinging on a "genetic relationship." Elsewhere, I called this "the toxic logic of protection":[19] the protector protects himself at the expense of oppressing the protected. In this case, provoked by his own transference, Freud must protect Schreber from excessive delusions, even at a distance (they never meet). Yet the reason for such disciplining "protection" is that Freud must suppress his own excess desire, "For otherwise *our explanations* [meaning: Freud's explanations] […] would assign *us* the ridiculous role described by Kant […]"[20] as that of the man who goes overboard with his desire. Freud casts the libidinal surplus (excess desire) into a denigrating Satanic handjob. He also attributes the whole affair to Kant, as if Freud wanted to distance himself from that excess desire even further.

Note that the Kantian handjob that Freud cites is opposed to Schreber's account in one important aspect. The Kantian picture is a gay threesome, which features Freud holding a sieve and Schreber giving a handjob. Curiously, the metaphor that Freud picks for his project exiles the central feature of Schreber's experience: femininity. This avoidance of femininity remains characteristic of Freud's interpretation as a whole. "I am not responsible for the monotony of the psychoanalytic solution,"[21] he proclaims while mapping the Schreberian pathologies onto an alleged desire for physical proximity to his father and, consecutively, repressed homosexuality. Hence, against Schreber's explicit and repeated claims, Freud does not even engage the hypothesis that Schreber might have gender trouble. Gender is solid, no questions asked – at least for Freud. Instead, he installs a father in Schreber's psyche in order to establish a "genetic relation" between divine intervention into Schreber's body and the feminine experience of Schreber's body. That genetic relation, the procreative relation between these two aspects, is supposed to be anchored in Schreber's father. Against Schreber's explicit statement, there is thus, in the Freudian narrative, no space for gender euphoria, no genuine Schreberian femininity nor a desire for it, no relishing in the experience of one's own feminized physicality. There is only sublimated desire for the father.[22] It is either the father, Freud seems to say, or a hotbed of sin, zoophilic handjobs, and disseminated, wasted sperm.

Why does Freud feel challenged by Schreber – so much so that he must drown out Schreber's experience as best he can? Here, the analogy with Kant comes full circle. In the *Critique of Pure Reason*, the namely passage deflects from the metaphysical indeterminacy of truth, hence, omitting a basic problem of the Kantian edifice. Freud, however, deflects from the indeterminacy of gender (*Geschlecht*) which designates a similar spot in his oeuvre as does truth to the Kantian project.

Gender as Libidinal Intelligibility

Schreber insists on the indeterminacy of gender:

> As is well known, in the first months of pregnancy, both sexes are created, and the peculiarities of the sex that does not reach development *remain* like the male nipples as rudimentary organs at a lower stage of development.[23]

The human body during gestation has an indeterminate gender – it may pan out in this or that direction. And that indeterminacy lays dormant in the adult body as the un-developed characteristics "remain ... rudimentary."[24] There is thus a trace of indeterminate gender in any adult body. And that trace allows for a path in the other direction:

> [T]he (external) male sexual organs (scrotum and male member) were retracted into the body and, at the same time the internal sexual organs were transformed into the corresponding female sexual organs. This may have taken place through a sleep of several hundred years, since a change in the bone structure (pelvis etc.) had to occur as well. There was therefore a regression or a reversal of the developmental process that takes place in every human embryo in the fourth or fifth month of pregnancy, depending on months of pregnancy, depending on whether nature gave the prospective child the male or the female sex.[25]

Technically speaking, this is not very far from contemporary gender affirming bottom surgeries, during which the penis is literally *invaginated*, namely inversed and moved into the body. When Schreber writes this passage in 1902/1903, there is no surgical procedure of this kind.[26] Consequentially, Schreber ascribes the procedure to divine intervention and hundreds of years of sleep. But nevertheless, Schreber's imagination captures the technique pretty astutely. And his basic point is anyway true: the gender of the human body is indeterminate, both psychologically (as pointed out earlier) and physiologically (as described just now).

Now, Freud himself famously points out in his *Three Essays on the Theory of Sexuality* that the infant's body is libidinally disorganized or "polymorphously perverse."[27] And there is a physiological component to this. Think of a baby elephant: even though they may *have* a trunk, they nevertheless do not know how to use it at birth and may in fact use it in various ways, with pleasure sometimes occurring and sometimes not. The same counts for the human body: upon birth, the *organization* of the body is not finished – how to use it, where desire is located, and how the infant relates to its environment are skills that are to be acquired. How does organization happen? By virtue of, for example, cultural prohibitions and social expectations.[28] Violent incursions and enticing seductions determine the sphere of possible expressions of infantile existence.[29] Joy, rejection, ignorance and encouragement from objects of love/desire/attachment (parents, caregivers, siblings, friends) are incredibly important in sculpting the young psyche in all respects, including gender. Adorno and Horkheimer describe the process analogically with the image of the feelers of a snail:

> Meeting an obstacle, the feeler [of the snail] is immediately withdrawn into the protection of the body, it becomes one with the whole until it timidly ventures forth as an autonomous agent. If the danger is still present, it disappears once more, and the intervals between the attempts grow longer. Mental life in its earliest stages is infinitely delicate. The snail's sense is dependent on a muscle, and muscles grow slack if their scope for movement is impaired. The body is crippled by physical injury, the mind by fear. In their origin both effects are inseparable.[30]

And inversely, if enticed and encouraged, the feeler may well move in particular directions and leave others behind. Thus, infant children are mostly libidinally amorphous, disorganized, indeterminate. Disciplining desire, however, is a process of embodiment – and of gender.

My suggestion is that gender is libidinal intelligibility. People want us to behave in this or that way. We may or may not like it. Yet in that assessment ("don't treat me that way!"), we conceive of ourselves *through* and in relation to the desires of others. Here then, we encounter ourselves through our libidinal intelligibility, the way others implicate us into their desires – and the ways in which we desire to be desired. Likewise, in self-reflection, be it mentally or through a mirror or images, we encounter ourselves *as* an other. That is to say, we encounter ourselves as an object of desire for what we want for ourselves. Here, we become libidinally intelligible to ourselves, including the necessary illegibilities.

Gender as libidinal intelligibility is hyper-stratified, plastic, and multi-dimensional. It has many shapes and forms. It functions as the message in a subtle system of omissions and allusions called "gender," understood as a poetic dance in the grammar of social reality. There is no expression of gender. Gender itself is that expression. From femme to daddy, from undercover brother through dapper girl to antifa enby to ace to doll and back, genders are often vernacular (meaning: locally specific) and directed at a particular audience. For the desires of people around me matter most to me, whether they would like me to be their friend or their lover or dead, etc. So, I inevitably adjust. Depending on who is looking, a gender says: "Hey you! Love me / fuck me / stay off me / ignore me / etc." And depending on where you are at, your gender may disseminate differently. Thus, Berlin Neukölln requires a sporty feminine simplicity that would never fly in downtown Manhattan. In any case, gender as libidinal intelligibility is in no way limited to or mappable onto a spectrum called "male/female." If you think it should not be called "gender" – I agree. It is libidinal intelligibility as an aspect of social intelligibility. Yet I will stick to the traditional term "gender" in order to preserve readability and textual flow.

Sexual orientations, among others, constantly blur into gender. For gender is a dimension of a more general social intelligibility, which is not primarily mediated through desire. It incorporates other aspects of social intelligibility, such as race, class, ability, sexual orientation, etc. In many ways, the distinctions between (!) sexual orientation, race, class, gender, and other categories are artificial devices, made to communicate our grievances to *the law*, the master, the authorities.[31] Yet we are friends, lovers, adversaries, and nemeses to each other, not judges and authorities.

Genders, however, have both libidinal reality (they reflect desires) and social reality (they function according to the vernacular grammars in place). Yet combinations and creative aberrations abound. Reality produces the desire to transgress as much as it produces the desire to submit. Gender as libidinal intelligibility depends on external factors as much as it depends on local particularities of the particular desires of particular people in particular contexts.

Gender, then, is first and foremost *intelligibility to the desire of an other*. Gender is a way in which we are known to each other's wanting, interest, lust, etc., (understood not necessarily in a sexual way, although sexuality plays a particular role here). Gender is *libidinal intelligibility*. This includes intelligibility to our own desire *as* someone else, perceiving ourselves *through* the others, *through* a mirror, *through* writing and re-writing ourselves. Consequentially, genders, just as truth, are inherently indeterminate. Cultural, social, and parental factors can establish a libidinal *paradigm* (such as heterosexuality). They can establish the "normal" or "originary." They cannot, however, determine the possible relations of a given libidinal constellation (a person, an infant, a couple, a group) towards that paradigm.

In relation to a paradigm, submission, subversion, denial, resistance, and more are in the cards. One may always desire to act or to be otherwise. One may always desire a different social position, always desire to be desired otherwise – and act accordingly. Genders continually manifest in ways that entail the potential for their own transgression. Schreber insists on that: gender is indeterminate and that indeterminacy can be pleasurable. We can enjoy the desire to be otherwise – the desire to transition.

Why Schreber Freaks Freud Out

What is Freud's deal with Schreber? Schreber is too close to home. As Daniel Boyarin points out, in the early 1900s, Freud is grappling with his own femininity in at least two ways: one is the alleged femininity of Jewish men in the anti-Semitic imaginary of *fin-de-siècle* Germany. The other is Freud's self-diagnosed hysteria, which goes along with desires for femininity or feminine desires, sometimes coded into homosexuality. Both, however, are linked.

Along these lines, Boyarin argues "[...] Freud [...] initial[ly] [engaged a] self-construction as homoerotic, as feminized [hence passive, receptive]."[32] I agree. Freud variously imagines himself as female or feminized. "In his 12 June 1895 letter to Fliess, Freud states that 'Reporting on [the psychological construction of defense] now would be like sending a six-month fetus of a girl to a ball.'"[33] Freud, in other words, is pregnant. In 1897, he writes accordingly that "after the frightful labor pains of the last few weeks, I gave birth to a new piece of knowledge."[34] On other occasions he fantasizes about his own menstruation,[35] or tells Fliess that he will "bring nothing but two open ears and one temporal lobe lubricated for reception."[36] Accordingly, Garner argues, that Freud seems to imagine his relationship to Fliess in particular as primarily passive/feminine, including in the *Interpretation of Dreams.*[37] Freud was also a self-diagnosed hysteric. Thus, on October 3, 1897, he envisions "resolving my own hysteria."[38] This would cast him as female and tendentially queer/gay in the eyes of his contemporaries.[39]

Boyarin continues, "But as Jewish difference became configurable not only as feminine but also as queer, and as queer solidified into an identity toward the end of the century, Freud would have been even more at pains to deny and repress anything that would seem to cast him as queer Jew."[40] Indeed, modern anti-Semitism is intricately linked to ideas about Jewish "difference" as inherently gendered.[41] Jewish masculinity in particular became associated with femininity in the European 19th century, often crystallized in linking circumcision to castration and hence effeminization. It is true that this alleged effeminacy of Jewish men in particular was then linked to homosexuality.[42]

Jewishness was thus increasingly pathologized. Boyarin argues that Freud eventually "panicked,"[43] faced with this melange of pathologizing homophobia and anti-Semitism juxtaposed with his own self-feminizing ideation. The result was, according to Boyarin, the Oedipal model of psychoanalysis: male children desire their mothers and develop hostilities toward their fathers. According to Freud, much of the later identity formation follows from this. Boyarin points out that the Oedipus complex is inherently heteronormative and hence (in his interpretation) exiles Freud's own latent homosexual leanings. But, I want to add, it also hard wires gender: by the time the child gets Oedipalized, its gender is already clear. It is not *by* the desire for the mother that the child becomes male. Rather, the child is already male. That is not to say that Boyarin was wrong. But it is to say that there is another layer to Freud's conversion to the Oedipal model: the stabilization of cis gender.

My simple point is that we should read the feminization of both homosexuality and Jewishness in European *fin-de-siècle* cultures in relation to an entirely normalized trans misogyny. Given Freud's own feminine leadings, it makes sense that he would want to stabilize cis gender in his invention of the Oedipus complex. Schreber's insistence on her femininity and her positive desire to transition echoes Freud's own desire of the same kind. In other words, there is a trans feminine dimension to Freud's own personality that had to be squashed in his analysis of Schreber. In an act of toxic protection, Freud pretends to protect Schreber from excessive delusions. But really, he mostly puts his own trans femininity to rest.[44] "All psychoanalytic theory was born from hysteria, but the mother died during the birth."[45] That mother was transgender Freud. She died of suicide. The tombstone declares: *Oedipus Rex*. But we can hear an echo of Freud's own trans feminine leanings in his fantasy of Schreber's Satanic handjob: it is really Freud's own trans desire, delegated to Schreber, mediated through Kant, screaming from the edge of repression.

It is the World that is Making Us Sick

Freud bends over backwards, even decrying the monotony of his own interpretative enterprise,[46] in order to omit the obvious: Schreber is [becoming] a woman. Gender is inherently indeterminate. Freud and his contemporaries find Schreber to be delusional. Yet, as I intend to show in this section, it is the world that is making her sick – a world that she is nevertheless taking pains to become intelligible towards.[47]

In today's terms, Schreber would probably reside somewhere on the trans spectrum. She is taking pains to justify her trans experience in ways that may be somehow (libidinally) intelligible to her environment. In fact, the first part of her autobiography is a philosophical treatise on the relation between God and the world. Here, Schreber commences from a distinction between immaterial souls and material bodies, where the term "nerves" sometimes designates the immaterial soul. At the time, this is less unintuitive than it may seem: famous philosophers such as Aristotle and Descartes, but also later vitalists, used the term "soul" partially in a physiological sense, describing the moving force inside both human and animal bodies.[48] Thus, we may interpret the Schreberian "nerves" in analogy to Freudian drives, the force of life or real causation itself. However, "God is [...] only nerve without body and thus akin to the human soul."[49] God is immaterial, just as the human soul is. Yet in contrast to humans, God has infinitely many nerves *aka* immaterial souls.

The basic plot of Schreber's memoir is as follows: God (pure immaterial soul) sometimes interacts with other material or immaterial things (human or non-human). Such interactions are called "rays" or "beams" (*Strahlen*). For reasons that Schreber speculates on but remains unclear about, someone (maybe her psychiatrist Flechsig, maybe God) tried to steal Schreber's soul. This attack caused Schreber to experience intensified nerve activity. God and other souls seem to be attracted by such intensified activity. Schreber's soul thus develops a magnetic force. That force threatens to swallow the whole world, including God. In order to reverse this process, another world must be born – and Schreber must do the job. For this purpose, Schreber must first become "the eternal Jew"[50] and be transformed into a woman. The combination of Jewishness and femininity has a long history in anti-Jewish narratives: Jewish men in particular have often been thought to be supposedly unmanly, hence, also not to be trusted. Boyarin notes accordingly: "European cultures represented male Jews as 'female'; […]."[51] Consequentially, there is a material connection between the histories of anti-Semitism and transmisogyny in particular, which we already touched on: 19th century Jewish masculinity had a trans-feminine flavor at least.[52] Consequentially, Schreber desires what Freud wants to escape: Jewish trans femininity.

However, the German man Schreber must transform into a Jewish woman in order to save the world. Apparently, God wants that transformation, which already manifests in Schreber's body as intensified pleasure. An early dream has Schreber enjoy the fantasy of being a sexually active woman.[53] And a particular psychotic break, if one may say so, setting in motion much of the initial drama of the memoirs, happens during a night marked by at least six orgasms.[54] In fact, Schreber envisions the blessedness of the immaterial souls (beyond physical existence) as the pleasure of continuous voluptuous desire.[55] Yet Schreber's transition is inhibited by the psychiatrist Flechsig and other external forces.[56] The reasons for this inhibition are complex. Yet the general picture should be clear.

An Inevitable Transition

Schreber experiences gender euphoria, the joy of self-recognition in the preferred gender.[57] She describes the link between her femininity and her (sexual) pleasure numerous times – and towards the end, the book contains a description of Schreber admiring herself in the mirror, topless with jewelry.[58] Schreber herself points out that she met the initial dream that consisted of her enjoying sexual intercourse as a woman with a very strong resistance: "This idea was so foreign to my whole sensibility; if conscious, I would have rejected it with such indignation that, after what I have since come to know, I cannot entirely dismiss the possibility that there were some external influences which gave me this idea."[59] Schreber's resistance against her own desire is so strong that she later comes to project the source of that desire onto an external force, which she will eventually come to identify as God.[60] In this initial dream, then, Schreber desires to be intelligible as a woman, to be treated like a woman during physical intimacy.[61] In this fantasy, the desire of someone else (a sexual partner) is directed towards Schreber *as* a woman – and that is what makes her a woman. Her gender is exactly her libidinal intelligibility.

Now, suppose that Schreber's desire to be desired as a woman (the desire to be a woman) was *very, very strong*. Yet the social inhibition, the culturally instituted obstacles against that desire in late 19th century Germany are not only insurmountable but also very much internalized into an image of male courage and honor within Schreber's own mental apparatus.[62] Consequentially, the desire must be exiled. Freud exiles his own trans desire to Schreber. Yet Schreber's own desire to be a woman is still stronger. "In any case, the soul-lust had become so strong that I felt the impression of a female body first on the arm and on my hands, later on my legs, my breasts, my buttocks, and all other parts of the body."[63] It does not seem very far-fetched that this struggle between an infinite force (Schreber's desire to be a woman) and an immovable object (the conservative social and cultural world of late 19th century German) simply drives her nuts. In order to find a balance between her desire and the social world around her, Schreber develops an elaborate system that eventually sanctions her gender euphoria. She says as much explicitly: "[N]either on the part of God's side, nor on my side, can there be any question of moral culpability."[64] The reason is that moral culpability only applies where the world is in order. But the intensified magnetic force of Schreber's nerves has kicked the world out of joint – hence all moral culpability remains suspended until the cosmic imbalance or queerness is fixed.[65] Consequentially, Schreber's femininity has found an outlet of epic proportions: her gender euphoria is OK because morality itself is out of balance. Furthermore, Schreber finally declares that she started embracing her desire to become a woman based on rational reflection (*Vernunftgründe*) in response to the repeated divine calling for her gender transition:[66] *resistance is futile, you will be transmogrified!* Or so the world seems to tell her. If reason is insight into necessity, Schreber is perfectly rational: she wants to be libidinally intelligible as a woman. Her desire articulates as an unchangeable necessity. This is the reality of her existence. Yet the world is not cut out for such recognition. As we learn from Freud, a gender transition is basically equivalent to Satanic sex, witchcraft, and zoophilia, hence the end of civilization as we know it. Schreber agrees: she experiences her desire to transition as the end of the whole world. And yet the desire persists against all odds. And where desire is not matched by a responsive world, the forces of desire will manifest regardless, often in destructive ways. Schreber spends years in psychiatric treatment, where she essentially experiences torture and regular abuse.[67] Now, as then, the lesson is the same: there is no external force that will break the will to transition. Rather than give up on her gender euphoria, Schreber sustains various suicide attempts.[68]

Putting her intellectual capacities to task is the only way to go. It is a ruthless forward defense with the means of science, philosophy, and empirical research. In fact, her *Memoirs* entail a whole metaphysics and a detailed phenomenological study of the pains of suppressed gender dysphoria in a situation of complete epistemic violence:[69] Schreber has no conceptual tools, no medical institution to turn to, no conceptual resources to draw from. The cis gender world has absolutely alienated her from her own experience. As a 19th century trans woman, Schreber is socially, epistemologically, and libidinally stillborn: there are no resources for her to express her social position, her desire, or her thoughts at all. She finds herself at a complete trans political dead end. Yet, in an act of extreme creative resistance, she generates a whole conceptual framework out of thin air, grabbing onto whatever resources she has at her disposal. She writes a book that has a single purpose: to make Schreber intelligible as a woman in the eyes of her contemporaries.[70] By doing so, her intellect and her desire are first opposed. But later on, they merge as rational insight into the necessity of her own transition. Consequentially, developed Schreberian reason, other than Kantian reason (see above), concurs with desire. And instead of merely reproducing reality (as Kant wants reason to do), Schreberian reason *generates* reality, generates a gender for herself, and, in turn, provides a key document for the understanding of psychosis and – from now on, maybe – gender. Of course, Schreber's ethical scream can only be heard as madness. *But it is being heard.* And it is inscribed into the archives of Western history as all that it can be inscribed as: a radical distortion of the resources at Schreber's disposal, a devastated call for a heterogenous world, a fundamentally and absolutely different social order in which Schreber could exist.[71]

The Transsexual Paradigm

To sum up: I read Schreber's memoir as a desperate attempt to be libidinally intelligible as a woman to an environment that simply does not have any model to understand what is going on. It is important to note, however, that Schreber's autobiography was written well before Hirschfeld coined the terms "transvestite" and "transsexual" and about 25 years before the first gender affirming surgeries at the Hirschfeld institute in Berlin. There was thus no possible way for Schreber to transition with the help of medical intervention. Schreber nevertheless explains the transition with reference to *physical* alteration: her nerves, her limbs, her genitals have been transformed or are in a process of transformation, her sensation is feminized, and God will, she says, eventually transform her physical appearance as well.

Schreber exists on the margins of what I call "the transsexual paradigm." I understand transsexuality to be the paradigmatic Western form of gender diversity. Within that paradigm, gender diversity is commonly understood as involving body modifications under the auspices of medical institutions. The medical paradigm of transsexuality remains inscribed like a photo negative into both the academic explorations of 21st century gender diversity and into the lived experience thereof. Both right-wing anxieties over surgeries on children and the need of many queer and trans people to distance themselves from the medical paradigm show that the medical paradigm is still going strong.[72] That is to say: gender diversity in Western societies is crucially understood as gender deviance in relation to, difference from, resistance to transsexuality.

The term "transsexuality" has been widely criticized for its medical history and the pathologization inherent in it.[73] Thus, Julia Serano rightly points out that reducing transsexuality to medical procedures objectifies the persons described, ignoring, among others, the social, psychological, libidinal layers involved. Such reduction also installs a classist veneer into the term, because medical procedures are not affordable or otherwise accessible to all.[74] Furthermore, thinking gender diversity through the paradigm of transsexuality seems to ignore non-Western models of gender diversity, deviance, and non-alignment which may well work in a completely different manner.[75]

I agree with these criticisms. Yet the current political climate in Western countries seems to be obsessed exactly with gender-related alterations of the human body, including its allegedly pathological nature and the alleged protection of "the children." I thus think it worthwhile to stop avoiding the term and start appropriating it instead. This appropriation has to do with the inherent cis-centric bias that marks "transsexuality" as a paradigm.[76] For more often than not, a cis body is taken as the measure to which a trans body is expected to conform. That is to say, it is generally assumed that a gender transition is intended to make you look or be "like" a *cis* man/woman.

It is in the context of this fantasy that some imagine transsexuality to be a threat. In this sense, little seems to have changed since 1979, when Janice Raymond wrote the infamous "transsexual empire," where trans femininity is an attack on (cis) feminine corporeality, spirituality, and sexuality themselves and not just on this or that aspect of this or that person.[77] This fantasy, which has affinities to Nazi ideology,[78] seems to motivate at least some, if not much of today's anxieties over so called "gender ideology" as well.[79] Thus, since the mid 2010s, church officials and right-wing politicians have increasingly pointed to "gender ideology" as a lethal threat to "the children" (heterosexual cis children I assume), "the family" (as it was re-invented mid 20th century), and everything that is allegedly good and worth protecting.[80] This fantasy of a threatening "gender ideology" is now a transnational phenomenon.[81] And transsexuality with its link to body modification is crucial to this right-wing demonology.[82] I thus worry that it is pointless just to repeat incessantly that not all trans people fit into the paradigm of transsexuality, that gender diversity is not a new phenomenon, and that trans people are not a threat but rather in need of protection.[83] These strategies cannot reach the demonization we see emerging as a transnational phenomenon.

In this context, it seems imperative to me to re-appropriate the term "transsexuality" rather than leaving it to the proclaimed enemies of so called "gender ideology." One step in this direction is to understand "transsexuality" not as a more or less adequate description of individual persons (hence, not as an identity) but as a paradigm, an inevitable point that friends and foes must relate to. Note, however, that beyond transsexuality as a social paradigm, there is no one thing that trans or transsexuality mean in any context and no-one can possibly determine its meanings without performing an exclusion that transsexuality inherently contests.

Yet the transsexual paradigm is the reason why "trans" and related terms are inherently fuzzy. They often function as the outside of the allegedly normalized, determinate embodiment of gender, aka "cis."[84] Recent studies show that the medical history of "trans" is complex and often contradictory.[85] And consequentially, it is often close to impossible to determine where the line between trans and cis and other related terms is situated. This relative indeterminacy, however, is not a result of bad reasoning, it is a symptom of a dysfunctional paradigm: the transsexual paradigm does not allow clear designations regarding who does or who does not belong into this or that set of people (trans, cis, transsexual, non-binary, transgender, themboy, afab, enby, etc., etc.). The reason is that the purpose of the paradigm is to *generate cis people* and *not* to generate coherent categories for non-cis people to live in. Consequentially, the paradigm is inherently fuzzy and allows for a plethora of people to attach themselves to it for a multiplicity of, at times, idiosyncratic reasons. Consequentially, and for the purpose of this chapter, I understand "trans" to mean gender diversity in the wake of the social paradigm called "transsexuality" (as explained above). That is to say, many people plug into the transsexual paradigm for various reasons. There are many transitions that cannot easily be absorbed into the paradigm of medicalized transitioning, be it because the transition happens without medical support, because the desired effects do not align with a certain model of gender, or simply because the transitioning person disidentifies from the paradigm of transsexuality – or all of the above or for other reasons altogether.

Yet in the case of Schreber, we can see what happens if there is no paradigm in place that can ensure some kind of social intelligibility: an incredible amount of force is required to generate the epistemic resources to provide *some* intelligibility (Schreber spends years in psychiatric confinement, spends years writing the *Memoirs,* and prints them on her own budget). And still, what transpires is just a crazy person. We can only imagine how many Schrebers did not manage to synthesize their experiences into anything intelligible, did not have the financial or intellectual resources to try and intervene into their social environment, and, hence, drowned in (epistemic) violence and cultural oblivion.

Transsexuality, then, is a bad paradigm. Yet it remains the vortex that provides much of the gravitational pull of contemporary gender politics. Instead of resisting this pull, we should use it in our favor, a wave that we ride, the wind in our sails. But do not walk around calling people "transsexual" while citing this text as a reference. My point concerns paradigms, not individual people.

In this paradigmatic way, Schreber must be read as a manifestation of the transsexual paradigm *avant la lettre,* before the term "transsexual" was invented and well before gender affirming surgeries had even been conceived, let alone successfully applied. Schreber's transition takes place within the confines of physical transformation in its relation to a medical framework (the psychiatry), yet without being intelligible as such. I already pointed out that Schreber finds herself in a situation of political, epistemic, and libidinal stillbirth: there was never a chance for her to genuinely understand herself, to act or to connect to others that may or may not be like her. In this sense, the transsexual paradigm comes with a kind of epistemic violence.

Gayatri Chakravorty Spivak makes a similar point regarding imperial epistemic violence:[86] she speaks of the violence of imperial narratives and institutions, of colonial eradication of pre-colonial life. In the colony, Spivak holds, resources for an understanding of oneself and of the world are always distorted by and towards the colonial force. The colonial framework frames everything, including the resistance against it and the self-understanding of the colonized. Distortion is originary, not derivative. This is the situation Spivak describes as "epistemic violence": all resources for an understanding of anything whatsoever point against the epistemically violated subject. Even the tools used for emancipation are inevitably harmful to the person or group using them. In this situation, Spivak says, displacement and distortion are all there is. All we can do is twist the dominant narrative. Truth is not an option. This is the exact situation that Schreber finds herself in – and it is still the situation of trans, inter, and non-binary people today. All epistemic resources that Western discourses have to offer are mediated through, sanctioned by, or responses to the transsexual paradigm, a medical discourse that has replaced all previous forms of trans, inter and non-binary meaning making.[87] Consequentially, Schreber uses the tools of philosophy, of empirical science, of phenomenological research, and of auto-fiction in order to become intelligible as the woman she anyway is. And clearly, her contemporaries can read this appropriation of violence only as distortion, as madness. Schreber herself, we could say, does not speak.[88] But she does her best to become a maximally distorted echo of the epistemic violence that shaped her – an appropriation of the transsexual paradigm.

Paradigmatic Transsexuality

Why should we read "about" Schreber today? Even if I am right and she was a trans woman *avant la lettre*, is this any more than a sad case of past brutalities against unhappy minorities? I do think so: Schreber may function as the model case for becoming gendered, for transitioning into *any* gender, be it trans, cis, non-binary, or something else.

Corporeal Indeterminacy

Leaving Schreber behind for the moment, I want to turn to *the* canonical work of queer theory: Judith Butler's *Gender Trouble*.[89] Strangely enough, right in the middle of the book, and unbeknownst to its various commentators, Butler provides an on-point description of gender transitions that can function as a model for a general theory of gender transitions (into cis, trans, non-binary, or other genders) beyond performativity. Even Jay Prosser, in his seminal analysis of *Gender Trouble* from a trans perspective in his *Second Skins,* takes it for granted that "the embodied transgendered subject does not occupy Gender Trouble in any substantial way […]."[90] And Viviane Namaste rightly criticizes Butler's mobilization of drag performances as an example of the citationality of gender in the third chapter of *Gender Trouble* as follows:

> The drag queens Butler discusses perform in spaces created and defined by gay male culture. Although Butler locates these spaces in relation to heterosexual

hegemony, she refuses to examine this territory's own complicated relations to gender and gender performance.[91]

It thus looks as though *Gender Trouble*, rather than cherishing trans lives, was *omitting them* in favor of cisgender performativity and a serious reductionism regarding the actual conditions under which mostly precarious people present their art.[92] It looks as though Butler was merely *appropriating* trans identities to make a point, effectively side-lining trans people along the way.[93]

And yet, I beg to differ. Here is the passage:

> Transsexuals often claim a radical discontinuity between sexual pleasures and bodily parts. Very often what is wanted in terms of pleasure requires an imaginary participation in body parts, either appendages or orifices, that one might not actually possess, or, similarly, pleasure may require imagining an exaggerated or diminished set of parts. The imaginary status of desire, of course, is not restricted to the transsexual identity; the phantasmatic nature of desire reveals the body not as its ground or cause, but as its *occasion* and its *object*. The strategy of desire is in part the transfiguration of the desiring body itself. Indeed, in order to desire at all it may be necessary to believe in an altered bodily ego which, within the gendered rules of the imaginary, might fit the requirements of a body capable of desire. This imaginary condition of desire always exceeds the physical body through or on which it works.[94]

It is easy to see that the focus on transsexuality as a mismatch between sexuality and body parts and the reduction of those body parts to "either appendages or orifices" introduces essentially *medical* binaries that are not only wrong, but, moreover, not necessarily common among trans people. Emma Heaney, for example, writes:

> [M]any trans feminine people experience a relation between their sex and their bodies that violates both the cis understanding of sex and the diagnostic narrative of trans femininity. There is a long historical archive that demonstrates examples of female identity that do not hinge on assigned sex or the possibility of sex change."[95]

In other words, Butler's image of transsexuality in this passage is cisgendered.

Nevertheless, the gist of the passages is remarkable: Butler's transsexual manages to transpose libidinal import onto non-existing organs. This transposition then functions as the motivation for "the transfiguration of the desiring body itself."[96] Note the crucial twist: the desiring body becomes *an effect of desire* and not its mere origin. This matches our analysis of Schreber: it is the desire for libidinal intelligibility as a woman that drives her gender euphoria and, hence, the physiological transition. Butler's point here, however, is of *general* nature and the transsexual is a paradigmatic case. "The strategy of desire is in part the transfiguration of the desiring body itself."[97] All desire (cis, trans, non-binary, and other alike), Butler tells us, is *in part* transsexual desire in that it shapes its own body.[98] Schreber is not an exception – she articulates the rule in an especially crisp manner. I will now go on to demonstrate that and how this transsexual "part" is in fact the beating heart of gendered embodiment itself.

Systematically, Butler's theory dovetails with Giles Deleuze's *indeterminacy of desire,* developed in *Difference and Repetition:*

> No one has ever walked endogenously. On the one hand, the child goes beyond the bound excitations towards the supposition or the intentionality of an object, such as the mother, as the goal of an effort, the end to be actively reached 'in realit' and in relation to which success and failure may be measured. But on the other hand and at the same time, the child constructs for itself another object, a quite different kind of object which is a indeterminate object or centre and which then governs and compensates for the progresses and failures of its real activity: it puts several fingers in its mouth, wraps the other arm around this in-determinate centre, and appraises the whole situation from the point of view of this indeterminate mother. [...] [However,] the real mother is contemplated only in order to provide a goal for the activity, and a criterion by which to evaluate the activity, in the context of an active synthesis.[99]

Deleuze argues that there is a virtual or indeterminate dimension of reality that exceeds actuality but is nevertheless inevitable. Reality itself is both actual and indeterminate. His example is a child that learns to walk. Walking, Deleuze says, does not originate within the child. Rather, the child is assisted by an "indeterminate" mother, meaning a mother who exceeds her actual physical existence. This indeterminate mother comforts the child throughout their first steps. The child "puts several fingers in its mouth" simulating the breast, "wraps the other arm around this indeterminate centre," simulating a comforting presence, "and appraises the whole situation from the point of view of this indeterminate mother"[100] – the child becomes (like) the mother by starting to walk. The maternal presence is reached *before* the now walking child reaches the "actual" mother – for (in Deleuze's picture) the presence of this *indeterminate mother,* a surplus mother to the mother in extended reality, enables the walking motion to begin with. This indeterminate mother exists besides and beyond her actual counterpart, yet she is vital for actual reality (the walking child) to become what it anyway will have been.

Now, in Deleuze's image, the infantile body is a given – two legs, several fingers, an arm, etc. But in Butler's version, a corporeal indeterminacy enables the transsexual to *become a particular body* in the first place. "The strategy of desire is in part the transfiguration of the desiring body itself."[101] Rather than merely going alongside the "actual" or "literal" body, Butler's corporeal indeterminacy substantiates the actual, physical body:

> "Indeed, in order to desire at all it may be necessary to believe in an altered bodily ego which, within the gendered rules of the imaginary, might fit the

requirements of a body capable of desire. This imaginary condition of desire always exceeds the physical body through or on which it works."[102]

Yet what Deleuze adds to the picture is that this force of an *other* (virtual, indeterminate) body is the essentially motivating engine of any corporeal movement at all. This includes the becoming of the body itself and thus erases the hesitant "in part" and "maybe" in Butler's formulation. In this sense, the transsexual experience is not a minority issue. It is a common experience: the fundamental organization of a body itself. For the desire to be this or that body or to be desired in this or that way is constitutive of particular physicality itself (being *this* body *right here*). There is no corporeality without desire. Desire is constitutive of human corporeality. Consequentially, gender as libidinal intelligibility is constitutive of each and every body – and with it, the indeterminate surplus body that motivates each individual attempt to engender, to be intelligible to this or that desire. "Transsexuality" is the name for a prohibited indulgence of this indeterminate surplus body, which we already encountered as the Schreberian handjob in Freud's analysis. In a less abstract way, "transsexuality" means "becoming a body." In the words of Andrea Long Chu:

> [N]ot getting what you want has very little to do with wanting it. Knowing better usually doesn't make it better. You don't want something because wanting it will lead to getting it. You want it because you want it. This is the zero-order disappointment that structures all desire and makes it possible. [It is the motivating power of indeterminacy.] After all, if you could only want things you were guaranteed to get, you would never be able to want anything at all.[103]

Becoming a body is always and necessarily oriented towards something that exceeds the present, that exceeds actual reality, that will never be actualized. Yet this un-actualizable element of reality is not an obstacle, it is not an absent aspect of reality that we should mourn or worry about. It is the inevitable *more than* reality of reality itself, the orientation of reality beyond itself, the motivating indeterminacy that we call "desire" when we sense it within ourselves.[104]

The transsexual paradigm says *do not be trans – do not indulge in the indeterminacy of your own body! And do not desire other bodies that point too far beyond themselves!* And yet the term "transsexuality" (in the same way as the Schreberian handjob) simultaneously gestures towards an inexhaustible surplus – though in a negative way. "Transsexuality" articulates a connection to that corporeal indeterminacy in the inevitable possibility of a transition: just as the Deleuzian mother enables a child to walk, this indeterminate, transsexual body enables our particular embodiment. Yet the pejorative, prohibitive term "transsexuality" simultaneously severs us from enjoying our indeterminate bodies by pathologizing them. In this sense, the term "transsexuality" works just like the image of "milking the goat" analyzed earlier: both interpellate a surplus desire that they simultaneously ask us to discipline. The transsexual paradigm wants us to believe that the enjoyment of our own corporeal indeterminacy *is sick*. But really, inversely, the prohibition of corporeal indeterminacy is making us sick. That is what becomes manifest in the exemplary case of Schreber. Yet eventually, she gives in to the enjoyment of her corporeal indeterminacy, she dwells in surplus desire.

More generally speaking, I understand "indeterminacy" as an irreducible surplus of reality which is nevertheless a dimension of reality itself. Reality points beyond itself. One reason is that repeatability is a necessary characteristic of all things – something that is not repeatable could not exist in the first place. A non-repeatable thing X would vanish in nothingness. There could be no memory of it (mental repetition), we could not put it elsewhere (spatial repetition), it could not persist (temporal repetition), we could not even think it (intellectual repetition). But if something can be repeated, then it points beyond itself – it exists *towards* its own repetition, never mind whether that repetition ever occurs or not. The same counts for reality itself. In order for the world to exist, it must point beyond itself. And this *beyond* is what I mean by an irreducible surplus, an inevitable indeterminacy as a dimension of reality. Indeterminacy, then, is existence that goes beyond presence, a surplus unassimilable to actuality.

Such indeterminacy is much less mysterious than one may think. The other side of a sculpture, for example, requires us to move around it. The sculpture is always *more than* whatever is experienced or even understood of it. In this way, the other side of a sculpture engenders its sculptu-reality *and inspires movement*.[105] The same counts for performativity and bodies: the fact that something escapes us, is *more than* can ever be captured, is a vital part of reality.[106] *There is always more-than.* Likewise, if you understand what a circle is, you understand that it could have any given circumference, any color, yet it would still be a circle. Such indeterminacy, however, is not restricted to experience: in each given circle (or any other object) there are infinitely many variants or versions of it – and that is because the indeterminate circle is itself a dimension of any actual circle. Likewise, for every natural number (1, 2, 5, etc.) there is another, indeterminate number which is larger than it. In this sense, the set of natural numbers is really indeterminate, that is, infinite. Now, transsexuality refers to corporeal indeterminacy – the sculptu-reality of the libidinal aspect of bodies, a causally effective, driving force *within* a body that is *more than* that body. Yet Western cultures rely on a crucial bias towards actuality or presence.[107] That is why the corporeal indeterminacy is denigrated into a pathology.

I already pointed out that Schreber insists on this indeterminacy when she points out that "the (external) male sexual organs (scrotum and male member) [could be] retracted into the body and, at the same time the internal sexual organs [...] transformed into the corresponding female sexual organs."[108] In Schreber's universe, the desire of someone else (God) shapes Schreber's body in ways that anticipate bottom surgeries. She thus insists on the susceptibility of the actual, physical body to the desire encapsulated in the indeterminate, virtual body. Later, that same insistence on one's corporeal indeterminacy will be pathologized as "transsexuality."

This is where Butler gets it right: transsexuality *enjoys* corporeal indeterminacy. It drives embodiment. This transsexual indeterminacy is like the Deleuzian mother:

motivator of actual corporeality rather than derivative of it. One might think that "transsexuality" is an old-fashioned name for this. Yet it captures the distortion (namely: a reduction of indeterminacy at large to gender identity in particular) and the denigration (a pathology, a slur) linked to the enjoyment of corporeal indeterminacy. *Do not become this corporeal indeterminacy*, the culture of alleged actuality tells us. The term "transsexuality" captures exactly this: we (all of us, *you too*) ought to submit to an "actual corporeality" sanctioned by cis-het-normative culture. The prohibition of transsexuality retroactively constructs an "actual," "cis" body – a body whose indeterminacy has been domesticated, a body that acquiesces into the confines of its allegedly pre-given actuality as prescribed by cultural institutions and social requirements. A normalized body, a docile body, a tamed body.[109] Reality, however, encompasses both – actuality and indeterminacy, embodiment as enabled by its own indeterminate transgression, indeterminacy as both embodied and debilitated through its realization, its literalization, its actualization.[110]

We can see this in the Freudian attempt to domesticate Schreber: the corporeal indeterminacy resurfaces in the image of the Satanic handjob, the gay threesome with a goat, and the affective reaction captured within it. I pointed out how and why Freud would feel provoked by Schreber's autobiography: Schreber insists exactly on the *indeterminacy of the human body*, the principle and inevitable possibility of a transition that Freud had to repress in himself. He thus displaces Schreber's corporeal indeterminacy onto a horror scenario: Schreber's femininity is completely omitted. Yet Freud transforms the indeterminacy articulated through it into a Satanic handjob as the epitome of total libidinal excess distorted into a mocking image of his own (Freud's) desire, twisted into culturally sanctioned terror. This is not an accident. Rather, it is a model. As we shall soon see, the repression of corporeal indeterminacy tends to re-surface elsewhere. Reality is both actual and indeterminate – and so are real bodies. If you try to reduce corporeality to actuality, indeterminacy is going to backfire. And in that sense, cis gender, in its attempt to domesticate indeterminate corporeality into the alleged reality of a "biologically given," is the real pathology – it generates monsters, namely in its displacements of corporeal indeterminacy onto anxious fantasies such as Freud's little orgy with a goat, or the Oedipal model of psychoanalysis.

In this sense, I want to suggest that we understand the term "transsexuality" as the mark of the originary displacement of libidinal organization, the fundamental deflection between indeterminacy and actuality that *creates the body*, rather than just taking it for granted (as Deleuze suggests) or using it as its objects (as it still echoes through the passage from Butler's *Gender Trouble*). Trans(sexual) libido is a desire in *adestination,* a desire without determined direction (or destination), forever going astray, driven by an indeterminacy that cannot be captured by any particular objective – driven by and despite its dysfunctionality. Yet this corporeal indeterminacy is a general feature of corporeal reality *in general* and not restricted to trans or non-binary people in particular. And in *this* sense, transsexuality is *original*.

Schreber however, existing at the margin of the transsexual paradigm, uses another term: she says that God wants to transform her into "the eternal Jew."[111]

Other than ideologies based on race, "[i]n modern anti-Semitism [the power attributed to 'the Jews'] is intangible, abstract and universal" or: indeterminate.[112] Consequentially, "jewishness" is another name for denigrated indeterminacy. That is why, to the present day, "[a]ntisemitism frequently manifests as a concern over putative Jewish hyper-power [indeterminate or infinite power]. [...] Jewishness is very much a marked identity—and the markers quite frequently center around beliefs about Jewish power, domination, or social control."[113] This fantasy finds a lethal manifestation in the Nazi project called "final solution," which Enzo Traverso and Moishe Postone interpret as the attempt at an eradication of *abstraction (or indeterminacy) as such,* projected onto a fantasmatic image of "the Jews," and identified with the ills of capitalism such as alienation, poverty, isolation.[114] Along similar lines, Joni Alizah Cohen points out that "[j]ust as the Jew becomes the concrete manifestation of the abstraction [indeterminacy of value] of capitalism [...], the trans woman becomes the concrete manifestation of the abstraction [indeterminacy] and denaturalization of gender."[115] It should be clear from our analysis so far that the indeterminacy of gender does not befall a body from a diabolically motivated outside, as both Kant and Freud might want us to believe. Rather, corporeal indeterminacy and, hence, transsexuality really live at the heart of gender itself. However, it is this link to indeterminacy in both Jewishness and transsexuality (and their link in trans femininity in particular) that also explains the recent surge in structurally anti-Semitic conspiracy fantasies concerning trans women that allegedly attempt to "groom" children by virtue of a "gender ideology" (see above). Anti-Semitism and hatred of trans people go hand-in-hand in that they phantasmatically exile and denigrate an indeterminacy ('abstraction') that lives in every one of us – though they act against different groups of people.

Cisgender as a Kind of Transsexuality

> The queered body takes a non-Euclidean geometric shape, like a complex manifold of curves and frictions.[116]

In his text "The Masculine Vaginal: Working With Queer Men's Embodiment At The Transgender Edge," Griff Hansbury shows how – in the terminology developed in the previous section – transsexuality permeates cisgender.[117] He does so from within his psychoanalytic practice, where he encounters what he calls "the transgender edge."

> As cisgender patients begin exploring the not-quite-cisgender aspects of themselves, we arrive at the place I think of as the *transgender edge,* a place where words that do not ostensibly belong to one's gender nevertheless get enlisted to describe sexual fantasy and experience. Insofar as it traffics in a denial that the difference between the sexes is immutable (and impassable), the transgender edge is a psychic space filled with grandiosity and shame, with envy and the fear of another's envy. How dare you try to have both?[118]

It is as though the cisgendered organization did fade out on the margins, was leaving loose threads occasionally, and sometimes did show significant residues of their transsexual engines in core moments of their libidinal organization:

> All gendered bodies are haunted bodies, inhabited by sexed parts not altogether relinquished, yet not fully recognized. Transgender people are not the only ones to experience gender dysphoria, if we think of *dysphoria* as feeling ill at ease, dissatisfied, or restless in the confines of one's prescribed gender role and bodily sex.[119]
>
> If my transmen patients, assigned female at birth, can have cocks, then my cismen patients can have cunts.[120]

Consequentially, we should:

> …conceive of the vagina and the symbolic Vaginal as multivalent, by turns feminine and masculine, depending on who is using it, in what style, and to what aim […]. When gender is treated as always multiple, the body might not matter much.[121]

Hansbury's work dovetails perfectly with what has been developed throughout the previous sections: the libidinal organization of *all* bodies is rooted in a certain displacement that I have suggested to call "transsexuality." This is *not* a minority issue. This transsexuality is a common issue, pertaining to the libidinal organization of bodies as such. This libidinal organization entails the active *creation* of these bodies – be it by means of hormone therapy, regular work outs at the gym, dietary habits, implants, self-destructive behaviour, particular sexual practices, or the most phantasmatic of all fantasies: the ideology of the "literal," biological body that we call "cis-gender."

To be clear: There is no such thing as an "original actual body" – not as corporeal material, not as a non-gendered "individual" essence, and not in any other way. Surely there is biology. But biology is nothing without the mobilizing force of indeterminacy, the natural surplus, the *more than* biology.[122] Inversely, some say, with RuPaul: "We're all born naked – the rest is drag." I disagree. Corporeality is always already adrift, fractured between the pull of the indeterminate and the push of naked actuality, materiality, biology. We are all born transsexual. The rest is transition.

I argued earlier that Schreber insists on the primacy of corporeal indeterminacy and its physiological surplus. She mobilizes it for her own transition – and freaks out Freud along the way. The reason is that in Schreber, Freud faces his own transgender edge, a remnant of his own violent transition away from Jewish femininity into white, bourgeois, cis masculinity. That is to say: everybody transitions into their gender, be it cis, trans, non-binary, or otherwise. And in cis people, these transitions often leave a transgender edge, loose threads where corporeal indeterminacy is still vibrant and can be mobilized for enjoyment or further transitions.

The excess desire captured in Freud's description of Schreber's satanic handjob is a reactivation of the libidinal potential stored in this transgender edge.

With Avgi Saketopoulou and Ann Pellegrini, we may say that "*all gender* is constructed out of the raw materials of what the other wants from (or for) us [gender as libidinal intelligibility]. Said differently, the other's invasion does not *determine* who we become. Rather, that invasion sets in motion the very process of our subjectivation; it is, rather, the response to this puncturing that consolidates as the ego, and also our experience of our gender."[123] But other than Saketopolou and Pellegrini, I do not think that "self-theorizing" is front and center in this process. The self is an effect of gender (and other kinds of social intelligibility) and not the site of its construction. Rather, just like a political revolution, a transition (never mind into which gender) is a collective effort. Returning to Wark, we may say that "[...] a political revolution is not the solution to anything. It merely enables the problem of organization to be posed."[124] The same counts for each and any transition, never mind into which gender, cis, trans, non-binary, and others alike: it poses the problem of *collective* organization of *this* body *and the world around it*. A revolution lives at the heart of any transition, never mind in what direction. How do I relate to others? How do they relate to me? Which institutions do we require, respect, refuse, rewire? How do I desire to be desired or not desired? Who should rather ignore me? Thus, every transition (cis, trans, non-binary, etc.) is inherently political because it poses the question of the organization of *collective desire*. What do *we* want? Yet posing the question does not in itself cause this or that effect. The question requires collective labor. In this way, hormone treatment or gender affirming medical interventions enable us to pose the question of collective organization anew and differently. But "as long as the answer is a drug, it's still capitalism, because that's how companies make money" (M. Wolf, personal communication, 2012). And as long as the answer is a pronoun, it is still capitalism – because differentiation enables cultural capital just as much.[125] Here, I agree with Jane Ward that "all genders demand work, and therefore all people both give and require gender labor."[126] Transitions pose that question of organization. But that organization must be worked out collectively – through labor and by everybody involved. Accordingly, Schreber writes her memoir *in order to become intelligible*. And she hopes that her contemporaries will put in the work and help her be the woman that she is. They refuse, Freud among them. Inversely, Freud uses Schreber in order to work out and confirm his own transition into his own cisgender by exiling his own transgender edge.

Consequentially, the problem of transsexuality will not be solved once everybody has access to gender affirming care and can change their legal name and gender at will. Transsexuality requires an encompassing collective re-modeling of human culture towards an emancipation of corporeal indeterminacy. Our corporeal indeterminacies function as engines that actively shape our actual bodies. They become most palpable in transsexuality. But this transsexuality, in fact, permeates all bodies alike – and may condense into forms of gender dysphoria even among cis people. What we know as "cis-gender" is really just the repression of original transsexuality as described in the previous section – the repression of the struggle between the actual and the corporeal indeterminacy, identification with another body, incorporation and mourning of bodies that are unlike our own bodies (bodies that we nevertheless become in some sense so as to cope with their loss). In his text, Hansbury presents the case of an analysand whose profound cis-gender-dysphoria can be processed in analysis by way of gentle confrontation with his *transgender edge*. That is encouraging. My point, however, is political: we should stop thinking of trans and cis as a clear-cut distinction and beware of giving in to the fantasy of an originally un-gendered, un-sexed body. Rather, we should understand human corporeality as originally transsexual, originarily displaced, in a primary friction between actual and indeterminate corporeality that creates the human body from within. In every body anew (cis, trans, enby, other), we hand down a long tradition of loss, mourning, incorporation, and iteration of irreducible transsexual displacement. A post-transsexual world is possible. But it requires more than just remodeling terminology and calling for legal rights and access to medical treatment. It requires an emancipation of corporeal indeterminacy and the pleasures involved in it *for everybody*.

Summary

Summing up: trans issues are, in general, treated as minority issues. I argue that transsexuality is *not* a minority issue, but a *common* issue, shared by all subjects of patriarchal societies. The term "transsexuality" is itself an expression of pure violence, but it holds special access to an emancipation of the indeterminacy that is articulated to be lost in this term. Transsexuality is the name for the prohibition of indulgence of corporeal indeterminacy that generates an actual body. We should not remain caught up in contesting the normalization of violence and critique of discipline by way of legal set ups, murder and threats, although of course that is a crucial part of our emancipatory politics and psychoanalytic practice. However, there should be another part to the project: *the emancipation of indeterminacy*. Originary transsexuality is key in this regard. Emancipation does *not* mean inclusion into neoliberal exploitation and bourgeois corporeality. It does not mean getting a job, a partner, a child (or two, or five) and disappearing into normality. Emancipation means a wholesale re-distribution of the libidinal organization wherever it occurs. It means a different (heterogenous, hospitable) relationship to indeterminacy, in our bodies and elsewhere – a relation that does not repress, nor exploit.[127] Emancipation means to use indeterminacy not as a nuisance that ought to be disciplined nor as a resource that must be exploited. Emancipation means to surf indeterminacy, to let it blow wind into our sails and generate a natural though unforeseeable surplus of political development.

We can take Schreber as our model: faced with maximized epistemic violence and minimal political resources, she generated a whole world, a whole conceptual framework, out of her sheer desire to transition. Clearly, the framework is marked by the violence that generated it and the way to emancipation does not lead into psychiatry. My point is not that we should go nuts like Schreber did. My point is that even in the face of the total dissolution of the world as we know it, we can still face down the violence and use that surplus indeterminacy of reality itself as our motivating force, drive, engine, and power house. Schreber did it. So can we. We should push for another relation to indeterminacy, to our own corporeal indeterminacy by all means – but keep in mind that what we really strive for is an emancipation of corporeal indeterminacy as a driving force of actual bodies and to liberate the indeterminate from the actual more generally. So then: put your fingers in your mouth, wrap the other arm around yourself, mobilize your corporeal indeterminacy to comfort you on the way, and *transition.*

Notes

1 Wark, M. (2022). "Dear Cis Analysts", Parapraxis. https://www.parapraxismagazine. com/articles/dear-cis-analysts.
2 Note that I am not payed for writing this article. But you are free to change that.
3 Wark, 2022.
4 I quote from the German edition. Translations are mine. Schreber, D. (2003). *Denkwürdigkeiten Eines Nervenkranken.* Munich: Kadmos.
5 I am, therefore, in critical conversation with recent psychoanalytic explorations of trans, transgender, transsexuality, non-binary, etc., such as: Saketopoulou, A., & Pellegrini, A. (2023). *Gender Without Identity.* New York: The Unconscious in Translation.; Hansbury, G. (2017). "The Masculine Vaginal: Working With Queer Men's Embodiment at the Transgender Edge." In: *Journal of the American Psychoanalytic Association, 65*(6), 1009–1031.; Gherovici, P. (2017). *Transgender Psychoanalysis: A Lacanian Perspective on Sexual Difference.* New York: Routledge.; Gherovici, P. (2010). *Please Select Your Gender: From the Invention of Hysteria to the Democratizing of Transgenderism.* New York: Routledge.
6 See exemplarily Nieder, T.O., Strauß, B., … (2019), "Geschlechtsinkongruenz, Geschlechtsdysphorie und Trans-Gesundheit: S3-Leitlinie zur Diagnostik, Beratung und Behandlung", *AWMF-Register-Nr.* [AWMF online], *138*(001), Section 4.2, 29–30.
7 Stone, S. (2023). "The Empire Strikes Back: A Posttranssexual Manifesto." In: *The Transgender Studies Reader Remix* (1st ed.). Routledge, pp. 15–30.
8 Freud, S. (1955). *Gesammelte Werke VIII.* London: Imago Publishing, p. 268.
9 Kant, I. (1900ff). *Gesammelte Schriften* Hrsg.: Bd. 1–22 Preussische Akademie der Wissenschaften, Bd. 23 Deutsche Akademie der Wissenschaften zu Berlin, ab Bd. 24 Akademie der Wissenschaften zu Göttingen. Berlin 1900ff. AAIV, 52.
10 I understand "bullshit" to designate a statement that resides outside or beyond the confines of truth and falsity. See: Frankfurt, H.G. (2005). *On bullshit.* [Online]. Princeton, NJ: Princeton University Press.
11 "It is a singular plural, which no single origin will ever have preceded. Germination, dissemination. There is no first insemination. The semen is already swarming. The 'primal' insemination is dissemination. A trace, a graft whose traces have been lost." (Derrida, J. [1981]. *Dissemination.* Trans. B. Johnson. Chicago: University of Chicago Press. [Quotation taken from p. 304.])
12 Federici, S. (2004). *Caliban and the Witch.* 1st ed. Brooklyn, NY: Autonomedia.
13 Kant, AAIV, 52.
14 Kant, AAVIII, 35.
15 Whether through God or through Schreber's psychiatrist Flechsig is at times unclear.
16 See exemplarily: Schreber, 2003, 193–194.

17 Freud, 1955, 268.
18 Freud, 1955, 268. (My emphasis.)
19 deLire, L. (2024a). "Can the Transsexual Speak?" In: *philoSOPHIA: Journal of Trans-continental Feminism*, 13.
20 Freud, 1955, 268. (My emphasis.)
21 Freud, 1955, 290.
22 See also Freud, 1955, 286.
23 Schreber, 2003, 40. (My emphasis.)
24 Schreber, 2003, 40.
25 Schreber, 2003, 40. See also 101.
26 Hirschfeld invents the technique and first applies it in 1930.
27 Freud, *Gesammelte Werke V*, 92.
28 Freud, *Gesammelte Werke V*, 92, 126, 144.
29 See, for example: Butler, J. (1999), *Gender Trouble*. London and New York: Routledge. p.100. (Original work published in 1990). Freud captures this as "castration complex," Lacan as the "*non/nom du pere*."
30 Adorno, T.W., and Horkheimer, M. (2002). *Dialectic of Enlightenment – Philosophical Fragments*. Redwood: Stanford University Press. (Original work published 1947.)
31 "[S]i Crenshaw a tendance á parler d'identités intersectionelles dans le cas des 'victimes' (juridiques) de la domination croisée, la raison en est que, pour elle, l'intersectionalité est utile comme un concept critique du *droit*, non pas comme un concept critique en général." Dorlin, E. (2009). "Introduction – Vers une Epistémologie des résistances." In: Dorlin, E. and Bidet-Mordrel, A. (Eds.). *Sexe, Race, Classe – pour une épistémologie de la Domination*. Presses Universitaire de France. See also: deLire, L. (2022). "Catchy Title – Gender Abolitionism, Trans Materialism and beyond". *Year of the Women Magazine*. https://yearofthewomen.net/en/magazin/catchy-title-1-gender-abolitionism-trans-materialism-and-beyond.
32 Boyarin, D. (1995). *Freud's Baby, Fliess's Maybe: Homophobia, Anti-Semitism, and the Invention of Oedipus. GLQ: A Journal of Lesbian and Gay Studies*, (2), 115–147.
33 Geller J. (1992). "(G)nos(e)ology: The Cultural Construction of the Other." In: Eilberg-Schwartz, H. (Ed.), *People of the Body: Jews and Judaism From an Embodied Perspective*. Albany: State University of New York Press. pp. 243–282, 260.
34 Freud, S. (1985). *The Complete Letters of Sigmund Freud to Wilhelm Fliess, 1887–1904*. Ed. and Trans. J. Moussaieff Masson. Cambridge: Belknap-Harvard University Press, p. 278.
35 Freud, 1985, 256; 270.
36 Freud, 1985, 904.
37 Garner, S.N. (1989). "Freud and Fliess: Homophobia and Seduction." *Seduction and Theory: Readings of Gender, Representation, and Rhetoric*. Ed. Dianne Hunter. Urbana: University of Illinois Press, pp. 86–109. (Text references pp. 95–96.)
38 Freud, 1985, 269.
39 Boyarin convincingly argues that the effeminacy of Jewish men was not entirely composed of anti-Semitic stereotypes: "The representation of the ideal male Jew as female [...] was not only an external one, one that originated in the fantasies of anti-Semites, but also an internal one that represented a genuine Jewish cultural difference. It is, moreover, while not untroubled, also not negative in its traditional cultural manifestations. In fact, this sense of self-feminization was one of the traditional ways in which male Jews defined themselves over and against the gentile world. Within traditional rabbinic Jewish culture, the feminization of the male, in part symbolized (or effected?) through truncation of the penis, was experienced as a positive phenomenon, as a positive sense of self identification and differentiation from the Romans (and their descendants)." (Boyarin, 1995, 131.)
40 Boyarin, 1995, 133.

41 Boyarin, D. (1997). *Unheroic Conduct: The Rise of Heterosexuality and the Invention of the Jewish Man*. Berkeley: University of California Press.; Geller, J. (2007). *On Freud's Jewish Body: Mitigating Circumcisions*. New York: Fordham University Press.; Gilman, S. (1991). *The Jew's Body*. New York: Routledge.; Gilman, S. (1993). *Freud, Race, and Gender*. Princeton: Princeton University Press.; Pellegrini, A. (1997). *Performance Anxieties: Staging Psychoanalysis, Staging Race*. New York: Routledge.

42 Boyarin, D., Itzkovitz, D., and Pellegrini, A. (Eds.). (2003). *Queer Theory and the Jewish Question*. New York: Columbia University Press.

43 Boyarin, 1995, 129.

44 deLire, L, 2024a.

45 Etienne Trillat, quoted in Showalter, E. (1993). "Hysteria, Feminism, and Gender." In *Hysteria Beyond Freud*. Oakland: University of California Press. pp. 286–344.(Quotation taken from p. 291.)

46 "I am not responsible for the monotony of the psychoanalytic solution" (Freud, 1955, 290).

47 Sentence by Juliet Meding in conversation.

48 On Plato, Aristotle and Descartes, see Wagner 1984, p. 53, Beavers 1989, Menn 1994, p. 73. On Aristotle in particular, see Dobbs-Weinstein 2014. For a general history of vitalistic interpretations of souls, starting with Descartes, see Normandin, S., Wolfe (2013), p. 6. For an alternative reading on Descartes, compare Jolley 1998, p. 26. On the early 19th century version of this, see Steigerwald 2013, p. 51, on the early 20th century, see Garrett 2013, p. 127.

49 Schreber, 2003, 10.

50 Schreber, 2003, 40.

51 Boyarin, 1997, 34.

52 For the continuation of that history in the 20th and 21st century, see: Bassi, S. and LaFleur, G. (Eds.) (2022). "Trans-Exclusionary Feminisms and the Global New Right" [Special issue]. *TSQ: Transgender Studies Quarterly, 9*(3).; Cohen, J.A. (2018). "The Eradication of 'Talmudic Abstractions': Anti-Semitism, Transmisogyny and the National Socialist Project." *VersoBlog.*' deLire, L. (forthcoming). "An Unfortunate Individual Case – Denazification and the Deconstruction of Value." In: J. Martell & T. Williams (Eds.), *Politica Comun*. Michigan Publishing.

53 Schreber, 2003, 28.

54 Schreber, 2003, 34.

55 Schreber, 2003, 39.

56 Schreber, 2003, 41.

57 See, for example, Schreber, 2003, 88.

58 Schreber, 2003, 122, 123, 193, 194.

59 Schreber, 2003, 28.

60 See also Schreber, 2003, 35–38.

61 Notably the gender of her partner remains undisclosed and there is at least one passage that may be read to point towards lesbian desire: when Schreber states that a naked woman attracts "both genders" (Schreber, 2003, 113).

62 See, for example: Schreber, 2003, 88; 120.

63 Schreber, 2003, 120.

64 Schreber, 2003, 45.

65 See also Schreber, 2003, 121.

66 Schreber, 2003, 121. (Vernunftgründe.)

67 See exemplarily Schreber, 2003, 43.

68 See, for example, Schreber, 2003, 32.

69 See also deLire, 2024a, 61.

70 Schreber, 2003, 7.

71 For more on the trans politics of heterogeneity and hospitality, see deLire, 2024a, 62.

72 For an in-depth study of transgender children, see: Gill-Peterson, J. (2018). *Histories of the Transgender Child*. Minneapolis: University of Minnesota Press. See also: Elster, M. (2022). "Insidious Concern: Trans Panic and the Limits of Care." *TSQ: Transgender Studies Quarterly*, 9(3), 407–24.

73 For a genealogy of hormones, see: Preciado, P.B. (2013). *Testo Junkie*. Trans. B. Benderson. New York: The Feminist Press.

74 "It is common for people to assume that being or becoming a transsexual involves some kind of 'sex change operation.' However, this is not necessarily the case. While some transsexuals undergo numerous medical procedures as part of their physical transitions, others either cannot afford or choose not to undergo such procedures. Indeed, attempts to limit the word 'transsexual' to only those who physically transition is not only classist (because of the affordability issue), but objectifying, as it reduces all trans people to the medical procedures that have been carried out on their bodies." (Serano, J. [2007]. *Whipping Girl – A Transsexual Woman On Sexism And The Scapegoating of Femininity*. Emerville: Seal Press. [Quotation is take from Chapter 1.]).

75 See exemplarily: Hinchy, J. (2019). *Governing Gender and Sexuality in Colonial India*. Cambridge University Press.; Saleh, F. (2020). "Transgender as a Humanitarian Category: The Case of Syrian Queer and Gender-Variant Refugees in Turkey." *TSQ: Transgender Studies Quarterly*, 7(1); Boellstorff T., Mauro C., Cárdenas M., Cotten T., Stanley E.A., Young K., Aizura A.Z. (2014). "Decolonizing Transgender: A Roundtable Discussion." *TSQ: Transgender Studies Quarterly*, 1 (3): 419–439. https://doi.org/10.1215/23289252-2685669Aristotle.

76 "Until now, discourses on transsexuality have invariably relied on language and concepts invented by clinicians, researchers, and academics who have made transsexuals the objects of their inquiry. In such a framework, transsexual bodies, identities, perspectives, and experiences are continuously required to be explained and inevitably remain open to interpretation. Corresponding cissexual attributes are simply taken for granted—they are assumed to be 'natural' and 'normal' and therefore escape reciprocal critique. This places transsexuals at a constant disadvantage, since we have generally been forced to rely on limiting cissexual-centric terminology to make sense of our own lives." (Serano, 2007, Chapter 8).

77 "All transsexuals rape women's bodies by reducing the real female form to an artifact, appropriating this body [the female form – femininity itself!] for themselves. However, the transsexually constructed lesbian-feminist violates women's sexuality and spirit, as well." (Raymond, J.G. [1994]. *The Transsexual Empire: The Making of the She-Male*. New York: Teachers College Press, 104. [Original work published in 1979.])

78 Cohen, 2018.

79 "Alongside its obvious anti-Semitic undertones, for example, the key anti-gender charge that gender ideology is yet another 'world program' unleashed by 'global elites' on 'normal families,' encodes demographic anxieties and fears about reproduction and ethnonational decline" (Bassi, S. & LaFleur, G., 2022, 316.)

80 See exemplarily: Bassi, S. & LaFleur, G., 2022.; Sosa, L. (2021). "Beyond Gender Equality? Anti-Gender Campaigns and the Erosion of Human Rights and Democracy." *Netherlands Quarterly of Human Rights, 39*(1), 3–10.; Sierakowski, S. (2014, January 26). "The Polish Church's Gender Problem." *New York Times.*; Schmidt, N. (2014, June 30). "Les ABCD de L'égalité: Un Abandon Symbolique. *Inegalites.fr.* https://www.inegalites.fr/Les-ABCD-de-l-egalite-un-abandon-symbolique.

81 Corredor, E.S. (2019). "Unpacking 'Gender Ideology' and the Global Right's Anti-gender Countermovement." *Signs: Journal of Women in Culture and Society*, 44(3), 613–38.

82 See, for example: Elster, 2022, 407–24.

83 See also: deLire, L. (2024b). "Nature is a Transsexual Woman – Lucretian metaphysics reconsidered." In: S. Nooter (Ed.), *Classical Philology, 119*(2).

84 Here I am thinking along the lines of Spivak, G.C. (1998). "Feminism and Critical Theory." In: *In Other Worlds – Essays in Cultural Politics*. London and New York: Routledge, pp. 103.

    For the trouble this produces in confrontation with non-Western models of gender in particular, see Towle, E.B., and Morgan, L.M. (2002). "Romancing the Transgender Native: Rethinking the Use of the 'Third Gender' Concept." *GLQ: A Journal of Lesbian and Gay Studies, 8*(4), 469–497. https://www.muse.jhu.edu/article/12222.; Saleh, 2020; Hinchy, 2019.

    For more general analyses of related problems, see: Bettcher, T.M. (2014). "Trapped in the Wrong Theory: Rethinking Trans Oppression and Resistance. *Journal of Women in Culture and Society*, 39(2), 383–406.; Dembroff, R. (2020). "Cisgender Commonsense and Philosophy's Transgender Trouble." *Transgender Studies Quarterly, 7*(3), pp. 399–406.; Valentine, D. (2007). *Imagining Transgender*. Duke University Press.

85 See, for example, Gill-Peterson, 2018, and Snorton, R. (2017). *Black on Both Sides*. Minneapolis: University of Minnesota Press.

86 Spivak, G.C. (1999). *A Critique of Postcolonial Reason*. Oxford: Harvard University Press. (Text references p. 219.)

87 For an ancient counter paradigm, see deLire, 2024b.

88 For more on the impossibility to speak for trans people, see deLire, 2024a.

89 Much of the second half of this text originates from conversations at and around Unbehagen NYC, for which I am eternally grateful. However, I handed in a version of this text to philosophy journal *Hypathia* and received mixed reviews. One reviewer responded with "I hate this article." But beyond this, the reviews were mostly ignoring my arguments. I protested on social media but nobody cared. I was left greatly discouraged. I wrote a letter to the editors of *Hypathia* but did not have the strength to send it as similar interventions from my side in other contexts were mostly ignored. As a consequence, the article lay dormant for years. Trans misogyny is real, in the academy and elsewhere. I am thus grateful to Vanessa Sinclair for the opportunity to publish a re-worked version in this volume.

90 Prosser, J. (1998). *Second skins: The Body Narratives of Transsexuality*. New York: Columbia University Press. (Quotation taken from p. 26.)

91 Namaste, V. (2000). *Invisible Lives – The Erasure of Transsexual and Transgendered People*. Chicago and London: The University of Chicago Press. (Quotation taken from p.10.)

92 See also: Heaney, E. (2017). *The New Woman – Literary Modernism, Queer Theory, and the Trans Feminine Allegory*. Evanston: Northwestern University Press. (Text references p. 259.)

93 Regarding Butler's reading of the death of Extravaganza in *Paris is Burning* in *Bodies That Matter*, Namaste comments: "Since Butler has reduced Extravaganza's transsexuality to allegory, she cannot conceptualize the specificity of violence with which transsexuals, especially transsexual prostitutes, are faced. […] More than simply denying Extravaganza's transsexuality, Butler uses it in order to speak about race and class" (Namaste, 2000, 13). I agree.

94 Butler, 1999, 90.

95 Heaney, 2017, 254.

96 Heaney, 2017, 254.

97 Butler, 1999, 90.

98 Could we even say that the transsexual is *especially successful* in this process?

99 Deleuze, G. (2004). *Difference and repetition*. Trans. Paul Patton. [New ed.]. London: Continuum. (Quotation taken from p. 99.)

100 Deleuze, 2004, 99.
101 Butler 1999, 90.
102 Butler 1999, 90.
103 Long Chu, A. (2018). *On Liking Women*. In: *N Plus 1*. https://www.nplusonemag.com/issue-30/essays/on-liking-women/. [Accessed 2024, March 29.]
104 For more on the relationship between desire and reality in this sense, see: deLire, L. (forthcoming [b]). "Erotics as First Philosophy – Metaphysics and/of Desire Between Aristotle, Avicenna, Cavendish and Spinoza." In: B. Gook (Ed.), *Libidinal Economies of Crisis Times*.
105 See Deleuze, 2004, 56.
106 For more on this, see: Cheah, P. (2008). "Nondialectical Materialism." *Diacritics*, 38(1–2), 143–157.
107 This "metaphysics of presence [may be understood] as the exigent, powerful, systematic, and irrepressible desire for [...] [the transcendental signified, which, at one time or another, would place a reassuring end to the reference from sign to sign]" (Derrida, J. [1974]. *Of Grammatology*. Trans. G. Spivak. Baltimore and London: Johns Hopkins University Press. [Quotation take from p. 49].) and thus puts to rest that "strange movement of the trace [here: indeterminacy]" (Derrida, 1974, 66). In this case, the transcendental signified is the actual reality of the (cis) body. Metaphysics of presence pretends that the indeterminate was subsumed under actuality. It has no life of its own, no non-human agency.
108 Schreber, 2003, 40. See also 101.
109 It should be noted that Butler performs this retroactive construction of the cis body throughout their work on mourning. Time and again, the introjection or incorporation of a lost object does – in their version – facilitate desire for the lost object, *but not desire to become that object*. Thus, if the mother is lost, why exactly should girls restrict themselves to desire *for* other females, rather than develop a desire *to become that other female* to begin with (or on top of that)? Here is an example of such an omission of the corporeal indeterminacy which retroactively inscribes an apparently stabilized cis body: "That the boy usually chooses the heterosexual would, then, be the result, not of the fear of castration by the father, but of the fear of castration—that is, the fear of 'feminization' associated within heterosexual cultures with male homosexuality" (Butler, 1999, 80). Needless to say, the fear of feminization *without quotation marks* is associated within heterosexual cultures with *transsexuality*.
     One page on, Butler continues: "Indeed, if the boy renounces both aim and object and, therefore, heterosexual cathexis altogether, he internalizes the mother and sets up a feminine superego which dissolves and disorganizes masculinity, consolidating feminine libidinal dispositions in its place" (Butler, 1999, 81). Yet again: why would this process not render the 'boy' in fact not a 'boy' after all? This omission of the corporeal indeterminacy and its inherent transsexuality may be observed in other Butlerian works on gender and mourning as well. Thus, in *Bodies That Matter*, Butler touches on transsexuality in distancing from Janice Raymond's general condemnation of all things *trans* in her *Transsexual Empire* – but only to mark "important differences" which remain otherwise indetermined: "Raymond, in particular, places drag on a continuum with cross-dressing and transsexualism, ignoring the important differences between them, maintaining that in each practice women are the object of hatred and appropriation, and that there is nothing in the identification that is respectful or elevating. As a rejoinder, one might consider that identification is always an ambivalent process" (Butler, J. [2011]. *Bodies That Matter*. London and New York: Routledge).
     Butler returns to the theory of mourning as constitutive of gender and sexuality in *The Psychic Life of Power*, yet on the 60 pages dedicated to the topic, the terms 'transgender' or 'transsexuality' and their relatives do not occur once (Butler, J. [1997]. *The Psychic Life*

of Power – Theories of Subjection. Stanford: Stanford University Press. [Text references pp. 132 – 200.]). Instead, Butler writes (and I will mark the omissions): "Drag allegorizes some set of melancholic incorporative fantasies that stabilize *gender.* Not only are a vast number of drag performers straight [and cis], but it would be a mistake to think that homosexuality is best explained through the performativity that is drag. What does seem useful in this analysis, however, is that drag exposes or allegorizes the mundane psychic and performative practices by which heterosexualized genders form themselves through renouncing the *possibility* of homosexuality [and of transsexuality], a foreclosure which produces both a field of heterosexual [and cisgendered?] objects and a domain of those whom it would be impossible to love [and to be?]. Drag thus allegorizes *heterosexual melancholy,* the melancholy by which a masculine gender is formed from the refusal to grieve the masculine as a possibility of love [and the refusal of the possibility to *be* a woman]; a feminine gender is formed (taken on, assumed) through the incorporative fantasy by which the feminine is excluded as a possible object of love [and, occasionally, as a possible way of existence], an exclusion never grieved, but 'preserved' through heightened feminine identification" (Butler 1997, 146). In this case, trans*masculinity* is absent from the picture – maybe even more than trans*femininity*. Passages like these may be found elsewhere in Butler's *Oeuvre* as well. I do, however, not think that Butler is simply making a *mistake* here. Rather, I believe that these omissions are *real* – they do actually happen like that *even to the best of us* (and Butler no doubt is one of those). An analysis of Butler's particular omissions on this issue could be useful in many regards, such as regarding the question of how homosexuality may be read in light of the original transsexuality that I am concerned with in the text: could it be that some heterosexuals compromise on loving a body that they allegedly cannot be? Is it possible that some homosexuals perform their rejection of transsexuality *even stronger* than heterosexuals do in and through their disavowal of feeling affection for that kind of body that they ought not to be? For matters of space, I will not investigate these questions any further here.

110   See also: Puar, J. (2017). *The Right to Maim – Debility, Capacity, Disability.* Durham and London: Duke University Press 2017, pp. 1–32.

111   Schreber, 2003, 40.

112   Postone, M. (1980). "Anti-Semitism and National Socialism: Notes on the German Reaction to 'Holocaust.'" *New German Critique, 19*(1), pp.97–115. (Quotation taken from p.106.)

113   Schraub, D. (2019). "White Jews: An Intersectional Approach." *AJS Review 43*(2), 379–407. (Quotation taken from p. 384.)

114   Postone, 1980, 129. For my take on this, see deLire, forthcoming.

115   Cohen, 2018. (Italicized in original.)

116   Hansbury, 2017, 1016.

117   For related arguments, see especially Saketopoulou & Pellegrini, 2023, but also: Gozlan, O. (2015), *Transsexuality and the Art of Transitioning: A Lacanian Approach.* London and New York: Routledge.; Stryker, S. and Currah, P. (Eds.) (2017).; *Transpsychoanalytics* [Special issue]. *Transgender Studies Quarterly,* 4, (3–4); Gozlan, O. (Ed.) (2018). *Current Critical Debates in the Field of Transsexuality Studies – In Transition.* London and New York: Routledge.; Gherovici, 2017.

118   Hansbury 2017, 1012.

119   Hansbury 2017, 1028.

120   Hansbury 2017, 1011.

121   Hansbury 2017, 1011.

122   I am reminded of Butler in response to her critics [which I amend for the current purpose]: "And if I persisted in this notion that [actual] bodies were in some way *constructed* [by and through their *indeterminate* counterparts], perhaps I really thought that words alone had the power to craft bodies from their own linguistic substance? Couldn't someone simply take me aside?" (Butler, 2011, ix).

123   Saketopoulou & Pellegrini, 2023, 26.

124 Wark, M. (2015). *Molecular Red: Theory for the Anthropocene*, New York: Verso. (Quotation take from p. 44.)
125 See deLire, 2024a, 54.
126 Ward, J. (2010). "Gender Labor: Transmen, Femmes, and Collective Work of Transgression." *Sexualities*, *13*(2), 236–254. https://doi-org.proxy1.library.jhu.edu/10.1177/1363460709359114.
127 For the difference between repressive disciplinary societies and exploitative neoliberal societies, see deLire, 2024a, 53, and deLire, L. (2023). "Beyond Representational Justice." *Texte zur Kunst* (129).

Bibliography

Adorno, T.W. and Horkheimer, M. (2002). *Dialectic of Enlightenment – Philosophical Fragments*. Redwood: Stanford University Press. (Original work published 1947.)

Aizura, Aren Z., Trystan Cotten, Carsten Balzer, Carla LaGata, Marcia Ochoa, and Salvador Vidal-Ortiz. 2014. Introduction: Decolonizing the Transgender Imaginary. *TSQ: Transgender Studies Quarterly* 1.3.

Bassi, S. and LaFleur, G. (Eds.) (2022). "Trans-Exclusionary Feminisms and the Global New Right" [Special issue]. *TSQ: Transgender Studies Quarterly,* 9(3).

Beavers, Anthony F. (July 1989), "Desire and Love in Descartes's Late Philosophy," *History of Philosophy Quarterly* 6(3).

Bettcher, T.M. (2014). "Trapped in the Wrong Theory: Rethinking Trans Oppression and Resistance." *Journal of Women in Culture and Society*, 39(2), 383–406.

Boellstorff T., Mauro C., Cárdenas M., Cotten T., Stanley E.A., Young K., Aizura A.Z. (2014). "Decolonizing Transgender: A Roundtable Discussion." *TSQ: Transgender Studies Quarterly*, 1 (3): 419–439. https://doi.org/10.1215/23289252-2685669.

Boyarin, D. (1995). "Freud's Baby, Fliess's Maybe: Homophobia, Anti-Semitism, and the Invention of Oedipus." *GLQ: A Journal of Lesbian and Gay Studies*, 2, 115–147.

Boyarin, D. (1997). *Unheroic Conduct: The Rise of Heterosexuality and the Invention of the Jewish Man*. Berkeley: University of California Press.

Boyarin, D., Itzkovitz, D., and Pellegrini, A. (Eds.) (2003). *Queer Theory and the Jewish Question*. New York: Columbia University Press.

Butler, J. (1997). *The Psychic Life of Power – Theories of Subjection*. Stanford: Stanford University Press.

Butler, J. (1999). *Gender Trouble*. London and New York: Routledge. (Original work published in 1990).

Butler, J. (2011). *Bodies That Matter*. London and New York: Routledge.

Cheah, P. (2008). "Nondialectical Materialism." *Diacritics*, 38(1–2), 143–157.

Cohen, J.A. (2018). "The Eradication of 'Talmudic Abstractions': Anti-Semitism, Transmisogyny and the National Socialist Project." *VersoBlog*. https://www.versobooks.com/blogs/news/4188-the-eradication-of-talmudic-abstractions-anti-semitism-transmisogyny-and-the-national-socialist-project.

Corredor, E.S. (2019). "Unpacking 'Gender Ideology' and the Global Right's Anti-gender Countermovement." *Signs: Journal of Women in Culture and Society,* 44(3), 613–38.

Deleuze, G. (2004). *Difference and Repetition*. Trans. Paul Patton. [New ed.]. London: Continuum.

deLire, L. (2022). "Catchy Title – Gender Abolitionism, Trans Materialism and Beyond." *Year of the Women Magazine*. https://yearofthewomen.net/en/magazin/catchy-title-1-gender-abolitionism-trans-materialism-and-beyond.

deLire, L. (2023)."Beyond Representational Justice." *Texte zur Kunst* (129).

deLire, L. (2024a). "Can the Transsexual Speak?" *philoSOPHIA*: *Journal of Transcontinental Feminism*, 13.

deLire, L. (2024b). "Nature is a Transsexual Woman – Lucretian Metaphysics Reconsidered." *Classical Philology,* 119(2).

deLire, L. (forthcoming 2025). *Property Property Property – Our Political Categories*, Brussels and London: Divided 2025.

deLire, L. (forthcoming [a]). "An Unfortunate Individual Case – Denazification and the Deconstruction of Value." In: J. Martell & T. Williams (Eds.), *Politica Comun*. Michigan Publishing.

deLire, L. (forthcoming [b]). "Erotics as First Philosophy – Metaphysics and/of Desire Between Aristotle, Avicenna, Cavendish and Spinoza." In: B. Gook (Ed.), *Libidinal Economies of Crisis Times.*

Dembroff, R. (2020). "Cisgender Commonsense and Philosophy's Transgender Trouble." *Transgender Studies Quarterly,* 7(3), 399–406.

Derrida, J. (1974). *Of Grammatology*. Trans. G. Spivak. Baltimore and London: Johns Hopkins University Press.

Derrida, J. (1981). *Dissemination*. Trans. B. Johnson. Chicago: University of Chicago Press.

Dobbs-Weinstein, I. (2014), "Aristotle on the Natural Dwelling of the Soul", in: Claudia Barachi (ed.), *The Bloomsbury Companion to Aristotle*, London, New Delhi, New York, Sydney: Bloomsbury Press.

Dorlin, E. (2009). "Introduction – Vers une Epistémologie des Résistances." In: E. Dorlin & A. Bidet-Mordrel (Eds.), *Sexe, Race, Classe – Pour une Epistémologie de la Domination.* Presses Universitaire de France.

Dyde, S. (2013). "Life and the Mind in Nineteenth-Century Britain." In: S. Normandin and C.T. Wolfe, *Vitalism and the Scientific Image in Post-Enlightenment Life Science, 1800–2010.* Dordrecht, Heidelberg, New York, London: Springer.

Elster, M. (2022). "Insidious Concern: Trans Panic and the Limits of Care." *TSQ: Transgender Studies Quarterly,* 9(3), 407–24.

Federici, S. (2004). *Caliban and the Witch*. Brooklyn: Autonomedia.

Frankfurt, H.G. (2005). *On Bullshit*. [Online]. Princeton: Princeton University Press.

Freud, S. (1905). "Three Essays on the Theory of Sexuality." In: J. Strachey (Ed. & Trans.), *The Standard Edition of the Complete Psychological Works of Sigmund Freud (SE)* VII.

Freud, S. (1955). *Gesammelte Werke V*. London: Imago Publishing.

Freud, S. (1985). *The Complete Letters of Sigmund Freud to Wilhelm Fliess, 1887–1904*. Ed. and Trans. J. Moussaieff Masson. Cambridge: Belknap-Harvard University Press.

Garner, S.N. (1989). "Freud and Fliess: Homophobia and Seduction." In: D. Hunter (Ed.), *Seduction and Theory: Readings of Gender, Representation, and Rhetoric.* Urbana: University of Illinois Press, pp. 86–109.

Garrett, B. (2013). "Vitalism Versus Emergent Materialism", in: *Vitalism and the Scientific Image in Post-Enlightenment Life Science, 1800–2010*, edited by Normandin, S., Wolfe, CT., Berlin: Springer, p. 127.

Geller J. (1992). "(G)nos(e)ology: The Cultural Construction of the Other." In H. Eilberg-Schwartz (Ed.), *People of the Body: Jews and Judaism from an Embodied Perspective.* Albany, NY: State University of New York Press, pp. 243–282.

Geller, J. (2007). *On Freud's Jewish Body: Mitigating Circumcisions*. New York: Fordham University Press.

Gherovici P. (2010). *Please Select Your Gender: From the Invention of Hysteria to the Democratizing of Transgenderism.* New York: Routledge.

Gherovici P. (2017). *Transgender Psychoanalysis: A Lacanian Perspective on Sexual Difference.* New York: Routledge.

Gill-Peterson, J. (2018). *Histories of the Transgender Child.* Minneapolis: University of Minnesota Press.

Gilman, S. (1991). *The Jew's Body.* New York: Routledge.

Gilman, S. (1993). *Freud, Race, and Gender.* Princeton: Princeton University Press.

Gozlan, O. (2015). *Transsexuality and the Art of Transitioning: A Lacanian Approach.* London and New York: Routledge.

Gozlan, O. (Ed.) (2018). *Current Critical Debates in the Field of Transsexuality Studies – In Transition.* London and New York: Routledge.

Hansbury, G. (2017). "The Masculine Vaginal: Working With Queer Men's Embodiment at the Transgender Edge." *Journal of the American Psychoanalytic Association,* 65(6), 1009–1031.

Heaney, E. (2017). *The New Woman – Literary Modernism, Queer Theory, and the Trans Feminine Allegory.* Evanston: Northwestern University Press.

Hinchy, Jessica (2019). *Governing Gender and Sexuality In Colonial India: The Hijra, C.1850-1900.* Cambridge: Cambridge University Press.

Jolley, Nicholas (1998). *The Light of the Soul: Theories of Ideas in Leibniz, Malebranche, and Descartes,* Oxford; online edn, Oxford Academic, 1 Nov. 2003, https://doi.org/10.1093/0198238193.001.0001

Kant, I. (1900). *Gesammelte Schriften* Hrsg.: Bd. 1–22 Preussische Akademie der Wissenschaften, Bd. 23 Deutsche Akademie der Wissenschaften zu Berlin, ab Bd. 24 Akademie der Wissenschaften zu Göttingen. Berlin 1900ff. AAIV, 52.

Long Chu, A. (2018). "On Liking Women." In: *N Plus 1.* https://www.nplusonemag.com/issue-30/essays/on-liking-women/.

Menn, S. (1994). The Origins of Aristotle's Concept of Ἐνέργεια. *Ancient Philosophy* 14(1):73–114.

Namaste, V. (2000). *Invisible Lives – The Erasure of Transsexual and Transgendered People.* Chicago and London: The University of Chicago Press.

Nieder, T.O., Strauß, B., … (2019). "Geschlechtsinkongruenz, Geschlechtsdysphorie und Trans-Gesundheit: S3-Leitlinie zur Diagnostik, Beratung und Behandlung", *AWMF-Register-Nr.* [AWMF online], 138(001), Section 4.2, 29–30.

Normandin, S., Wolfe (2013). CT., "Vitalism and the Scientific Image: An Introduction", in: *Vitalism and the Scientific Image in Post-Enlightenment Life Science, 1800–2010,* edited by Normandin, S., Wolfe, CT., Berlin: Springer, p. 1.

Pellegrini, A. (1997). *Performance Anxieties: Staging Psychoanalysis, Staging Race.* New York: Routledge.

Postone, M. (1980). "Anti-Semitism and National Socialism: Notes on the German Reaction to 'Holocaust.'" *New German Critique, 19*(1), pp. 97–115.

Preciado, P. B. (2013), *Testo Junkie,* translated by Bruce Benderson, New York City: The Feminist Press.

Prosser, J. (1998). *Second Skins: The Body Narratives of Transsexuality.* New York: Columbia University Press.

Puar, J. (2017). *The Right to Maim – Debility, Capacity, Disability.* Durham and London: Duke University Press.

Raymond, J.G. (1994). *The Transsexual Empire: The Making of the She-Male.* New York: Teachers College Press. (Original work published in 1979.)

Saketopoulou, A. and Pellegrini A. (2023). *Gender Without Identity.* New York: The Unconscious in Translation.

Saleh, F. (2020). "Transgender as a Humanitarian Category: The Case of Syrian Queer and Gender-Variant Refugees in Turkey." *TSQ: Transgender Studies Quarterly*, 7(1): 37–55. https://doi.org/10.1215/23289252-7914500.

Schmidt, N. (2014, June 30). "Les ABCD de L'égalité: Un Abandon Symbolique." *Inegalites.fr.* https://www.inegalites.fr/Les-ABCD-de-l-egalite-un-abandon-symbolique.

Schraub, D. (2019). "White Jews: An Intersectional Approach." *AJS Review, 43*(2), 379–407.

Schreber, D. (2003). *Denkwürdigkeiten Eines Nervenkranken.* Munich: Kadmos.

Serano, J. (2007). *Whipping Girl – A Transsexual Woman On Sexism And The Scapegoating of Femininity.* Emerville: Seal Press.

Showalter, E. (1993). "Hysteria, Feminism, and Gender." In: *Hysteria Beyond Freud.* Oakland: University of California Press. pp. 286–344.

Sierakowski, S. (2014, January 26). "The Polish Church's Gender Problem." *New York Times.*

Snorton, R. (2017). *Black on Both Sides.* Minneapolis: University of Minnesota Press.

Sosa, L. (2021). "Beyond Gender Equality? Anti-Gender Campaigns and the Erosion of Human Rights and Democracy." *Netherlands Quarterly of Human Rights,* 39(1), 3–10.

Spivak, G.C. (1998). "Feminism and Critical Theory." In: *In Other Worlds – Essays in Cultural Politics.* London and New York: Routledge.

Spivak, G.C. (1999). *A Critique of Postcolonial Reason.* Oxford: Harvard University Press.

Steigerwald, J., (2013). "Rethinking Organic Vitality in Germany at the Turn of the Nineteenth Century." In: S. Normandin and C.T. Wolfe, *Vitalism and the Scientific Image in Post-Enlightenment Life Science, 1800–2010.* Dordrecht, Heidelberg, New York, London: Springer, p. 51.

Stone, S. (2023). "The Empire Strikes Back: A Posttranssexual Manifesto." In S. Stryker & D. McCarthy Blackston (Eds.), *The Transgender Studies Reader Remix.* London: Routledge. pp. 15–30.

Stryker, S. and Currah, P. (Eds.). (2017). *"*Transpsychoanalytics*"* [Special issue]. *Transgender Studies Quarterly,* 4(3–4).

Towle, E.B. and Morgan, L.M. (2002). "Romancing the Transgender Native: Rethinking the Use of the 'Third Gender' Concept." *GLQ: A Journal of Lesbian and Gay Studies, 8*(4), 469–497. https://www.muse.jhu.edu/article/12222.

Valentine, D. (2007). *Imagining Transgender.* Duke University Press.

Wagner, Steven J. (1984), "Descartes on the Parts of the Soul", in: *Philosophy and Phenomenological Research* Vol. 45, No. 1 (Sep., 1984), pp. 51–70 (20 pages), International Phenomenological Society, https://doi.org/10.2307/2107326.

Ward, J. (2010). "Gender Labor: Transmen, Femmes, and Collective Work of Transgression." *Sexualities,* 13(2), 236–254. https://doi-org.proxy1.library.jhu.edu/10.1177/1363460709359114.

Wark, M. (2015). *Molecular Red: Theory for the Anthropocene.* New York: Verso.

Wark, M. (2022). "Dear Cis Analysts." *Parapraxis.* https://www.parapraxismagazine.com/articles/dear-cis-analysts.

Chapter 8

Sissy Dance $1

The More and More of Gender[1]

Griffin Hansbury and Avgi Saketopoulou

In a scholarly yet playful conversation, the authors explore why analytic thought about trans remains so intransigently difficult. They propose that countertansferential responses to trans patients manifest not just in clinical work but also as blockages to psychoanalytic theorizing. They draw on extensive experience treating trans and non-binary patients, on teaching and supervisory work, and on analytic scholarship to think about why and how theorizing on trans stalls. Whereas in the social realm trans bodies are often hyper-sexualized, in metapsychology and the consulting room trans is notably desexualized. What is the cost of that and why does it occur? The authors locate the problem in the disaggregation of gender from the sexual, arguing that not only has this separation outlived its (once exigent) metapsychological utility, but that it is itself a defense against the anxiety of polymorphous perversity and psychic bisexuality that trans bodies can awaken in analysts of all genders, and especially in cisgender analysts.

AVGI SAKETOPOULOU:	We have planned to have a conversation about trans this morning, about the pressure the category of trans has put on psychoanalysis, and about the theoretical and clinical challenges it introduced. Our particular focus is on cis analysts' countertransferential anxieties when working with trans patients. But as we are sitting down to start, I am kind of wanting to bring us in from another angle, somewhat unorthodox as perhaps is most fitting when talking about non-normative experience. I am thinking of the video you posted yesterday on your social media, "Sissy Dance $1." How would you feel about using that as a starting point?
GRIFFIN HANSBURY:	Let's do it. I'm curious to see where this takes us.
AS:	Shall we describe the video for our readers? I will also link it here for whomever wants to look it up. I suspect we'll be discussing it extensively, so I hope our readers get to see it.[2]

DOI: 10.4324/9781032624129-9

GH: Last night, when biking home to the East Village in Manhattan, I noticed a person sitting on a milk crate by a pile of trash bags on the corner of St. Mark's Place, which was, until recently, a center of counterculture for several decades. She appeared to me to be trans, assigned male at birth (AMAB), middle-aged, and White, and she was dressed all in pink, in a miniskirt and tight top, with pink bows in her hair. She had a cardboard sign on which she'd written the simple offer: Sissy Dance $1. Of course I had to stop. I said hello and introduced myself, telling her that I was trans, to let her know I was family, though she didn't seem to care. I gave her two dollars, because one did not seem like enough, and then she told me to take out my camera and film her, which I did. When I asked her name, she replied, "Sissy Pussy Cunt." And then she began her dance.

AS: There is so much in what you are saying already that strikes me as significant in thinking about encounters with trans – and we haven't even talked about her dance yet. What struck me about your video per se is that it refuses everything that has to do with the dignified trans discourse, making no overture to respectability politics: it is pure queer pleasure, which is connected to the pleasure of the sexual as well. By sexual I don't refer to genital sexuality (that is, sexuality organized around genitals) per se, nor I am referring to intercourse. I am alluding to Laplanche's "sexual" (1987), a neologism in its original French that aimed to capture the polymorphousness of infantile sexuality and which Freud argued is the object of psychoanalysis (1905). (In English *sexual* is usually italicized to highlight its distinctiveness from sexuality per se.)

First, there's the exuberance – in her and in you. Some of it is in her body, in how she moves in a way that luxuriates in something, though what exactly is not clear. We know that it has to do with gender, but words fail. Perhaps clarity, as far as her performance is concerned, is not even the point. Then, I am struck that she asked for one dollar, and you gave two; there's another kind of abundance there, connected to the psychic economy of the sexual, which is not an economy of conservation but has to do with the "more and more" of experience (Saketopoulou, 2019, 2020b), a dimension of "more life" (Corbett, 2008), as opposed to the economy that psychoanalysts are usually preoccupied with, which is how to prevent things from becoming "too much" (Benjamin & Atlas, 2015).

Of course, you are not her analyst and she is not your patient. But it strikes me as interesting because in our professional conversations analysts are quite worried that the trans subject goes too far, acts impulsively and without deliberation, is too dysregulated, may be too overstimulating – that's where the respectability of the trans subject that seems otherwise well positioned comes in. That respectability is then used to institute a "proper" trans subject that gets levied against less transnormative subjects. But that's not the economical standpoint from which you join her. You join her from the opposite economical viewpoint, we might say, jumping into her over-the-topness with an over-the-topness of your own. It's that moment, I would argue, that signals to her that you are of kin, not only your formal introduction as being trans yourself. Her "more and more" does not scare or put you off.

GH: I was excited to see her. I'm writing a book about New York during the pandemic, called *Feral City* (2022), about how the city is re-wilding during this time, as "deviants" are returning to the streets after many of the hyper-normative gentrifiers fled the city in the early days of the coronavirus pandemic. (I'm using "deviant" in the sociological sense, to mean someone who violates social norms.) I moved to what was a punk-bohemian neighborhood in the early 1990s as a young queer trans person to be around other deviants, but many have been priced out or policed out, so when I see one – and one so wonderfully exuberant – it's like encountering a fellow rare bird, from my own lost world, which I've been mourning, or maybe refusing to mourn, which I think of as a kind of resistance to cultural erasure.

AS: The word "excited" with which you just started does a lot of work here, it seems to me. The issue of "excitement," as in "the body's excitability" and the notion of "excitation," has been with us since early Freud (1895, 1905). And yet, generally speaking, it remains hard for psychoanalysis to think with excitement and excitability, to think, that is, about excitability not as the failure of self-regulation but as experience's springboard, and the springboard, as well, of a range of invigorated gender positions.

So I am delighted to think about this with you in relation to Ms. Sissy Pussy Cunt and the notion of re-wilding, of wilding again. To me, this is a straight line back to Freud's *Three Essays on the Theory of Sexuality* (1905) and to the notion of polymorphous perversity. Though, perhaps, not a straight but a jagged, queer line. This forward-moving backward-time may be understood in the après-coup (Laplanche, 2017) as a movement towards more gender. Some of our colleagues seem concerned that trans epitomizes the destruction of gender (Aisenstein, 2018; Chiland, 2000), but, in fact, what we see, both inside the clinic and without, is just more of it. Perhaps it's not an accident, then, that your language, much like her body in the video, is awash in sexuality. This contrasts beautifully with another concern anxiously expressed by some colleagues (like David Bell [Blass, Bell, & Saketopoulou, 2021], Roberto D'Angelo [2020a], and Susan and Marcus Evans[2021]), that the aim of trans identity is to desexualize, to take the heat out of sexuality by turning it into the docility of identitarian politics, aka gender (Blass, Bell, & Saketopoulou, 2021).

GH: Re-wilding does involve temporality, a moving forward and then back, spiraling into a new kind of liberatory space. To be feral means to be wild (or descended from wildness) and then tamed, and then to go wild again, with the experience of having been tamed, domesticated. So, the new wildness also contains those memory traces.

When you say that trans is seen as desexualized, you're referring to the old "trans people are really homosexual" argument that, by transitioning, unhappy gays make their attractions "straight"; for example, a lesbian transitions into a straight man and is assumed to be sidestepping whatever conflicts he has about homosexuality. This argument, as you've pointed out in other conversations, omits the reality of gay and other same-sex-attracted trans people (Blass, Bell, & Saketopoulou, 2021). Not to mention the frequent phenomenon of many trans men who once identified as lesbians and then, after transition, identify as gay men, maintaining a same-sex object choice, but on the flipside. (Trans people who identify as gay/lesbian before and after transition, where the sex/gender of the desired other flips, enable us to think about homo, the sameness of homosexuality, as the exciting factor here, an unexplored angle on the phenomenon. But I can also imagine the analyst who interprets that shift as a maneuver to make heterosexual genital sex manageable.) Instead of desexualizing, I think you and I see trans as an experience that often expands the sexual possibilities, so I'm curious why, in your opinion, some analysts see trans as "taking the heat out of sexuality."

AS: I think it has to do with how identity can work to leech out sexuality by coming to rest on rigid forms that no longer permit drive movements. An understanding of oneself that is singular and inflexible can organize someone in excessively bound, rigid ways. I think we all see this in our practices with cisgender patients and I have seen it in trans patients as well. I don't see it as a property of transness per se, though. In fact, because we live in a transphobic culture, trans people are oftentimes put in the position of having to produce fortified self-narrativizations, to present self-understandings to the clinicians on whom they rely for care (including medical care) that are durable over time and which presume a "core" gender identity. Trans patients are expected to tell their stories over and over again, and in the same way, as proof of the validity of their existence. Psychoanalysis makes those demands too, though it does so more implicitly. Certainly, Ms. Sissy Pussy Cunt's engagement with you sidesteps those snares; she delights in showing you her body, a sexually gendered body perhaps because she senses you place no such demand on her. And she is quite sexual in her flirtatious enticements of you. We see both the sexual and sexuality in her performance.

That part of the video actually made me want to ask you about a particular decision you made. Sissy Pussy Cunt is partly dressed in her underwear, inviting us to look at her genital area; and your camera lens does not avoid it. At times, it even makes it the focus point. It seemed to me that that's something worth thinking about because a focus on a trans person's genitals can be problematic in an objectifying sense. This is especially the case when genital morphology (by birth or surgery) is used as supportive (or disproving) of the person's "real" gender (Salamon, 2014). Analysts are especially anxious, I find, about the trans body in this way. As if the body holds the final verdict on gender. But in your filming of Sissy Pussy Cunt, you don't go to the genitals as a way of confirming or disconfirming her gender, you are not looking for evidence supporting her claim, you go there in another vein. A more sexual vein it seems to me. Can you say a bit about that decision?

GH: Sissy Pussy Cunt's dance was certainly sexual; she was getting off on performing for me and my camera. She was moving her hips quite a bit and I understood this was an important part of our exchange and that she was requesting my focus to include this part of her body. I felt excited by the surprise of her, this unusual, bold, and joyful creature who'd suddenly appeared in my orbit, as if from the past. Such an appearance doesn't happen very often. The affective landscape of New York City, and formerly countercultural neighborhoods like mine, in particular, has been tamed, domesticated, over-policed both formally by the actual police and informally by hyper-normative bodies that discipline those of us who might step out of line. They perform as straightening devices, to use a term from the queer feminist theorist Sara Ahmed (2006). So here was someone defying that device. She was absolutely queer, a crooked line, delighted by herself and by delighting me. For others, she might stimulate anxiety and, because of that, the police will likely shoo her off the corner. What is being shooed away in that act? What is it that people are being protected from? I'm thinking of the disorientation that many analysts have described when working with trans patients, a bodily anxiety that feels like falling out of gender and the ground giving way (Hansbury, 2017b). It can happen even before the patient walks into the consulting room for the first session. The presence of a trans body isn't necessary for the anxiety to start. Just the idea of a trans body is enough to set that cascade of anxiety in motion – and I suspect the mystery of trans genitalia is part of that tumult. What do you think is happening there?

AS: I would think that one factor is the anxiety that comes up for many cis analysts around the challenge trans patients pose to the binary (Posadas, 2018). And as you (2017b) and Jack Pula (2015) have also suggested, I suspect that some envy, perhaps, arises for the cis analyst. We see in our literature that analysts oftentimes have a fantasy that the trans patient gets to have it all, that trans individuals are trying to inhabit both genders, and that their very trans-ness marks their unwillingness to relinquish and/or inability to mourn. Kubie's extremely influential paper "The Drive to Become Both Sexes" (1972) made some of these claims, and Corbett (2011) has very beautifully countered them. Kubie's paper was written a long time ago, but I routinely hear such ideas when I present on trans or supervise colleagues today. Personally, I have not found this to be true clinically. Trans patients have to contend with mourning all kinds of things. My experience leads me to hear the idea that trans patients don't have to mourn as having more to do with the cis analyst's fantasy than anything else.

But, and this is very much along the lines of what we've been thinking with in relation to your video, I think that trans patients also introduce a disturbance on another level: they disturb, in the sense of agitating, not just gender but also sexuality. Their polymorphousness, the fact that their bodies are not expectable but may surprise, can stir up sexual affect. The much commented on preoccupation cis people have with trans persons' bodies is not just a gendered concern but also, and perhaps primarily, a sexual one. I have always been surprised that that is not discussed more in our literature.

GH: What I understand you saying is that in the presence of the trans body, with its perhaps unknowable genitals, some unpermissible sexual feeling or desire will arise in the cis person who is preoccupied; in this case, the analyst. The trans body is experienced as destabilizing the sexuality of the analyst; for example, lesbian cisgender analysts have discussed the concern that they might be attracted to formerly lesbian-identified patients who transition to male (Suchet, 2011), and straight cisgender male analysts have described a similar concern when working with trans women (Torres, 1996). What would such attractions mean for the stability of the analyst's sexuality – and gendered position?

AS: An erotic countertransference to a trans patient could certainly stand to scramble the analyst's sexual orientation per se. If a cis female analyst becomes attracted to a trans female patient, does that make her gay? We can imagine several such permutations that unsettle an analyst's "stable" sense of hetero- or homosexual orientation. Perhaps this is one reason why we hear about so many different types of countertransferential responses to trans analysands but we don't, at least not yet, have much writing on erotic transferences/countertransferences in trans/cis analysands-analyst dyads.

But I am not only thinking about sexual orientation per se. The very many thoughts analysts entertain, and are oftentimes fixated on, about trans patients' bodies – for example, has the patient had genital surgery, what kinds of medical interventions have they had, how has that changed their body morphology, etc. – that brush up against the sexual, are also, it seems to me, laced with the erotic. In some way, they all function as incitements to think about a gendered sexual. Here's an example: a few years ago, I presented to an audience of analysts my work with a trans girl. My seven-year-old patient had never shared with me that she was trans; I can't go into the details in depth here but she "revealed" it to me by lifting her skirt in a session to "expose" her "bulge" to me (see Saketopoulou, 2014). Such a gesture certainly gives an analyst a lot to think about. In the Q&A a colleague asked me whether the patient's genital was erect when she lifted her skirt; to me that query, however it's arrived at theoretically, conveys a sexual charge. In other words, the question appears as if it's a question about the child's eroticism (which is not an invalid query), but fails to ask after the countertransference of the person asking it. Is the analyst's own infantile sexuality stirred up? To be thinking about the patient's genitals and their state of tumescence is de facto erotically charged (Dimen, personal communication, 2015). How could it not be? This would be an entirely uncontroversial statement to make in the case of a cis patient (i.e., if an analyst was wondering if her patient had an erection, we would also be wondering what the analyst's affective relationship to thinking of her patient's erection might be). But it seems to me that when it comes to our gender-diverse patients' bodies, it is hard to think of the analyst's questions as also being about sexual reverie. In the case I was discussing there is, of course, the additional prohibition of a child's sexual body since my patient was so young. But I have seen this scotoma happen with adult trans patients as well.

GH: From that perspective, it's the analyst who is "taking the heat out."

AS: Exactly. When I supervise work with trans patients, for example, I find that it's oftentimes the analyst who can't allow herself to think, for example, about erotic countertransference in a cis-trans dyad. I wonder if you have noticed that as well.

GH: It's certainly been absent in my supervision with cis clinicians who work with trans patients. My thoughts turn to the ways that trans people, in the wider culture outside psychoanalysis, are often treated as sexually nonviable and therefore nonthreatening; although this might mostly apply to the treatment of trans men, while trans women have been depicted, certainly in the media, as sexual threats. I don't think the cisgender psyche, to vastly oversimplify, knows what to do with trans people and sex.

Your question also makes me think about some of the responses to my paper on the masculine vaginal (2017a), which is about a cisgender gay male patient who, in sexual play and fantasy, refers to his anus with the words *pussy* or *cunt*. One of the repeating responses I get to the paper when I present it to analytic audiences is the question: is the patient fantasizing about having a vagina or does he really think he has a vagina? And the question always stumps me. It feels like the wrong question.

AS: I don't know if this is what you have in mind, but having been present at times you've been asked this question, it's felt like a foreclosure of some sort of thinking about what your patient is trying to do with his "cunt," as opposed to whether he can test reality vis-à-vis his anatomy. This is actually very connected to what we've just been discussing because what your patient wanted to do with his "cunt" was very sexual.

GH: Right, the question arrives like a thud, the slamming of a lid on a boiling pot. To extend the heat metaphor. My own thoughts shut down whenever this question is asked and I find it difficult to think.

AS: The insistence on whether your patient was fantasizing about his anus as a vagina or really thought he had a vagina reminds me of what Winnicott advises us regarding transitional space, namely that we do not "challenge the baby to… answer to the question: did you create that or did you find it?" (1969, p. 713). He taught us that trying to situate the creative gesture on either side of the reality divide is to concretize, even squash it. This squashing seems to me to relate to another countertransferential problem that many analysts struggle with, which is that we can become unimaginatively concrete in the presence of a trans body. Here's an example from our literature: in a recent paper, an analyst working with a transmasculine (assigned female at birth [AFAB]) patient insists on using the word "vagina" to refer to the patient's genitals even as the patient protests that usage (D'Angelo, 2020). To the analyst, the word "vagina" is not gendered (that is, he does not understand himself as doing gendered violence to his patient) but an anatomically correct one. Such naming, this analyst writes, establishes that the dyad will speak truthfully, and in so doing, will refuse the patient's efforts to "control" the analyst's mind. The patient, as anyone who has sat with a trans patient would expect, is made quite uncomfortable by the analyst's unyielding insistence.

To me there is a perplexing concreteness in the analyst's decision, almost as if it is word choice itself rather than the long and arduous work of analysis that will underwrite how the treatment proceeds vis-à-vis "reality."

GH: When I read the paper to which you're referring, I identified with the patient and felt his discomfort, having been myself on the receiving end of a cisgender analyst's need for certainty and "reality." Trans people are often accused of being overly concrete when it comes to gender – we reify gender, acting out on the physical substance of the body (Bell, 2020) – but so many trans people (dare I say all, when you scratch the surface?) occupy a much more fluid relationship to the body than might be readily apparent, including those who identify as binary.

It's the analyst's preoccupation with genital "reality" that constricts the analyst's thinking space, as you point out, and yet it's often the transgender patient who is blamed for that constriction, which some analysts experience as control and coercion. D'Angelo's patient, like many transmasculine, AFAB patients, asks that they both use the word "genitals" instead of "vagina" for that part of his body, but D'Angelo experiences this as "complying with pressure" from the patient. He describes feeling "cornered" and censored by what he calls the patient's "autocratic control of what could be spoken," coerced into perpetuating "what seemed like a deceptive agreement that his genitals were not what they were."

This mirrors the current discourse around trans in the wider culture, especially in the United States and Britain, in which some cisgender people describe feeling controlled and censored by transpeople, forced to perpetuate what they think are falsehoods about trans bodies and genders, i.e., that they are coerced into accepting trans women as women and trans men as men, and therefore should be permitted in single-sex spaces, like public restrooms, that best fit their identities. The whole controversy seems to come down to who gets to define reality itself, and the cisgender anxiety, once again, lands on the trans person's genitals, most anxiously on the transfeminine penis, which gets cast as a sexually dangerous and uncontrollable object that should not be permitted access to female spaces. In both of these scenarios, it's the cisgender person who is concretizing the trans person's experience of gender, over focusing on the "reality" of the body, i.e., thinking something like: he looks like a man but he's really a woman and you can call it a genital but it really is a vagina. Do you think this hang-up comes down to language? So much of it gets presented as a fight for the freedom of speech.

AS: It has certainly been discussed this way in the literature. I am thinking of Jill Gentile's recent paper where she puts it this way: "Freedom of speech… [is] the freedom for all subjects to be included in a robust speech community in which the eruptive movement of desire, the improvisatory action of libido, can be sustained without collapse into fixed ideas, vicious binaries, or ideologically confining gender categories" (2020, p. 179). The argument oftentimes becomes the hot potato of who is being overly concrete (Pellegrini & Saketopoulou, 2019). As you noted, the charge is that it's the trans subject who concretizes the space afforded by fantasy and by psychic bisexuality by shutting down multiplicity, i.e., by transitioning medically instead of holding down the fort of psychic bisexuality *in fantasy*. This idea that multiplicity is to be upheld only in the domain of the symbolic is what I appreciate in this part of Gentile's thinking. We need to put pressure on the idealization of the symbolic, because symbolic economies are not equitably distributed across different subjects and those who are marginalized are always already left outside the symbolic order. The symbolic, in other words, is always already imbricated in normativity, it issues from what has already been imagined, lived, psychically represented. To be able to "think trans," "do trans," and "work with trans" individuals psychoanalysis needs to journey outside its usual borders and to use, and craft, tools beyond those already at our disposal. Analysts who worry that their freedom of speech or of thinking is constricted by the mere existence of trans patients seem to be reacting exactly to that need for novelty, except that this need for expansion is defensively experienced as a form of being controlled.

This is not what I saw in your video, and why it so delighted me. Ms. Sissy Pussy Cunt, in her own performance and as she is delivered to us by your gaze, encompasses possibilities too varied and too rich to make it through the bottleneck of psychoanalysis's conventional symbolic thinking and of binary psychic representation.

GH: There are other ways that I, or another person encountering her, could have responded to her. When I asked her name and she said Sissy Pussy Cunt, I could have rejected that and insisted on knowing her "real" name.

AS: By "real," you mean the name by which she calls herself, right? Instead of Ms. Sissy Pussy Cunt?

GH: Yes, I mean her everyday name, maybe not her legal name, but the one her friends call her by. I've been on the receiving end of such demands many times, both as a trans person, of course, where it is too often an unfortunate inevitability, and also as a person assumed to be cisgender. For many years I have written about New York City under the pen name Jeremiah Moss, and for ten of those years I did not disclose my everyday name – I don't say "real" because a pen name is also real. I found that people generally had two non-neutral reactions to my choice to maintain privacy. Many so enjoyed the mystery of not knowing my full identity, they did not want to know. Knowing, they told me, might spoil the fun. Others, however, were bothered by it. They seemed to feel entitled to know what they called my "real" name, and my refusal to disclose it stimulated hostility in them, along with the suspicion that I must be hiding something criminal. They could not play with me; it wasn't fun at all for them. They had to have "reality" – and to get it, they felt a need to invade me.

One journalist for a very powerful newspaper went so far as to send the question to the paper's research department. They triangulated a few pieces of biographical information I had shared, searching through voter registration and birth records, until they found my identity. Discovering nothing actually criminal, they dropped the matter. The journalist, who seemed shaken by what transpired, told me that the level of scrutiny I received was equal to the way they would treat a mass murderer. He said it was as if I'd "walked into a movie theater and shot it up with an automatic weapon."

AS: It is so interesting to hear about the level of anxiety this "not knowing" generated, the threat it seemed to mushroom into, and how that sent him down the path of a search for "truth."

GH: What, exactly, is the imagined threat? And this had nothing to do with my being trans – it was about having another, private name that I chose not to disclose. Trans people do have other, private, less than easily knowable/thinkable parts, whether those parts are names, or genitals, or experiences of gender and sex, that aren't obviously accessible and legible. So, we get the transphobic trope of the transgender pretender, the trans person who is seen as deceiving the cis person, tricking them into queer sex with the "wrong" body. Maybe analysts, too, feel tricked into feeling what they don't want to feel with trans patients. In the general culture, this dangerous way of thinking about trans has too often led to cis violence, including the murder of trans people, overwhelmingly the murder of trans women by men who claim to feel deceived. On the other hand, there are people who enjoy not knowing, or at least don't feel threatened and enraged by it.

Maybe it comes down to the capacity for negative capability. Recently, a patient – who is queer, but not trans – gently pushed back on a line of inquiry I was pursuing. Sensing my need to know, to understand a connection between her past and her present, she told me, "Being okay with not knowing is a decolonizing gesture." I liked that and it has stayed with me, including its inverse, that not being okay with not knowing can be a colonizing gesture, an urge to put the self into the other, and to thereby replace the other. I'm interested in what motivates the people who don't just want to know, but who demand to know, and who insist that knowing is essential. And, for that matter, even possible.

AS: This demand to know is, from a psychoanalytic viewpoint as well, problematic; it prioritizes the analyst's preoccupation with mastering the other over genuine curiosity. And it can have a totalizing effect. To me, the wish to "know" is not problematic if held gingerly, as a "wish" that could generate a curiosity that is supple, a querying that can follow the path the other travels as opposed to forcing one to take the particular path the demand to "know" imposes. What you are speaking about is something that resembles more an authoritarian impulse: knowing here works more like possessing, like a conquering that does away with the strange (Davis & Dean, 2022), in the other and in oneself. It's easy to see how that can then galvanize an insistence on "truth," "truth" being what one possesses and can then impose on the other. It could be a word, for example, that inscribes reality (like, D'Angelo's "vagina"), the body's material surface (the "women-born-women" argument we hear in some transphobic feminist discourses), or what's written on a birth certificate.

What you are saying is that one's own creation is also worth dignifying with "truth status," something that we should expect psychoanalysts would know better than anyone else perhaps.

This returns me to Winnicott's urging that we not ask the baby "did you create that or did you find it?" The question is itself a cold shower to the process of play. Your not asking Ms. Sissy Pussy Cunt her "real name," your not insisting on identity or pronouns since they don't preoccupy her, is not because you disrespect her, but precisely because of your valuation of her. This includes how you are receiving her sexual effervescence, something that I think analysts are especially anxious about with trans patients. We may even say that her gender is not something you tolerate or accept, but something you participate in. Gender, for Ms. Sissy Pussy Cunt, and for us all, is not a property of the subject but something that materializes in the space between us and others, both personal and relational. In your video of you and Ms. Sissy Pussy Cunt, gender is what happens in the space between her performance and your recording.

GH: I was thinking of Winnicott, too, specifically the Squiggle Game, when we were talking about names. Do you keep the play going or do you foreclose it?

AS: That's so succinctly and crisply put. Thank you for that. The question would be: how does the analyst keep the play going rather than drag her own "reality" into it, which can often shut the play down.

GH: After her dance, I asked Sissy Pussy Cunt (I notice, by the way, that you're adding "Ms." when you mention her) about her pronouns. She said, "I like female pronouns, but I don't make a big deal out of it. I mean, it's obvious anyway, isn't it?"

AS: That's an interesting observation, about my sometimes calling her Ms.

GH: I wondered where it came from, if you were being respectful by giving her a title, if you felt the need to elevate her.

AS: I think of Ms. Sissy Pussy Cunt as more campy, as an additional layer.

GH: The once-famous line from Janet Jackson's song "Nasty" comes to mind, where she says, "My first name ain't baby, it's Janet. Miss Jackson if you're nasty." Actually, in my memory of how you addressed Sissy Pussy Cunt, I thought you called her Miss.

AS: What could that have meant? Miss as opposed to Ms. – I am curious where your thoughts go.

GH: There's the slippery elision of letters, as the title Miss is so close to the word Sissy, but I also think Miss, as a youthful title, better suits her playful girlishness, like little Miss Muffet in the nursery rhyme, sitting on her tuffet of sidewalk trash, uncensored and unrestrained. This brings us back to the feral, queer child of polymorphous perversity.

Miss Sissy Pussy Cunt is doing gender raw and unprocessed, she's not learning about it from *Ms.* magazine, she doesn't try to fit in with respectability politics.

Since my associations went to Miss Muffet, I have to say something about spiders. I've long been fascinated by spider phobias and the way they've historically been interpreted by psychoanalysis as representations of queer genders and sexualities, penis and vagina blended together in a single genital object (the phallic legs, the mother's hair-covered vulva); the spider is often said to represent a confusion of eroticized body parts (nipple is penis, mouth is vagina, and vice versa), as well as bisexuality, the primal scene, and cross-gender wishes (Sperling, 1971). Spiders then are very transgender – and very creative. In the nursery rhyme, the spider doesn't do anything aggressive. It simply comes along and sits down beside Miss Muffet. In vintage illustrations, the spider is often drawn as a friendly character, doffing a top hat in greeting. It is saying, "hello." Maybe it wants to play. But Little Miss Muffet is frightened away. I bet the spider wouldn't scare Miss Sissy Pussy Cunt, who wears her own spideriness openly on her body.

That's a bit of a digression, but it makes me think of what we've been talking about here, about the way some cisgender analysts need to assert the "reality" of the genital, to state this is a vagina and nothing else, denying the spidery, shape-shifty malleability of transgender – and much queer – embodiment. It's a vagina and a penis and a vagipenis and a penigina, or whatever unnamed, neo-named, yet-to-be-named shape it takes, symbolically, for the trans person who lives with it and in it. Of course, this can be frightening for those (trans and cis) who see only the spider's monstrousness and not its creativity. Can the fear be felt and named? Or will the observer/analyst defensively hold tight to their tuffet, their piece of ground, that which grounds them?

AS: I like what you say about the neo-named body parts, and about how that can be frightening. The term reminds me of McDougall's work on neo-sexualities (1986), sexualities that would otherwise seem perverse but which are, instead, inventive solutions. But this neo-naming is also a risk isn't it? In the sense that if something can be renamed, it means its meaning is malleable, which endangers our previous understandings of it and the ways they grounded us. We can see how such a crisis point can be responded to not with curious or delighted receptivity but concretely, by a swooping in (for example, the insistence on "vagina") that aims to restabilize. "Reality" can then be the promised, orienting North Star that promises to shake anxious analysts out of transitional, play space and onto "solid" ground. In the short run it's organizing, but in the long run it's a disappointing way out of the disquiet.

Talking about rigidity and malleability, I was also wondering if we might think together about what's come to be referred to as "detransitioning," the term used for someone who transitions and then, for varied reasons "returns" to their original gender assignment.

GH: Yes, let's. What are you thinking about there?

AS: There are burgeoning conversations about detransitioning at the moment, about what drives it, and an emphasis on developing ways of anticipating who might detransition. For many analysts, I find, much countertransferential anxiety is staked on the fear that the patient will regret their transition. And, further, that this regret was preventable, caused by the analyst's failure to sufficiently probe and analyze what anxious analysts see as the patient's "gender conflict." If the dyad had done that work, the argument goes, and the dynamic issues had been properly addressed, the need for transition would have been eclipsed and the person would have been spared the back and forth.

My clinical experience tells me that there are many reasons why people detransition, that it's not a singular phenomenon. But I also find that many analysts are very (perhaps overly) concerned about their patients deciding to transition in case they later discover that they have taken the wrong path and have to retrace their steps, some of which may not be medically reversible. I am not minimizing the complexity of such possibilities but want to note that other decisions that patients routinely make during the course of a long analysis, like, for example, whom the patient marries, or whether they'll have children, are also very consequential and irreversible, but are not met with the same level of regulatory anxiety (Corbett, 2011) in the analyst. Of course, we sometimes feel that a patient is choosing a problematic partner, or is not ready to have children, etc., but we don't tend to regard it as our responsibility to foretell if the patient is heading in the "right" direction, we do not imagine ourselves to have at our disposal such powers of prediction. Certainly, when the patient divorces or their kid suffers we don't see it as a failure of the analysis per se. When it comes to trans though, the stakes seem to feel different to many analysts, as if the analyst's job is now more concretely oriented towards a "good outcome." When colleagues consult with me on patients who are considering transitioning, they are often relieved to hear me tell them that the question of whether the patient should or should not transition is not a responsibility they can reasonably take on.

GH: Right. We don't hear about analysts having this level of anxiety about hetero- and gender-normative decisions like marriage and pregnancy, experiences that irrevocably change one's life and, in the case of pregnancy, one's body, and that also involve decisions about the lives and bodies of other people. If any major life choice would benefit from analysis beforehand, it's the choice to bring a vulnerable, completely dependent new human into one's care. So why are the stakes so much higher when it comes to a trans individual's transition? Not that this isn't a major decision – it certainly is, and has to be weighed with thoughtfulness – but why the extra charge?

And why do many analysts imagine we have the power – and that we should have the power – to know what is "right," and to safeguard the patient from making a decision they will later regret? I think about the linear structure of the concept of detransition, the formulation that a patient moves into and through transition, from point A to point B, and then, feeling regret, returns back to point A. But what if, in many cases, so-called detransition is not so linear, and does not move backwards, but forwards into some other gendered/sexed landing place? I'm thinking here about patients assigned female at birth who go on testosterone and then go off, and then maybe on again, who are trying to find a comfortable gender spot in which to land. Many don't describe their going off testosterone, or retaking feminine or non-binary pronouns, as going backwards. They describe it as arriving at some place new – a place that, by the way, may shift again, as gender experience can do throughout life.

AS: Indeed, I have some patients too who seem to be working something out in these movements. There is also, of course, the fantasy in the background that one will land on a single gender "outcome," but what if gender is not something we coagulate, but something that can be in constant evolution? What would it mean if, as analysts, we tried to track and understand what gender movements mean or try to do, rather than become so wedded to the gender category itself and where it lands?

I don't want to trivialize the sense of responsibility that comes with clinical work, or to diminish the depth of anxiety that some analysts experience in working with trans patients. To some degree, a feeling of responsibility for our patients is unavoidable in our profession. And certainly, working with gender has some particularities that, in my opinion, require a particular knowledge base and countertransference attentiveness, which adds further difficulties to clinical work, which is hard as it is. I do wonder, though, if clinicians have not accepted too easily and too uncritically the role of gatekeeper that has been assigned to us by the medical establishment. I am not referring here only to the matter of writing letters for hormone therapy or for medical interventions. I am also asking if we have not too readily accepted the charge to "know" the patient's gender correctly, when all we can ever really do is accompany our patients on a journey one dimension of which is gender's vicissitudes.

GH: I definitely think the imposition of the role of gatekeeper, which comes from the requirement to write letters in support of a patient's starting hormones or having gender-confirming surgery, exerts a tremendous force on clinicians, myself included. In essence, the letter requires us to state that we know, i.e., know the patient's "true" gender, know that the patient's decision is correct, know that the patient won't feel regret. That concrete object, the official letter, an attestation with our name printed on it, like a contract, doesn't it strike the charge to "know"? Years ago, I thought I'd gotten around that pressure by crafting a letter that establishes informed consent instead of stating a diagnosis of gender dysphoria, and that worked for a while, doctors accepted it without question; but then health insurance companies got into the game and started requiring a diagnosis, which is another way of saying, "I know." I provide such letters in service of my patients' needs, but it makes me uneasy. How can I possibly know what the future holds for any patient decision, whether it's transition, marriage, pregnancy, career change, whatever? I cannot protect any of my patients from feeling loss and regret.

That said, the desire to protect our transitioning patients from making the "wrong" decision doesn't belong only to cisgender analysts. I also feel the anxiety of needing to know, to be certain, and to protect my trans patients from regret. I have two patients at the moment, both AFAB, both just starting testosterone and contemplating top surgery. With one, I don't feel this anxiety, and with the other, I do. I keep asking myself: what is the difference? The first one was already identifying as male when he started working with me, while the other was identifying as female when we began, and I think it's likely that I became attached to the female identity of this patient and that I am having trouble letting it go. My own feelings of loss are getting stimulated as they (the patient is currently using they/them pronouns) transition into a shape I cannot yet – and admittedly feel some resistance to – imagine, though I am working on that.

AS: Noticing this attachment to your patient's female gender seems important, important in the sense of your being able to observe it in yourself, to track your own response. In some utopian universe, we hear all material in a disinvested way, some analysts would argue; but this is rarely, if ever, possible, true, or even desirable. In your practice, how do you work with an observation of this sort? I mean, now that you've registered that you have an investment in your patient's female identity what do you do with it clinically?

GH: I am working on making space in my mind for this patient's boy self, to imagine him coming into being. You've written about the importance of mentalizing the trans patient (Saketopoulou, 2014), and that is how I think of it. Simultaneously, I'm also saying goodbye to the young woman I've spent years working with – and the way I felt and experienced myself in relation to that young woman, which has to do with how I experience and express my own gender. Here I don't mean, necessarily, the young woman who sat before me session after session, but the young woman I thought of in my mind when I thought of this patient, the young woman who occupied a space in my mind, space that intersects with time, moving back in the past and forward into the future. Isn't this the way a parent thinks of their child, holding both past and future? Can I allow the new shape of this patient to take up that occupation? Can they (or he) also coexist in my mind spatiotemporally, across time and space?

This patient, too, has a complicated and conflicted investment in what we're calling their girl part. We're in that together right now, talking about this girl part and what she's experiencing as the patient moves further into their transition. Does the girl want to go along for this ride? Does she have other desires and feelings that are not aligned with transition? Is she someone who can or should be mourned? This patient can tolerate that exploration and is open to exploring it. They can ask themself questions like, "Is my desire to transition related to some internalized misogyny?" We can wonder together if transition is a way to separate psychically from their mother, to assert a necessary boundary, and then we can ask the question, "So what if it is?" So what if transition is doing a lot of important psychic and relational work that is not specifically about gender?

AS: I think I know the kind of process you are talking about. And I am appreciative of your bringing the analyst's mourning, not just the patient's, into our conversation. I am thinking of Loewald (1960) here who writes very evocatively about what the parent imagines, and makes room for, in their child. That imagining has to be held gingerly, to enable exploration rather than constrict it. And I am also thinking of the many helpful interventions from queer authors (for example, Stockton, 2009) who urge us to think about what happens when the parent imagines in a direction that is gendered differently than what the child becomes.

We could track that thread further, but I also want to pick up on the very difficult and complex questions you are exploring with your patient: the relationship between their trauma and gender. It makes me think of a patient of mine who has been recently wondering if their gender's formation is related to their sexual trauma history, and how. And if so, what, if anything, does that mean about their gender experience? These are very sensitive matters, which I feel can be tackled helpfully in our work, as seems to be the case in yours with your patient, because these lines of inquiry have arisen in the patient organically out of our work, they don't come from the analyst's theory or personal investment in the patient's gender being this or that. I suspect that for your patient too, the question, "What does this have to do with my mother?" (a preeminently psychoanalytic question, I might add) can be explored without the patient feeling defensive because you are not jumping on it too quickly, and because they don't need to be worried that you'll quickly then rally around trying to "fix" their gender, to restore it to some imagined "originary" state. The question "What if there is a connection between your mother/your sexual assault and how your gender has morphed?" is a very capacious one if it's arrived at by the patient through the work and not pressed on the patient by the analyst. What this also means is that the analyst needs to relate to it as a question rather than as a conclusion.

GH: Right, the patient knows, or maybe senses, that our goal is not to "cure" them of being trans and that capaciousness is felt and trusted enough that it can provide room for many questions that might not otherwise be askable.

With this patient, I've also been noticing, as we go further into our exploration, that they are experiencing what might be examples of a kind of – I'll call it transgender après-coup –looking back and understanding afterward that they were having trans experiences in childhood that they did not, at the time, think of as trans, or think much about at all, perhaps because these experiences were unthinkable, and that only now, through the lens of their current understanding, can be known. For example, they're remembering feeling childhood discomfort when wearing a dress, or telling their mother, "I'm really a boy," or fantasizing about male names in secret. These were not previously disclosed in our treatment and the patient recalls them now with a sense of wonder and relief. They have a kind of "filling in the blanks" feeling.

In the current discourse around what's being called rapid onset gender dysphoria (ROGD), parents and clinicians are concerned about adolescent AFABs identifying as male and transitioning without any apparent history of cross-gender expression. The majority of the parents in the original study (Littman, 2018) said their child's coming out as trans came "out of the blue without significant prior evidence of gender dysphoria" (p. 11). The parents remember female children who loved wearing bikinis and makeup and engaging in princess play, and they don't remember these children refusing to wear dresses or wanting to play with boys' toys. Part of that might be a blind spot on the part of the parents, for sure, but part might also reside in this unthinkability of the gender dysphoria and desire. These are some questions I'm playing with, wondering about, because I'm also curious about patients who don't recall dysphoria in childhood and yet come to identify as trans, with or without adult-onset gender dysphoria.

AS: I think this is a really fascinating matter. I am also very interested in psychic time and the workings of the après-coup in particular. Certainly, in some instances someone looks back and realizes that their gender complexity was always there, deferred to the future and discoverable only in looking back because it was so prohibited in real time by the parent who didn't want to know (see the Pellegrini discussion in Garfinkle et al., 2019). But I have recently also become interested in another way of thinking about this question: if only so much of the unconscious makes it through the bottleneck of representation, and if what becomes represented can take only a certain number of forms (what is already available in the socius; Aulagnier, 1975), might it be possible that as the world gets bigger and new forms of translational possibilities become available to us, gender may be stitched anew through the workings of the après-coup (Saketopoulou, 2020a)?

In this way of thinking, gender is not a "true core" that was there all along but which could nevertheless not be discovered or permitted in one's childhood because of parental or social prohibition. Neither is it a futural possibility that enlarged social freedoms afford us in the sense that one can just select more genders in the way neoliberalism promises a richer array of gender choices. Gender is, instead, a translational form, a way of crafting a self (though here, too, words fail; by "crafting" I am not referring to a conscious "choice" of one's gender but to an unconscious process). Under certain conditions – i.e., certain crises of representation if you will (Scarfone, 2015) – these stable forms of who we understand ourselves to be, for example, our gender, can come undone. This is a putting of oneself in question. This state, unsteadied and unsteadying, is succeeded by a redoing of identity, which, in all likelihood, will also be a neo-doing, a doing differently. This neo-doing, of course, will be knitted through new translational materials that have emerged in the interim (between the first identity and the second), stimulated by new "sexual ideas," as Laplanche called them (2017). One such example is the developing discourse on trans and the proliferating conversations around different gendered possibilities. The new genders arrived at in this neo-doing would not be "genuine" or "true" (as in, "I was always trans but didn't know it" or "I was always trans but couldn't be out"), but new constructions, which would ideally work better than the older ones. By saying that a newly arrived at gender would not be "genuine" or "true," I am not suggesting the new gender would be fake or false – at least no more than any gender is also not "true" or "genuine," including, and perhaps especially, cis genders that understand themselves as being "natural." I am saying, rather, that it would be an idiomatic concoction, which also heavily leans on the cultural surround's updated gendered possibilities. What can make the gender one arrives at – as opposed, say, to one that is assigned to us at birth – feel prized may not be the gender position itself (whether one is trans or femme or twink), but the fact that it's been arrived at on one's own, that it's a personal construction crafted by the subject herself. We can imagine many dynamic scenarios where that kind of agency could feel critical.

This way of mapping temporality onto gender would permit us, it seems to me, to take into account all the rapidly shifting discourses around gender, including the developing medical, hormonal, and digital technologies that seem to envelop it, while also retaining space for personal freedom. Detransitioning could then be seen as a new neodoing, as yet a new translation, rather than as one that seeks to correct a previously failed one, a shedding of a second skin of sorts that no longer works, rather than as a failed experiment from which one has to backtrack. What comes after detransitioning is not a return to the "original" gender, but a new gender. Laplanche (though not in reference to gender specifically) insists that evolutions of this sort are not about coming full circle back to a starting point, but about moving in three dimensions, in a spiral (2017).

GH: And perhaps also in the fourth dimension of time as well. In this conceptualization of stitching gender anew in the workings of the après-coup, I hear you offering a way out, for both analyst and patient – a way out of the anxiety we've been talking about, a way out of the sense of failure, the regret discourse, and what is often framed as an inevitable gender catastrophe.

Viewed through this lens of detransition as a new translation and not a mistake, individuals who transition and then alter their course would not be doomed to experience that alteration as failure, with all its attendant self-loathing and disaster. When gender is unleashed from concrete truth, we are free not to "know" it, in the sense of certainty; we can, instead, move with it.

The idea of new translational materials offers an alternative to the "social contagion" model put forth by Littman (2018) and taken up by many others, including psychoanalysts, to explain why, at this moment in history, we're witnessing an increasing number of young people opting to transition, especially young people assigned female at birth, a population with numbers that have historically lagged behind trans people assigned male at birth. This increase may be alarming to some, but perhaps should not be surprising in a time of rapidly developing new sexual ideas and gendered possibilities – ideas and possibilities that invite and permit new genders that are not organized around traditional binaries and do not follow the old linearities, i.e., do not necessarily progress from A to B and then stop, as if the stopping place of male or female, man or woman, could ever be stable.

AS: I really like your phrasing, to be free to not know gender, to decolonize gender as your patient framed it. This is another way of thinking of gender as fluid, not fluid in the sense of hovering between the masculine/female dipole, but fluid over time and not necessarily even having a final destination. No translation, after all, ever does. Which translations and genders will survive, and how they will fare, is something that can be determined only after the fact. This way of looking at gender can help shake the anxiety of "mistaken" transition, to move us more towards thinking about evolutive processes. To me, gender is always best understood as propositional, a translation always subject to further breakdowns and reformulations.

GH: This all brings my thoughts back to where we began in our conversation, with re-wilding and the feral, the temporal, spiraling movement of going forward and then back, from wild to tame and then to another kind of wild, in which the "back" is actually forward, into a space that remembers and retains something of the middle space that was passed through. Without equating one position with "tame" and the other with "wild," without even declaring two opposite positions (language, once again, fails us), could we imagine some detransitioners as occupying, potentially, feral genders – genders (and bodies) that were one way, and then another, and now contain both/all in a new formulation?

AS: That's elegantly articulated, thank you. And thank you also for pointing out that we, too, have traveled in a spiral in our conversation, revisiting the same themes, but also evolving them.

We could keep talking, but as I look at time, and our word count, I realize we are nearing the end of our conversation for now. I want to tell you how much I appreciated our talk – and your bringing Sissy Pussy Cunt to our attention.

GH: I appreciate your bringing her into the conversation.

AS: She has no idea how generative her dance has been for us.

Thinking Further: In the Après-Coup

GH: After we handed in this paper to our editor, you got in touch to let me know about an experience you had presenting the material to a group of analysts. You and I had a conversation about it, and it seemed important to include it here. Do you want to explain what happened?

AS: Yes, and thank you for revisiting this with me. You and I ended our conversation with talking about how thinking evolves in spirals, and what we are doing now seems to follow that path, without our having anticipated it would. In any case, a few weeks ago I was teaching a short class on gender to a group of analysts. Among other texts, I asked the participants to read the draft of our conversation (up until this postscript). An interesting issue arose from one of the participants who said that his primary reaction to the video was to feel concerned about Sissy Pussy Cunt's safety. His worry, which others shared, was that she might be assaulted. It was not clear if the idea was that she could be sexually assaulted or otherwise attacked, and while he was clear that he did not find himself feeling critical of her, he did also say he felt sad *for* her, sad that she had to dance for money. He did not say this, but I did wonder if there was another question in there as well – what else, other than money, she had to dance for, i.e., your attention (or anyone else's for that matter).

GH: She definitely seemed more interested in my attention than in my money. I wonder why this analyst, and probably others who did not speak about it, felt what sounds like pity for Sissy Pussy Cunt, along with a wish to protect her from an imagined danger. What is not being felt when pity and protection come to the fore?

AS: It appears as if something about her pleasure, excitement, enjoyment is being either evacuated or overlooked. I have been thinking a lot about this sadness that he described, the notion that there was something to be sad for in Sissy Pussy Cunt, or something to be concerned about (safety, assault). On the one hand, trans people are, we well know, at increased risk for physical harm, so the concern raised is not at all unreasonable. On the other hand, however, I wonder if this "wish to protect" (what in our field could be framed under the "do no harm" dictum) may be a more knotted kind of protectionism than it first appears to be. I say "knotted" because the "do no harm" dictum can become its own diktat that, in the interest of care, exerts a different kind of regulatory pressure: some forms of queerness are okay (perhaps the drag queen who entertains a bride-to-be and her guests at a bachelorette party), but others are not (those that cannot be as easily assimilated into the mainstream). This concern comes up with other forms of non-normative relationships around gender and sex; for example, I am thinking of sex workers I treat, who routinely bring up others' preoccupations with "worrying" about them and their safety.

GH: I also hear it from patients who engage in BDSM and other sexual practices that people in their lives, including previous therapists, "worry" about and consider dangerous. When I've presented and published material about these sexual practices, a common response from fellow analysts is that I am not anxious enough, not worried enough, and I should be more protective of the patient. To be the analyst who does *not* react with abundant anxiety to a patient's "dangerous" sexual activity is to risk being seen as negligent, a bad analyst who does not (magically) put a stop to the behavior, as if that were possible or even desirable. It makes me wonder if the "worried" analyst wishes to be protected – from the anxiety, as well as the loss and envy, she might feel when engaging with the polymorphousness of the patient's queer sexuality. I think of the police shooing Sissy Pussy Cunt off the corner. Their regulatory function is not to protect her, but to protect normative others from her – and what she might stir up. When you told me about your class, we talked about my enjoyment of Sissy Pussy Cunt's dance, and I asked you what the analysts thought of me, my camera, and my dollars. In my question, I was feeling a related risk, that of being another kind of "bad analyst," the kind who, on his off-hours, behaves as a voyeur.

AS: In fact, quite the opposite happened. In this group of progressive analysts, you were seen as the eminent trans analyst whose observations were interesting and useful. I did wonder in retrospect, though, if something more complex might have been at work. As the eminent analyst, you are the trans-normative subject: White, educated, published, dollared. Might Sissy Pussy Cunt, then, embody the abject trans subject in need of our protection, endangered from others, and endangering herself? To say this differently: is there a splitting operation at work here? The good trans subject, the eminent analyst Mr. Hansbury; and the abject one, Sissy Pussy Cunt, dancing in the street for money, over-sexualizing herself and imperiling her safety.

GH: I feel ambivalent about being split from my own trans abjection, my own capacity to disturb the normative order. As a trans person who is assumed to be cis, and who has become more acceptable over the years – as I have improved my station and as society has grown more accepting of trans people, especially those of us who "pass" for cis (and who are White, educated, dollared) – I feel the loss of my queer visibility, with all its transgressive power, in the eyes of the normative other who accepts me as the good trans subject.

I keep wondering where you fall in the split, the eminent analyst who cowrote and presented this material, and at the same time watched with pleasure the video of Sissy Pussy Cunt's dance. You were also the one who suggested we bring her into our paper.

AS: I really appreciate that question. In our field, I am often read as straight and even some analysts who know I am queer somehow "forget" it. Further, my gender is almost always read as straightforward when it is actually much more labyrinthine (which constantly reminds me how little we really think about genders we read as cis). But it is precisely because of how my queerness is inflected (through my sexuality and my gender), as well as my immersion in particular queer subcultures, that your video stood out to me, why it drew me in. It is true that I was the one who asked you to talk about it; I did so because I felt that discussions about queerness generally, and transness in particular, that align with respectability and leave out pleasure and abjection ultimately leave analysts unprepared to work with the range of queerness our patients bring to us. Part of what I saw in your filming of Sissy Pussy Cunt, I now realize, was an opportunity to shift clinical conversations from approaching trans subjects in general, and trans women in particular, as exclusively in need of "help" or "safety," to register the particular forms of joy and exuberance that can undergird trans living.

For me, this focus issues from my immersion in queer subcultures and, especially, my early closeness with trans women, some of whom are sex workers, whom I have seen wrest pleasure out of abjection in ways that are not defensive, and that are not necessarily imperiling. These pleasures include the pleasure of camp and of community. That joy can be constellated out of difficulty – specifically the difficulty of transmisogyny – is neither a new idea, nor is such wresting unique to trans people; however, to contest these pleasures because we, as analysts, do not understand them, do not share their aesthetics, or worry they are de facto dangerous, may make *us* dangerous to our patients.

GH: That's well put, thank you. As always, we could keep talking, spiraling and unspiraling, but this seems like an important note on which to end. Until the next turn of our après-coup.

Notes

1 First published in: *Psychoanalytic Review*, 109(3), September 2022, 227–256.
2 https://youtu.be/5AkVv22Sop0.

Bibliography

Ahmed, S. (2006). *Queer Phenomenology: Orientations, Objects, Others*. Durham: Duke University Press.

Aisenstein, M. (2018, November). Αμφισεξουαλικότητα [Bisexuality]. Paper presented at the Hellenic Psychoanalytic Association, Athens.

Aulagnier, P. (1975). *The Violence of Interpretation: From Pictogram to Statement* (A. Sheridan, Trans.). Hove, UK: Brunner-Routledge.

Bell, D. (2020). "First do no harm." *International Journal of Psychoanalysis*, 101(5), pp. 1031–1038.

Benjamin, J. & Atlas, G. (2015). "The 'too muchness' of excitement: Sexuality in light of excess, attachment and affect regulation." *International Journal of Psychoanalysis*, 96(1), pp. 39–63.

Blass, R.B., Bell, D. & Saketopoulou, A. (2021). "Can we think psychoanalytically about transgenderism? An expanded live Zoom debate with David Bell and Avgi Saketopoulou, moderated by Rachel Blass." *International Journal of Psychoanalysis*, 102(5), pp. 968–1000.

Chiland, C. (2000). "The psychoanalyst and the transsexual patient." *International Journal of Psychoanalysis*, 81(Pt 2), pp. 21–35.

Corbett, K. (2001). "More life: Centrality and marginality in human development." *Psychoanalytic Dialogues*, 11(3), pp. 313–335.

Corbett, K. (2008). "Gender now." *Psychoanalytic Dialogues*, 18(6), pp. 838–856.

Corbett, K. (2011). "Gender regulation." *Psychoanalytic Quarterly*, 80, pp. 441–459.

D'Angelo, R. (2020a) "The complexity of childhood gender dysphoria." *Australasian Psychiatry*, 28(5), pp. 530–532.

D'Angelo, R. (2020b). "The man I am trying to be is not me." *International Journal of Psychoanalysis*, 101(5), pp. 951–970.

Davis, O. & Dean, T. (2022). *Hatred of Sex*. Lincoln: University of Nebraska Press.

Evans, M. & Evans, S. (2021). *Gender Dysphoria*. London: Karnac.

Freud, S. (1895). "Project for a scientific psychology." In J. Strachey (Ed. & Trans.) *The Standard Edition of the Complete Psychological Works of Sigmund Freud (SE)* I. London: Hogarth Press. pp. 281–391.

Freud, S. (1905). "Three essays on the theory of sexuality." In J. Strachey (Ed. & Trans.) *The Standard Edition of the Complete Psychological Works of Sigmund Freud (SE)* VII. pp. 123–246.

Garfinkle, M.S., Gentile, J., Litowitz, B.E., Pellegrini, A., Sheehi, L., Wilson, M., & Zeavin, L. (2019). "What can I say? Contested words and contested thoughts in the contemporary moment." *Journal of the American Psychoanalytic Association*, 67(4), pp. 655–697.

Gentile, J. (2020). "Transgendering speech: Discussion of Farley and Kennedy's 'Transgender Embodiment as an Appeal to Thought.'" *Studies in Gender and Sexuality*, 21(3), pp. 173–181.

Hansbury, G. (2017a). "The masculine vaginal: Working with queer men's embodiment at the transgender edge." *Journal of the American Psychoanalytic Association*, 65(6), pp. 1009–1031.

Hansbury, G. (2017b). "Unthinkable anxieties: Reading transphobic countertransferences in a century of psychoanalytic writing." *Transgender Studies Quarterly*, 4, pp. 384–404.

Hansbury, G. (2022). *Feral City: On Finding Liberation in Lockdown New York*. New York: W.W. Norton.

Kubie, L. S. (1972). "The drive to become both sexes." *Psychoanalytic Quarterly*, 43(3), pp. 349–426.

Laplanche, J. (1987). *New foundations for psychoanalysis* (J. House, Trans.). New York: The Unconscious in Translation.

Laplanche, J. (2017). *Après-coup*. New York: The Unconscious in Translation.

Littman, L. (2018). "Parent reports of adolescents and young adults perceived to show signs of a rapid onset of gender dysphoria." *PLoS One*, 13(8), e0202330.

Loewald, H. W. (1960). "On therapeutic action." In *Papers on Psychoanalysis*. New Haven: Yale University Press. pp. 221–255.

McDougall, J. (1986). "Identifications, neoneeds and neosexualities." *International Journal of Psychoanalysis*, 67, pp. 19–30.

Pellegrini, A. & Saketopoulou, A. (2019). "On taking sides: They/them pronouns, gender and the psychoanalyst." *Psychoanalysis.today*, https://www.psychoanalysis.today/en-GB/PT-Articles/Pellegrini167541/On-taking-sides-they-them-pronouns,-gender-and-the.aspx

Posadas, M. (2018). "Tiresias and his trouble with ambiguity of gender." *Undecidable Unconscious: A Journal of Deconstruction and Psychoanalysis*, 5, pp. 93–106.

Pula, J. (2015). "Understanding gender through the lens of transgender experience." *Psychoanalytic Inquiry*, 35(8), pp. 809–822.

Saketopoulou, A. (2014). "Mourning the body as bedrock: Developmental considerations in treating transsexual patients analytically." *Journal of the American Psychoanalytic Association*, 62(5), pp. 773–806.

Saketopoulou, A. (2019). "The draw to overwhelm: Consent, risk, and the retranslation of enigma." *Journal of the American Psychoanalytic Association*, 67(1), pp. 133–167.

Saketopoulou, A. (2020a). "How the world becomes bigger; implantation, intromission and the après-coup: Discussion of House." In P. Sauvayre & D. Braucher (Eds.), *The Unconscious: Contemporary Refractions in Psychoanalysis*. New York: Routledge. pp. 174–184

Saketopoulou, A. (2020b). "Thinking psychoanalytically, thinking better: Reflections on transgender." *International Journal of Psychoanalysis*, 101(5), pp. 1019–1030.

Salamon, G. (2014). "The dignity of belief." *Undecidable Unconscious: A Journal of Deconstruction and Psychoanalysis*, 1, pp. 113–118.

Scarfone, D. (2015). *The Unpast*. New York: The Unconscious in Translation.

Sperling, M. (1971). "Spider phobias and spider fantasies: A clinical contribution to the study of symbol and symptom choice." *Journal of the American Psychoanalytic Association*, 19, pp. 472–498.

Stockton, K.B. (2009). *The Queer Child, or Growing Sideways in the Twentieth Century*. Durham: Duke University Press.

Suchet, M. (2011). "Crossing over." *Psychoanalytic Dialogues*, 21(2), pp. 172–191.

Torres, M. (1996). "Transsexualism: Some considerations on aggression, transference, and countertransference." *International Forum of Psychoanalysis*, 5(1), pp. 11–21.

Winnicott, D. W. (1953). "Transitional objects and transitional phenomena – A study of the first not-me possession." *International Journal of Psychoanalysis*, 34, pp. 89–97.

Winnicott, D. W. (1969). "The use of an object." *International Journal of Psychoanalysis*, 50, pp. 711–716 Notes

Chapter 9

Dragging Psychoanalysis

Geoffrey Hervey and Lara Sheehi

Psychoanalysis has had little to say or theorize about the queer subculture and practice of drag. This chapter showcases multiple conversations facilitated by a psychoanalytic doctoral trainee and multiple drag artists. The conversations were transcribed and are presented here with a lead-in conversation by two clinicians – a mentor and her former student, who was the one to lead the drag conversations. The chapter, in its form and collaborative creation, attempts to challenge this particular oversight of queerness while also highlighting the psychoanalytic richness within the drag artform.

The Frame

Geoffrey Hervey:	This is a Friday that I've been looking forward to. This is actually my last business item of the day. So, what a wonderful lead into my weekend.
Lara Sheehi:	Awesome. Well, since it's business, let's jump right in!
Geoffrey:	Yeah, this little bit of pleasure, and I guess that's the nature of drag.
Lara:	Exactly. So, let's just start there – this is a piece about drag and you had the brilliant idea of calling it "Dragging Psychoanalysis." I know we're switching roles here, which feels very much part of the spirit of role play, playfulness, and queering a process. As we lead our readers into the transcripts, I wanted to make sure to give you space to talk a little bit about the title, the concept, the everything of how we got here.
Geoffrey:	I think for me the origin of the book, the way I understood it, was looking at queerness and psychoanalysis as the primary focus. And for me, one of the biggest components or cornerstones of my queerness is drag, ever since I became a semi-professional drag artist. It really has changed that aspect of my identity regarding gender and sexuality.

DOI: 10.4324/9781032624129-10

That is just for me personally, as Geoffrey, the individual. But thinking about academia and knowledge production, to me, drag is an aspect of queerness that is often, despite a lot of strides in contemporary times, underrepresented – or at the very least, singularly represented. And that feels exponentially so in the context of academia and psychoanalysis. Now, I'm still a fledgling in psychoanalysis. I'm still developing that skill. But even with the rudimentary knowledge that I had at the beginning of this project, I definitely had a sense that there's a lot to get into psychoanalytically speaking, when it comes to the art form and practice of doing drag. So that's where the subject came in.

With the title, you know, again, this is something that has been underrepresented, and I don't think that's by accident. I wanted to do a little play on words, which is very queer, very drag. I mean, how many drag names are puns and plays on words? I wanted to make a little bit of a dig towards psychoanalysis by having the voices of actual practitioners, actual artists, speak to their own experiences. By making the space in a very unorthodox way with this process, even with what you and I have done in structuring this chapter, we kind of are "dragging" psychoanalysis a little bit. Because, like, why haven't you done this before? You should have. There's clearly a lot to pull from, and we're doing it.

Lara: Yes, yes. There's so much that happens in these transcripts. And I say that both in terms of the material, the content that happens, but also the relational spaces that we, as readers, are brought into, what you all have created and animated so fully. This is what immediately jumps out of these transcripts and that is the part I find myself attuning to and wondering how it felt for you. For me, experiencing it as a reader – I wasn't somebody in these live conversations, which was a decision that you and I made actively and intentionally – it felt like I was invited in on the process of making, of being witness to this active producing of knowledge, and the material and knowledge being about intimate relationship building and making. That is psychoanalysis and dragging psychoanalysis.

Geoffrey: You know, using "producing" is a funny and accurate word, because I felt like a show producer trying to put this together. Managing drag queen schedules, especially multiple schedules, it is quite a task, but fortunately we were able to make it happen, speaking to the meta of it all. The relational space is where I found the experience that I had in, you know, facilitating these listening groups, these circles, it felt like we were transported to the green room. We/I were backstage before or during a show, and these are the conversations that we have, the understandings we come to, us just kikiing[1]; we *get* it. Like you said, the material is there, but there's an immaterial understanding that I think was also present, and it seems as though even you as a reader – and as someone who, well, maybe you have done drag and I just don't know – still felt. That was my experience of it as well, I felt seen in an important way.

But obviously we weren't in the backstage of some venue, this was Zoom, these are all Zoom calls, so it kind of was shifted in that sense. I think another shift was I was having to do a bit of drag myself. All the calls that we did, the question that a lot of the participants asked when I reached out to them was, "Do I need to be in drag for this?" And I was like, "Oh, you don't have to. It's up to you. Like, frankly, you can have your camera off for all I care. It's mostly just us talking." But I felt like for me, even though I didn't have a stitch of makeup on, I had to get into group facilitator drag. And academic drag as well. I was having to engage in these conversations and these understandings that I embody. I know these things in a very informal and fun and performative way, and while that was the content and that was the material, my meta process of it as it was happening was also being attuned to the idea of me as scholar, me as drag scholar, and I'm trying to *do* knowledge production. So, it was an interesting process. There was a lot of immaterial things that were happening.

Lara: I love how you are distilling the experience for us, through drag. I'm struck at the same time by the way in which this setup that we decided on, invites us to think in real-time about the splitting off of parts, and makes us think about roles and identity; questions of taking up space and how much of us can be present. You all had very deep emotional and philosophical conversations around identification, affective investments, capitalism, body autonomy, and about gaze and legibility. And within that all, you're saying that as a facilitator there was a question around technique, almost, where you felt there is a difference between "me as the artist" and "me as the facilitator" here. If we're thinking about drag as a site of knowledge production, psychoanalytic knowledge production, too, what is asked of us if we are engaging psychoanalytically? How does one think about the space of drag as a mode of production itself, not just as a place where psychoanalysis as a method or theory gets overlaid or imported? I am thinking through these questions vs. the typical reactionary position of "here we are, *applying* psychoanalysis to drag, and that's how we get psychoanalytic drag," or psychoanalysis in drag.

Geoffrey: Yeah, there is a thought that I wish I had said in a lot of these groups, which is, "You all are doing psychoanalysis!" I wish I could have told them that. They are doing psychoanalysis because they are excavating their interior worlds, not just individually, but together in the process. One, by nature of doing drag, but also by the nature of participating in these recording sessions. And I really enjoy the idea of thinking about what is split off because I think that's part of why I frame this as: "I was in scholar drag doing this." Because to loop back to the earlier question about the title and my decision to orient this book chapter around these conversations – I am from Tennessee, and in this past year there was a lot of very virulent and targeted anti-trans and anti-drag legislation in my home state and across the United States as a whole. A lot of this happened very shortly after I left to come to begin my doctoral degree. I felt like I left my home right before it got very unsafe for a lot of people in my community that I know and hold dear.

One thing that I was trying to reconcile, and I think this endeavor helped me reconcile, was the question of why these two aspects of self felt so split off from one another. Why can't there be room for both to exist? You have me really thinking about what gets split off. For me, my role, my drag, because of history and systems of power and structures of respectability, I think a lot of my sensibilities and aspects of self are things that have been split off. In doing this, enacting it, I felt like there was room and an ability to merge those things. So now I actually have been able to really incorporate this creative aspect of self, my drag, into my work as a clinician.

Lara: I want to drill down on this further; when I talk about aspects of ourselves, or yourself being split off, I want to also highlight that I am not talking about it in an abstract or in a theoretical way. I am talking about it as a literal demand, as precondition of being in certain spaces, especially in our field. I feel the need to highlight that, because in dragging psychoanalysis, there is also a way in which I make a commitment to making known the coercive processes that happen and may go unnamed and unseen. Processes that are central to the making and remaking of subjectivities of psychoanalysts in service of social reproduction. And this is especially the case when – and because you are in training, I want to make sure that is noted – these are not passive or innocent processes of splitting, and oftentimes they are also not unconscious, when the splitting we are speaking of often is. What I am thinking about instead is the conscious disciplining of people, tacitly, or through directly communicating that there are parts of you that are not welcome in spaces where psychoanalysis "happens," in training spaces.

The communication that there are parts of you that are "not professional," or there are parts of you that the field may be "fine with," but that belong in other spaces, hidden spaces, which eerily matches the political discourses and actions you just highlighted, where you have these crude laws that would truly make it impossible for people to practice or perform drag in public. Those are often the instances that we go to because they are so obvious. And yet, because I am interested in the textures of ideology and how it comes to be lodged within us, I am also interested in animating the subtle, but just as violent, ways that transmute into the discourse we have been witnessing, the moral panic: "Do whatever you want to do but not in front of my children." And here I am thinking of how the spectre of the child is always used as a front to discipline and dictate fascistic ways of managing spaces, disciplines, and professions, with the intent also to depoliticize and de-sexualize bodies and people.

Geoffrey: In the name of saving those children. Right. That's the figure of the child. Lee Edelman made a couple of points; that is the bastion, that is immutable, right? So much can be justified, all sorts of tyranny, or a fascist sentiment, or dictatorial, controlling action can all be done in the name of the children. Now, not the actual queer children that do exist – those children are not cared about – but the fictional child that is endangered by us.

Lara: Yes. This feels like a very important point because of the act of all of you coming together under these circumstances, against the backdrop of this violence, to make meaning in a way that is also very visible – codifying it in print.

Geoffrey: Right. And like you are saying, the play on words: we're dragging psychoanalysis on one hand, we are being provocative and evocative. On another hand, we are saying: you must see this, you have to engage this. I'm thinking about another dimension to "We are dragging it:" we are putting psychoanalysis in drag. We made it fierce.

Lara: And that is much more the psychoanalysis I, and many others, want to be a part of. There's also something incredibly important about making psychoanalysis cash out on all the promises that the theory and the practice has made, and in that way, you're *dragging it there*.

In your conversations, you all are laying a challenge: do you believe in your theory or do you not? Because what I saw in these transcripts that our readers are going to engage is psychoanalysis *happening*. There is intimacy, there is desire, there is identification, there are contradictions, there is relationality. There is expansiveness, there is outward struggle, there is playfulness.

Geoffrey: 100 percent spot on. I really resonate with that reading as well. Like us dragging it there. I didn't realize how many avenues this title can hold, and that's the power of drag. I am also thinking about, to add on to what you just said, sort of putting the proof in the pudding as it relates to "Dragging Psychoanalysis." One thing I am glad I made clear in these recording groups is, by nature of doing this, all these people are part of knowledge production, right? This is something that, I don't want to say is formal, but it *is* real. This is something we are making meaning out of, we are making it. We are uplifting and making meanings that have existed but have not been recognized and have not always been heard or seen.

I get so much joy in thinking about the people reading through this and being able to tap into something that they probably would not have been able to otherwise. The participants also were able to speak up and speak to these things that they might not have ever been able to. Actually, I know for a fact that they have never been able to because that is the feedback that I consistently got, in addition to the desire to do something like this again.

Lara: Very powerful. I want us to talk a bit about how we came to decide on this process and how we even talked through the sticking points, the contradictions of, for example, "What is it for me to be part of this as a queer person, but not a drag artist?" As somebody in the field, somebody who was already in relationship with you, in psychoanalytic space with you in classrooms and mentorship. I wanted to speak to how we came to create this together and negotiated what it would look and be like, understanding that it was also curated just like a performance, without it being a replacement for an organic relational process.

Geoffrey: Thinking about the logistics and the intentions behind this process, it makes a lot of sense of how it came to be what it is. I think the word "conversation" comes to mind. It is what we did from the beginning, what I did with the participants, and what we're doing right now. Even if it was scheduled, we are having an organic exchange. That part seemed to be our real priority, and it made a lot of sense to me. And again, thinking about the different hats that I'm putting on and the different drags that I'm embodying in those conversations with the participants, I was a facilitator and now look at me! I am now the participant and an author.

It felt very important from the beginning to be doing this in a way that was a conversation that felt natural and *accessible*. This may be my own personal biases speaking, but I think oftentimes there is a high barrier to entry when it comes to academia, and specifically psychoanalysis. To the point of dragging psychoanalysis, taking it there, having this be a conversation-oriented piece and project was one way to do that. It was important for this to be as accessible as possible even just in terms of the legibility of the content.

Lara: That comes through in the richness and robustness of these exchanges. And to me, it feels like they trouble this notion that somehow psychoanalysis is not always already there vs. having to be imported. I am not speaking to or about the institution of psychoanalysis or institutionalized psychoanalysis, but rather the practice and method of psychoanalysis: who owns the contours of that? Where does it happen? Where do we imagine psychoanalytic processes unfolding?

And where are the spaces in which psychoanalysis is happening that never occur to us? For me, in these transcripts, it is right in your face. I feel that folks will engage these transcripts, and both be fully engrossed and recognize the depth that is present – a depth that psychoanalysis as an institution had no hand in.

Geoffrey: I have done qualitative research before. I have done line by line analysis for themes, and this isn't that – I'm happy about that. It is so rich. I think that's the word that I can use.

Lara: Is there anything else you would want our readers to be oriented to as they engage alongside or with these conversations?

Geoffrey: Yeah. I think one thing that is coming to mind for me is the idea of embodiment. It's a very easy thing to think about when thinking about drag as related to psychoanalysis. I hope it is made clear that obviously drag is an art form, and these are characters for some. I do not mean this only for all the participants in this chapter, but more broadly speaking. And that also, for a lot of people, drag is their life. It is not like a lot of other art forms where there is some other product that is separate from you. It quite literally is you. But it also isn't. It is a beautiful and wonderful contradiction. That is something that I would love for the readers to sit with as they are reading. There are aspects of self that are present and related to a real, tangible human being that you are reading. These are actual real people. Drag is a lot broader, even broader than whatever came to mind when I said the word drag just now. And odds are you are probably in drag, even as you are reading this, in one form or another.

Introducing...

Geoffrey aka Sin Clair (@sin.clair.x_x): I feel a genuine connection to my name: I asked my mom what my name would have been had I been assigned female at birth (AFAB), and she said she would have named me Sinclair. I was like, "Oh, well, that's a cute name," and I like sinning, so: Sin Clair. And I put the "black" in "black magic."

Karli Marx (@thekarlimarx): Karli (she/they in drag) is a mental health professional, drag performer, and advocate for queer rights. She is interested in psychology as a liberatory science, fostering queer spaces and creative expression.

Ani So Exotic (@anisoexotic): Ani So Exotic is the FLYING Bollywood Barbie, always serving a chaotic, crafty number, and making the audience gooped and geeked! You can find her in the DMV listening to K-pop and flipping her wig (praying it doesn't fall off again).

Saga Wolf (@lesagawolf): In the spotlight, Saga Wolf emerges. In the kaleidoscope of identities, this nonbinary Guatemalan-American rises, bedecked in the resplendence of their Indigenous roots, crowned in the luminosity of bearded drag royalty. With every sequined step, they dance through the intersection of cultures, weaving a tapestry of pride and power in the vibrant realm where self-expression reigns supreme.

Gin Toxxic (@gin_toxxic): Performer, and an inspiring sex educator, helping spread awareness on sexuality and gender in a safe, relatable, and understandable space. Hoping to make the world a better place for everyone to love freely.

Dollya Killz (@theeee_sean): I'm somebody who likes to make people laugh and entertain a crowd. Then again, you can't do what I do and NOT be entertaining!

Lana Mars (@official_lana_mars): Lana Mars is an entertainer based out of Knoxville, TN, and is a cast member at Club XYZ. She is a former Miss Gay Knox County Newcomer and a former Miss East Tennessee.

MiSTER SiSTER (@meitvl): Baltimore's Girlboyant Drag King and Conceptual Plaything.

Syren7 (@syren.7): Syren7 is DC's sweatiest incubus icon. Her specialty is showing skin, but also showing her heart and her mind through drag.

Coqueta (@coqueta_official): La más perra, Coqueta is a Salvi mami and the winner of SiSSi Cycle Six in Nashville, TN.

Kali Fuchis (@kalifuchis): My name is Kali Fuchis in my feminine form and Niccolo Roditti in my masculine form. I am a co-director of the LGBTQ Youth Center of Durham and passionate about people's access to spaces for expression, human development, and community.

Domingo (@domingosaintx): Domingo is a non-binary drag artist and musician from Washington, DC. Their work is centered in club kid ideology and performance art, while tempering their religious iconography with sex and subversion. Catch them singing jazz in leather or performing other people's music in their signature vampy style. Domingo has been performing in DC for seven years, and as a result has politicized much of their platform to give space to queer artists of color who are emerging in the scene.

Dragging Psychoanalysis

Group 1

Sin Clair:	You know, there are not a lot of art forms or professions like drag. It's kind of unique in that way. And to the point of uniqueness, I want to pose the question to you all: how do you as an individual drag artist approach drag? From your physical bodies, to your minds, to what you want to present to the world?
Ani So Exotic:	The word I've been using to describe things I really like recently has been, like, "cunt"...[2] I was like, "Oh, that's, you know, it's like, that is perfect to me." I think it's perfect to me in the way that it, like, embodies the characteristics of who I want myself to be in the future, whether that's physically or like in a more... I think of things in kind of like a physical world or like a deeper world, kind of like what's beyond the surface in terms of like, who

you are as a person and like your thoughts versus, like, how you appear. So in, like, both ways, I feel like drag allows me to manifest a version of that, maybe like an alternate dimension, future version of that. I just want to be like that perfect version of, like, myself in my head, like the version of my future self that I see. For me, Ani So Exotic is me from an alternate dimension where I was a girl, and I go into that alternate dimension sometimes and we switch spots and she has a fun time here, but she's like, "This place is not for me." Then she gets out.

Karli Marx: I live and love that, and spring-boarding off that: we've kind of referenced it a few times throughout this, but I want to, like, explicitly connect this like *cunt, slay* feeling or fantasy, like all these kinds of ethereal things we're using to describe what we go for in drag. It's, I think, like feeling the fantasy and just naming what we have in our minds, just like the fantasy of where we want to be when we get in drag. And we do the work to make that or to bring that into reality, to translate this thing from our fantasy into the material world.

Sagawolf: I agree with that. To add, I think it's a two-pronged approach because that's me as a person trying to do that when I get to the stage. But to answer SinClair's question, the purpose is the gag of it all, the surprise, the shock value, the sublimation of my characters and how that is just intercepted differently, and you didn't see it coming. So that's on stage, and based on that response is how I feel validated. That's how I feel my drag or my art – good or whatever, whatever we want to put it as – is the answer to me. However, in relation to what was stated first: I'm working on the part that everyone's talking about right now, which is the first part. You getting yourself into that fantasy, which I think is harder done than said, for sure. I'm a full-figured person, I'm curvy, and most people don't expect that to be sexual, or expect that to be "diva." They don't expect that, so when you're giving yourself permission to do that, again, you're empowering others and yourself to feel like, "I can do that too, and I should be liberated just as much as you are."

Gin Toxxic: At least for me, my whole point in drag is to become this sex symbol, is to be like sexualized. But not just in a physical way, like, "Oh, look, look, her body, it's hot." But like, at least in my experience, I think for a lot of us, sex was always an issue that wasn't really talked about in the household… and so growing up, I've always been like, "No, like we need to talk about it." We need to have these discussions… so, and that's why I perform in the little thing I do, or like my songs are very much of a sexual nature because I want people to seek, to see and know being sexual is okay. If it's consensual, it's okay. Like, we are sexual beings. We do have sex. We do have questions about our body and other bodies, and that's okay to have. We need to stop the stigma of: "sex is bad" or "sex can only be between a man and a woman that are both cis;" it can be for everyone and anyone who wants to enjoy in that topic. And to bounce off Saga, I do love the gag of it all: when I do a reveal, and I'm like wearing just basically pieces of a chain and they're like, "Oh my God, how dare you?" (*mimes astonishment*) – and that's what I love about it. Like, yes, look at my body. Look at me being sexual on stage and… what I do is consensual. Like, I want you to sexualize me. I want you to ogle my body because that is what I want to bring to the table. I want you to be comfortable in being uncomfortable with that situation, if that makes sense. And as a trans woman, it is hard to be and be comfortable in your own body. So to see another trans performer just going, giving it all on stage is like, wow. Like, I might not be where I am physically, but I can be there mentally. I can be there emotionally until I reach that physical goal with myself. And everyone's goal as a trans person is different. You know, someone can just be okay with not having any operation or not having hormone therapy, but someone else might feel differently. So it's definitely that way, of just the bridge of let's just all love our body in the journey it's in right now.

Karli Marx: Yeah, I like all these comments and they have been really helping me think about how I wanted to phrase this, but I think as the artist, we get to kind of explore these parts of ourselves that are so often disciplined out of us, and so what the audience then gets is getting to bear witness to that exploration that we're undertaking on the stage. And they get to see us either being playful with it or really, like. deep diving and being gritty with it and just doing the things that we're told not to do. And so the audience then sees that and they get to be, like, "Oh my God, I can explore these parts of myself, too. I can, like, see this other person embarking on their own journey, and that can liberate these, like, parts of me that I've had to keep under lock and key, like all the way over here." I can bring those back into my life to, like, integrate them. So, for me that is like a symbiotic relationship between the audience and the artist.

Sin Clair:

This is the good stuff, and this is why we're having this conversation. I'm glad both personally and broadly speaking, that we're having these things being said, especially so to the point of sex and sexiness and sexuality. Because for me, that's one of my main goals in drag. (*raises a finger*) Look hot. (*raises another finger*) And make money. And so, I really think that when we talk about sex and sexuality, especially as it relates to drag as well as body image, I think that's where the mind and body can merge. If you all feel comfortable – since this can be quite sensitive material, please feel free to engage as much as you feel comfortable doing so: what does drag do for you in your body image? How do those two things interact?

Ani So Exotic:

Ruined it! To be honest, because I can kind of talk forever on this, I'll try to see if I can, like, concisely say my topics. When I first started drag, I was like, "Oh, I'm going to like, use my natural body. I'm not going to pad. It's really going to be me feeling the fantasy." For me, feeling it in drag is like a mental thing; I don't have to, like, necessarily get in drag to fully feel it. Obviously, when I get in drag and I look at myself in the mirror, there's like an extra click there. But, like, for me, it's definitely just like a mental thing. I'm just like, "I'm slay now," and then I am. But, like, for body image wise, like at first people didn't like that. Like, I was getting negative feedback. People were like, "You should pad." I was like, "Ooh." And this causes me to not feel good about myself. I feel like I need to think that about myself because now I, like, lost a ton of weight since I started drag. All people say to me is, "Oh, you're so skinny." "Wow, like you have such a nice body." And it's like, okay, what? Can you come up with something else now? Losing weight for me wasn't necessarily in an unhealthy way or in a problematic way, but it was from my meds. So, it's like, it's not really my choice, you know what I mean? I have so many complex issues on this, and sorry, that was kind of all over the place. But I really don't like what drag has done to my body image.

Sagawolf:

I can, to add to that, I can somewhat agree with a lot of things you said relating to the whole body, especially the last sentence. But in regards to drag right now as a fuller figure person, I have the luxury that sometimes I don't need to pad, but I don't have shoes that properly fit. I can't really serve you a heel properly because they don't fit properly. And as someone who can dance and who has a background in Latin ballroom dancing, I lose my dance ability. So, I feel like what I'm strong at is no longer what I'm strong at, it is where I'm weak. And so when I'm doing a drag king number, there's no expectation on heels. I can wear whatever I want. If I'm wearing a kitten heel as a drag queen, depending on the act, it could work. But you know, there's going to be the naysayers and the commentary from the popcorn stand. So, you can do a performance on how you think you can best deliver your talent. I will add also, there are not many plus-size queens that are highly thought of in ways that are not either mammified or a joke, mainly just ignored. And I don't like being mammified.

Sin Clair: The way people respond to fatness is mind boggling. And I think part of what you're getting at is also, it's not in isolation either. It's connected to so many things like racism and colonization.

Sagawolf: Right. Fatphobia is a primary symptom.

Group 2

Sin Clair: Thank you all so much for agreeing to do this and introducing yourselves to one another. I think that that really helps locate all of us, where we are and where we're coming from. And I guess that's sort of where I would like to start with this. First question is: where are we coming from as it relates to drag? If you all can remember or recall, what sort of brought you to drag?

Dollya Killz: My gosh, I can go. So well, of course I started drag – I started getting interested in drag when I was like 15. This is going to sound really cringy, but of course, I started watching RuPaul's Drag Race and, you know… yes, I was watching Drag Race. And of course, you know, that's how I learned what drag queens were, that's how I learned who RuPaul was and things like that. And then I did start making friends out in the drag scene who do drag themselves. And that's when I met Lady London and Monica Vernonza, and that's when I learned what drag really was. And that it's not just what you see on TV. And then when I was like 16, almost 17, is when I was like, "All right, you need to take this seriously." Like, if you want to do this, take it seriously. So that's what I'm trying to do now, take it seriously. Even though I'm not much of a serious person.

Lana Mars: My first exposure to drag was probably 2013. It was at this old bar that used to be by our campus called The Carousel, where I was introduced to the very first drag queen I've ever met in my entire life. Her name is Anastasia Alexander. I work with her today, which is amazing, but at the time I didn't really know what drag was. That was kind of, like, my first exposure to it. And so the following year, during Sex Week at my university, I volunteered to be one of the performers. And so that was when I first dipped my toe into drag. Someone did my makeup for me, and all I wore was like a cheap wig and some bra and panties and called it a day. And then I did that on and off with the yearly Sex Week shows until around 2017, when I graduated with my bachelor's. And then I suddenly had all this free time on my hands because I was taking a year off from school. So, I decided to take it a little more seriously. I started performing at talent nights at what used to be the Edge, and then eventually I – after doing a couple of shows at talent nights, I managed to start my own show out in Maryville, Tennessee, and eventually I ended up getting on cast at Club XYZ, and that is where I just kind of went into treating drag more professionally, more as a job during the pandemic. It was definitely a way for me to pay the bills. So, that's kind of been my journey into it.

MiSTER SiSTER: I'll say for me, I have a background in comedy, so I had some familiarity with performing, because before COVID, I was doing stand up, and I also had started my own sketch comedy team and we did some live shows and competitions and stuff, so I was no stranger to being on the stage. But drag was kind of something that I started doing in my house. It was actually my 22nd birthday. I had some friends over. I was housesitting for my parents, who let me have some friends over, and we all just like – I was like, "Everybody get in drag." Like, I didn't even know what it really meant for me. I was just like, "I want to know what I would look like if I was a boy." And I just had all my friends do that. And we all just, like, smoked and like, danced around in my parents garage. Then, like, I kind of sat with that for a while, and I've always kind of been passionate about photography and photo editing. So,

I started sort of just doing drag looks in my – my room-mate had moved out, and I had, like, a full room. So, I kind of used it as, like, an art and photo studio. So, I just kind of started getting in drag in my house and, like, tak-ing pictures and playing around and editing the photos and seeing what happened. I left my house in drag for the first time just to go to a concert. Like, I was like, I want to like – I went to a Poppy concert and I was like, "I think this is the time and place." And I did it. And it was terrify-ing and liberating.

Things got a little bit more tricky when it came time to look for a stage that would have me. I did – I will be very frank about the fact that I did face a fair bit of gate-keeping. I won't name names, but there was a drag queen that my girlfriend at the time had reached out to on be-half of me. She had gone to high school with this per-son. And that person basically said, like, for some reason, like, people just don't want to book drag kings. They're not really interested in it. They're not ready to perform like queens are. They're not really in search – like people aren't searching for them, people aren't booking them. Mind you, this is someone that books their own shows, so they fully could have fucking booked me. But they basi-cally were like, "I would try looking in, like, Philly or New York instead maybe." And I was basically just told, like, the scene here isn't an uplifting one for you. You're not going to find a stage. And it was really hard for me to find a stage just because, you know, like, I was reaching out to the various people in the area, being like, "Hey, I'm looking to do this." And everyone was looking for people who had some experience already. And it wasn't really a newcomer stage, especially for a king.

I'm still oftentimes the only one in the green room, but my first time actually getting on stage was, I found there's a group called Pretty Boy Drag, and they have like an Open King Night every now and then. And so I signed up for that show. The first time that I saw one of their shows, I made myself a volunteer and got to dance on stage and stuff, and I showed up in full drag. I was like, "Y'all are about to know me." And then they gave me a shot. And yeah, I've been at it since then and just kind of headlined and hosted my own like eight-hour show on Saturday.

I know if I knew drag kings existed, like, earlier, like, everything would have shaken out really fucking differently for me and everything would have happened at a much more accelerated pace. But the most touching thing that happened to me is, I have this one act that starts with me with, like, these massive tits, and at the end, like, I'm like flip flopping them around or whatever, and at the end, like, they pop off. And I have top surgery scars. And there is this one show that I did – I'm getting chills talking about it, but these two guys came up to me and they were like, "Can we take a picture with you?" And I was like, "Yes, sure." I didn't think anything of it until like they lifted their shirts and, like, showed their top surgery scars, and that, like, in a picture is like, that is why I need to be doing this. Like, that is why, because people need to see it and people need to be seen and people need to know that drag is not just what you see on TV. Drag is everything and nothing. And drag is all of it. So, that's the long and short of it.

Syren7:   For me, I think, like, gender expression – I honestly feel like drag has been a part of my life for as long as I can remember. I was a theater kid and a quiet kid in high school, so I'd always been like, performing even in, like, middle school. Yeah, for as long as I can remember. I think my inspiration for drag has always come from, like, female villains and, like, dark femininity. And I ended up doing HIM from *Powerpuff Girls* as my first ever performance a little under a year ago. It was October of last year, and I've been performing like inconsistently ever since because I think, like I said, the first half of my drag adventure would just be me like exploring and growing. And then I do plan on taking it seriously from, like, here on out. I had a friend from high school tell me about the first show that I did. I think the hosts of that show, I don't think she does that show anymore, something a little bit wild happened, so she does not host that show anymore, and yeah, yeah, that's kind of my little drag adventure as of now. I'll be one year in October, I think the end of October.

Sin Clair: My goodness. Thank you all so much for sharing that because I, I honestly think that a lot of what you all describe, and there's so much in what every single one of you said, but the one sort of through line that I keep thinking through, it's not something that you all said explicitly as much, but I'm thinking about queerness. I think there's so many ways in which queerness manifested in what you all were saying, whether it was like the gate-keeping that MiSTER SiSTER mentioned or, you know, the representation, for better or for worse, of Drag Race that Dollya mentioned, or just internal gender expression, like Syren7, or the realities of like work and labor.

MiSTER SiSTER: I would be curious to know how other people navigate whether or not to bring it up in a more professional context. Like, I don't have – I feel like drag should be on my resume, but I don't have it on there. And I feel like I almost don't want employers, or people that are at a place I'm applying to, to know about it. But it is a huge way to see what I'm about and what I'm capable of. So yeah, I guess navigating it professionally is – and like how I present myself online in a drag context.

Syren7:   I will say, I can definitely agree with the fact that – umm… Syren takes up a lot of my money. (*laughs*) She runs my checks up and down, left and right. I think that right now I'm taking a break from drag, and it's definitely to start spending more time taking care of myself… Yeah, I think drag, it has its impacts, but I think overall I've taken the good and kind of like thrown out the bad. Like, I'm fine with whatever happens from here on out, and if I'm not getting certain bookings, I'll live.

Lana Mars: So, to speak to what Syren just said: it took a long time for the money from drag to balance out, because I almost quit in 2019 because I was a grad student then and my stipend was $900 a month and my rent was so much of that. So, like at the end of the month, I had like maybe $50 to spend on drag. And like every time you go out on stage, they want to see something new. So, like, you know, how on earth are you going to make that stretch? I think the way that I conceptualize drag is this, like, very, like, postmodern kind of art form. Like we… the language of drag is built on references, it's built on parody, it's built on creating new meanings out of, like, existing ones; drag is also the triathlon of being an artist. You have to make your own mixes, learn how to sew, learn how to dance. There's so many different art forms that come together to basically make a Frankenstein of a performance art piece that you put onto the stage. One of the benefits that I got out of doing drag was one of the categories in pageants is interview. And so, prior to my most recent job, I had never actually done a job interview. Most of the jobs I ever had in my life kind of fell in my lap. So, I recently applied all the things that I learned from drag into getting a job interview there. We have to do so much in drag where we have so many skills anyways. So, if you don't want to talk about it bluntly, you can be like, "Oh, I work as a host or a hostess and I host events, or I DJ." There's so many skills when you break drag down because at the end of the day, that's what it is.

Dollya Killz: I actually also want to add on to what Syren and MiSTER SiSTER said. First, Syren: I'm also on a little "no drag" moment right now because this shit is expensive, okay?! And I think people understand that doing drag is fun; it's amazing to do, but it's work. It's things you do. You do have to be very skilled in a lot of things to be considered a successful or a good drag queen. I have an interview on Wednesday where I'm like, "Do I bring it up?" Because they asked you like, "What do you do outside of work?" Or like, "What do you do that might keep you away from work?" And I would answer with that because it keeps me away from work. I think people that understand that, like, doing drag is where it is fun. It's amazing to do, but it's work.

Sin Clair: I am so grateful that you all kind of organically raised this point about drag, money; not "drag money," but drag and money. (*laughs*) And my thing, because I think one thing that often does not get said enough – and I think MiSTER SiSTER and Lana, all of you really have sort of phrased this in one way or another – drag is work, and arguably at a certain level drag is a job.

I think that this is an issue that happens in a lot of creative fields, whether it's writing or painting or singing and, you know, etc… But, you know, with drag, we are our art. And when it becomes not just an art but our job, that can be pretty taxing. And, you know, to the point of like working and labor. I do think that we can't not recognize the fact that we live in a capitalist society in which we do have to work and provide and produce in order to live. Unfortunately, and I feel like I'm picking up on some mental health effects of those contexts and of those circumstances, both financially, but also mentally and emotionally, particularly in what pieces of self get split off and we are pressured to disavow.

Dollya Killz: It's like there's always, when you're a queer person, there's always that fear that something bad could happen to you but you don't ever think it is going to happen to you… And like, that's a fear we shouldn't have to have. That's not something we should be thinking when we leave the house every day. So, of course, it's scary and it's a little… it's worrying. But I wouldn't change my life at all. I love being queer. I love being who I am.

Group 3

Sin Clair: Domingo, I think for a lot of us, our access point to drag, it all starts with a name. And I would love for you to share where your name came from, and what does it mean for you?

Domingo: Yeah so, Domingo, in a very gendered romance language, is already so masculine sounding. And the way that my, like, government legal name is Jésus, has some sort of… a lot of like biblical value to it that I have come to full circle, from like resenting to trying to exorcise away from me, to then coming back around to it, almost like embracing it as, like, satire in a way. So, like "Domingo" means "Sunday," and Sunday is the Lord's Day, whatever. And, like, my party that I host every month at DC9, which is a punk bar, is like a Sunday tea dance.[3] And it's just, it makes sense that it's my drag name. I have a Sunday ritual. I create rituals instead of spaces. I like to think of it that way. I consider every performance to be a work that liberates us, that liberates the people watching. I am a survivor of religious conversion therapy, which I try not to leave out of this kind of conversation, because as dark a matter as that is, it's such a big part of, like, why I do drag. So, there's something very esoteric that romanticizes my religious trauma by having Domingo as my name.

Sin Clair: I really appreciate your usage of the word ritual, both here in this conversation and also in your drag as a whole, especially as someone who likes to fancy themselves as a witch. And I kind of want to just open this question to all of us right now. And like, what about drag feels like a ritual for you? For me, it's literally, like, getting ready. That feels like a ritual for me.

Coqueta: Fuck that part, I hate getting ready. I wish I could just close my eyes and, like, wake up and look beautiful. (*laughs*)

Sin Clair: (*laughs*) Like a Sailor Moon transformation sequence!
Coqueta: Yes, exactly that!

Kali Fuchis:	The first 30 seconds of the performance is ritual for me, which is why I really love an opening thing to a song. I know a lot of people love to do, like, just the song, but that's kind of like – I feel like Dragon Ball Z, you know, like there are different versions that I go into. Like the first one is getting ready. But I feel like again, my performance is important for me especially because I organize shows. A lot of people are like, "Oh, you must love organizing;" I'm like, "Hell no!" I do that because I went to school for it. And so, like, that's my time and energy given. Performing is for *me*, it's like, that is exactly why I do what I do. The mixes are for me, the songs are for me and for the audience; it's literally what *I* want. And I know it will transport me to that next level. And so hearing people, like, at the end of a song and after my opening sequence, what I'm doing is allowing myself to get into this like second state of Kali, like I'm already, I already am Kali, but this other ritual of doing an opening part before the song allows me to really feel that in the way that I'm not able to access outside of that. Like, not explicable in any other way. When I think of these mixes and I think of these transitions, it's like these eruptive moments that allow me to feel that level of intensity that I know I wouldn't be able to do otherwise. You leave it all out on that fucking stage, and I think that is why I really love getting into drag as the performance art.
Sin Clair:	100%. I really hear you on, like, the performance part of it; I think all of you – well, at least Kali and Coqueta know, and Domingo, now you will know, that for me, my least favorite part of drag is getting ready. But my absolute favorite part is the performance. And I think all three of you can agree – and I'm actually going to talk my shit a little bit right now – but I think all of you can agree, I'm a fucking fierce performer. I love being on stage. I do, I really do. And yeah, for me that's where the transformation really happens. Like, yes, the lashes, the wig, the lip gloss, all of that. But when I'm on that stage, I become SinClair. SinClair is me. And it's not just… it is for me, but I also get to have that received and seen by other people, too. I am a chronically social person, and I need people to like me. And so I decided to be a drag queen. (*laughs*) I really appreciate the word ritual, that really speaks to me a lot. So much of what we've been talking

about in this conversation has been about the feelings that drag evokes within us, from us as the doers, the subjects. But I think, as we all know, drag can evoke a lot of feelings in other people. And so I kind of want to pose the question to you all: why do you think drag brings out so many feelings, such strong feelings in other people?

Domingo: For me, at least, my knowledge of the whole culture of this is, is like human satire and being able to laugh at ourselves in extreme ways and in extremely obscure ways and, and satirize sort of like human emotions, experiences, trauma, beauty, like exaggeration, like we are clowns and jesters of the human experience, right? And so I think whenever we go on stage, people are either looking at a reflection, like we're a fucking disco ball, and they're looking at themselves when they look at us, and they're like, "Wow, you just set me fucking free. I didn't know I could do that with a beard. I didn't know I could feel this weight of the song. I didn't know I could want to be what you are like." There's a very personal thing going on with each person. They're having this sort of like – and I don't mean narcissistic in a bad way because it is a very basic human trait that we all possess to some extent; it's like people see themselves in you, or they see you as, like, a deliverer of a message, like a messenger as somebody or something. And so they're either having an out-of-body experience because they see themselves in you, or they're looking at you for the pedestal that you're on. Either one is very powerful, but I feel like those two things are happening in those kinds of situations.

Coqueta: I was just pretty much going to say a similar answer. For me, I think it has a very psychoanalytic view. I think a very basic human experience is that we see each other in other people and also see what we don't, what we are not in other people as well. And I think for some people that are, like, really, really, really, really into drag, they will go out of their way to tell you, like, you look beautiful or, like, I remember one thing that I always got commented on when I did bearded drag was, like, women coming up to me and being like, "Oh my God, you have hair like me." Which is such a silly comment, but I mean, it is literally just, like, such an honest thing to say because I mean, it was genuine, right? Like I think people, like, do like to see themselves in drag performers a lot. And there's often a lot of gratification that comes in feeling the applause

	and feeling the gratitude and the admiration from other people in your own community. I think many of us have not felt that at all in our regular lives outside of drag.
Kali Fuchis:	I feel like when people find newness, like, I think it's kind of, like, that, right? Like a lot of times, people have fear of queer folks because they've never met a queer person, or they have fear of trans people because they've never met trans folks. But, like, when people see drag, it invokes in general, like, a baseline of "Yes, this is entertaining," but when you see high drag, you see something that's more connected to that person intimately. Which is why the first 30 seconds of a performance feels like a ritual for me, I really love the opening. There's the attention of it all. Once you get past the uncomfortability of all the eyes on you, you're like, "Yeah, I'm literally sickening[4]."
Sin Clair:	I mean, every drag queen needs a healthy dose of narcissism. Yes or no?
Coqueta:	Yes. Some have too much, then they get delulu. But yeah.

Glossary

1 Kikiing: ballroom/Black LGBTQ slang for chit-chat and gossip.
2 Cunt: slang for powerful high femininity or confidence.
3 Tea dance: social dance events organized on Sunday afternoons in the US gay community, originating in New York in the 1950s and 1960s.
4 Sickening: fierce; to be entertaining or impressive in a grand fashion.

Chapter 10

Erotophobia

Or, Isn't Everyone A Pervert?

Gila Ashtor

Sex and Sexuality Today

I confess to being continually surprised that what "queering" psychoanalysis often amounts to is a queer psychoanalyst telling other psychoanalysts that queer = sex, and any theory or technique which is insufficiently attentive to sex is necessarily inattentive to queerness, or that any theory of sexuality that does not revolve around bodily sex is guilty of "sex-squeamishness." I am often even more surprised to hear that this idea was developed in queer theory, when what distinguished queer theory from the discourses preceding it was precisely the repudiation of simplistic equations such as queer = x (where x signifies a particular identity, desire, or genital activity). Queer was revolutionary because of how forcefully and unapologetically it disrupted stale and reductive trajectories of desire, daring to tell feminism that essentialism was more dangerous than whatever emancipation it secured. Think, for a moment, about Eve Kosofsky Sedgwick's breathtaking claim that for her – a literary critic widely regarded as the founder of queer theory – genital sex is boring relative to the other ways she experiences her sexuality.

> 'As far as 'having sex' goes, things couldn't possibly be more hygienic or rou-
> tinized for me. When I do it, it's vanilla sex, on a weekly basis, in the mission-
> ary position, in daylight, immediately after a shower, with one person of the
> so-called opposite sex, to whom I've been legally married for almost a quarter
> of a century. I've learned to like it, you know, I have orgasms and it feels good,
> but it's not what I think of as sexual... Does that,' she asks her therapist, 'make
> any sense to you?'(1999, p. 44).

We do not know what her therapist makes of this, but we do know what Sedgwick does – a body of queer theoretical writing that puts pressure on the normative con-flation of sex with sexuality and continually elaborates queerness as precisely that place (in theory, in life) where no easy equations prevail.[1]

Ever since queer theory emerged – roughly in the 1990s, and generally tied to the simultaneous publication of Judith Butler's *Gender Trouble* (1990) and Eve Kosofsky Sedgwick's *Between Men* (1985)[2] – the field has been grappling with the

DOI: 10.4324/9781032624129-11

meaning of sexuality and its relationship to sex. The history of these questions is too long to recount here, and indeed, retracing that history is a microcosm of queer theory itself, but one way of understanding these debates is as between an "expansive" and a "narrow" view of sexuality. According to the expansive view, queerness describes an enlarged realm of sexuality that is unmoored from the usual anchors of anatomy, genitality, and kinship structure, a term that could apply to sex but is not reducible to it. The narrow view, by contrast, sees queerness as indissociable from sex, as representing a more radical, destabilizing, anti-relational experience of sex. My delineation of these two competing views can make it seem as though these two positions are clear and unambiguous and that queer theorists align comfortably with one or another view, but in actuality, the situation is messier; most theorists do not explicitly locate themselves on this spectrum, and many popular polemics are confrontations between different positions that do not recognize the conceptual source of these differences as such.

That said, as it plays out in queer theory, one way to conceptualize the relationship between these competing positions is as a majoritarian vs. minoritarian view, whereby the expansive view of sexuality prevails in most queer writing while the concrete view bemoans its relative unpopularity. At least this is the impression one gets from reading advocates of the concrete view for whom queer theory will never really be queer until it restricts the meaning of sexuality to *actual* sex. For these critics, the problem with queer theory is that the expansive position overwhelmingly dominates queer discourse, and since this expansive position undermines the centrality of bodily sex, queer theory as we know it is disinterested in sex. Or, as Tim Dean, one of the most vocal advocates for a concrete view, has written, "there is an open secret about sex: most queer theorists don't like it" (Dean, 2015, p. 614). According to this view, "there is something about sex… as erotic practice – that many scholars in Queer studies find oddly aversive" (Dean, 2015, p. 615), and therefore even while queer theory promotes itself as a discourse devoted to radical sex, it is, for Dean, nevertheless and surreptitiously guilty of a "sex-squeamishness" (Berlant & Edelman, 2015, p. 725) that does not take seriously the messy, embodied, anti-identitarian potential of sex. Among queer thinkers, Dean has become one of the most insistent proponents of the concrete position, in large part by promulgating the "hatred of sex" diagnosis which alleges that, "sex, a source of intense pleasure, is actively hated" (Davis & Dean, 2022, p. 1). Why? Because "something internal to its mechanism renders pleasure difficult, paradoxical, and always potentially *un*pleasurable for those troubled creatures we call human. At the root of hatred of sex lies the problem of pleasure" (Davis & Dean, 2022, p. 17).

Now, what does any of this have to do with psychoanalysis, especially since Dean never engages with the field of clinical psychoanalysis directly? As this chapter will show, whilst Dean may not address practicing psychoanalysts or even be particularly concerned with the clinical applications of his "hatred of sex" diagnosis, recent calls to assimilate queer theory into psychoanalysis have mostly replicated Dean's diagnosis, in many cases accusing psychoanalysis of the same crimes queer theory is guilty of (selling out sex for the hygienic ruse of identity). What's more, even while Dean's indictment is rarely cited explicitly, his version of the "real" queer theory as one which puts sex (and only actual sex) at the center has been imported and superimposed onto psychoanalysis wholesale. Consider, as exemplary of this trend, the recent conference on "Sex" organized by members of Division 39 of the American Psychological Association (APA). According to the call for papers, psychoanalysis has committed an egregious betrayal of sex by actively suppressing the radical potential of "bisexuality," "perversion," and "radical desire." Not only has sex been "largely moved to the periphery of psychoanalytic psychotherapy" but "sex has been severed from clinical theory, to make psychoanalysis less subversive, apolitical" because it would rather sell its soul to the puritans and neoliberals than confront the discomfort and disorganization that "sex" represents. Moreover, although some have made excuses for this situation, the "ousting of radical desire" is neither innocent nor accidental but the result of an untreated (and until now, undiagnosed) hatred that has festered and made itself complicit with "Nazis, capitalists, colonizers, and homophobes who have used psychoanalytic theory to justify ideologies of hate and dispossession under the guise of clinical expertise" (2024).[3] Echoing Dean's sensational trope that everyone is secretly averse to the "physically satisfying" and "psychically disturbing" pleasure/unpleasure of genital sex (Davis and Dean, 2022, p. 17), the conference alleges that "sex" – not desire, not otherness, not even sexuality – is what is most derided and "abjected" in contemporary psychoanalytic discourse. In another example of this phenomenon, consider a recent essay entitled, "No sex please, we're psychoanalysts" that explicitly repeats the title of Dean's own essay, "No sex please, we're American," just swapping out "American" for "psychoanalysts" (Pellegrini, 2023). As one would expect from an article that expressly repeats Dean's title and only changes who, specifically, is being accused, Pellegrini indicts clinicians for a field-wide aversion to sex, citing Saketopoulou's queer intervention as a much-needed, radical antidote to this entrenched "defensiveness." Indeed, within psychoanalysis, Saketopolou has been among the most vocal promoters of Dean's "hatred of sex" diagnosis, popularizing his thesis (that we all hate sex because we all hate pleasure) and that any paradigm which strays from this view belies its "sex-squeamishness" and so betrays sex all over again (Christinaki, Narayanan & Saketopoulou, 2023).

While the recent attention to sex has been invigorating for the field,[4] and the demand to take queer theory seriously is both urgent and essential, the uncritical adoption of only one version of queer theory – and the narrower, concrete position at that – is limiting and problematic. Whether intentionally or unwittingly, it reduces all of queer theory to a particular and minoritarian view (even as it rarely acknowledges this context) and obscures a robust tradition of theorizing queerness that has, as its starting point, a deliberate and strenuously cultivated *uncertainty* about what sex actually "is." As Berlant and Edelman write in their defense of the expansive view, "Dean seems certain about it: sex is embodiment, or what he calls 'bodily desire,' without considering for a moment that desire may not spring from the body alone" (Berlant & Edelman, 2015, p. 626). That is, not only does the "hatred of sex" diagnosis rely, for its coherence, on a steady definition of *what* "sex" as the hated object "is," and not only does this disregard one of queer theory's principal aims – to question the relation between sex and sexuality, desire and genitality, gender and sex – but in soldering sex to the body alone, and even then, only certain bodily experiences (intense, ego-shattering ones), it characterizes anyone who deviates from the narrow, pure, definition of sex, as secretly hating it. Here is how Dean impugns Berlant and Edelman – arguably among the most rigorously self-critical queer theorists – of such reprehensible deviation: "It is hard not to see the authors' love of abstraction as simultaneously a disavowed hatred of sex. Abstraction enables the maintenance of a hygienic distance from the messiness of embodied desire. Hatred of sex likewise manifests itself in the form of a preoccupation with affect – of 'affectivity'" (Dean, 2015, p. 621). Here, a concern with "affect" or worse, "feelings," is nothing but a fancy deviation from the "messiness of embodied desire" and abstraction is just a defense against being embodied. Rebuking theorists for being "abstract" about sex is a bewildering charge, given that all of language – and theory especially – is an abstraction compared to the "messiness of embodied desire," but this kind of incoherence is entirely typical of the "hatred of sex" diagnosis: since any expansion of sexuality beyond sex is motivated by hatred, it follows that everyone who talks about sexuality in relation to anything *but* the body and bodily responses, hates sex and wants to evade and destroy it.

While the narrow view of sex has its admirers within queer theory, the temptation of psychoanalysis to adopt only the most salacious versions of queer theorizing results in a model of subjectivity that lacks psychological complexity and depth. As this chapter will show, such an uncritical adherence to the concrete view – that sex = intense pleasure, embodied in the individual – is problematic for three major reasons: it (1) isolates sex from the rich and vexed interpersonal and interpsychic context in which it often occurs, (2) limits sexual experiences to a very narrow set of physical–genital activities, and (3) designates as pure "sex" only those kinds of encounters which override the instinctual economy of need-satisfaction, in effect saying that only sex which is "perverse" or "deviant" qualifies as real sex. Everything else is just hatred and defensiveness, which can only be overcome by admitting that we secretly hate pleasure, but since most of us will not change our hatred into love (because we are too attached to normativity), there is no hope for us; the least we can do is stop pathologizing the real heroes among us by calling them perverts.

That this argument for a narrow view of sex is routed through the radical reformulations of Jean Laplanche amplifies the clinical stakes of these questions, especially since it is Laplanche, more than perhaps any other contemporary psychoanalyst, who explicitly, unequivocally, and consistently calls for sexuality to be "enlarged" (Laplanche, 2011). Indeed, not only does Laplanche use the phrase *"enlarged* sexuality" to specify his innovative de-instinctualization of sexuality, but his entire model of psycho-sexuality depends on the astringent delineation of two separate and categorically distinctive economies, "instinct" and "drive," in which sexuality can be shown to behave differently than instinct. Not only does the concrete view utterly erase the word "enlarged" from Laplanche's references to sexuality, but doing so seems symptomatic of broader efforts to undermine the challenge that "enlarged sexuality" poses to the narrow conceptualization of sex.[5] In what follows, this chapter will explore Laplanche's model of "enlarged" sexuality and, particularly, his careful parsing of the different economies of instinct and drive. According to Laplanche, "enlarged" sexuality "absolutely goes beyond genitality, and even beyond sexual difference",[6] meaning that not only is "sexuality extremely mobile as to its aim and object" but it is fundamentally and categorically outside the economy of instinct (Laplanche, 2011, p. 142). By elaborating the important differences between these regimes, Laplanche is able to show that sexuality exists anywhere that it functions like a drive (and not an instinct), thereby expanding the realm of psycho-sexual life beyond familiar activities and zones. This "enlargement" of sexuality complements queer theory's expansive position, and it is this chapter's hope that a more complex, multi-dimensional picture of queer theory, and a more rigorous, radical reading of Laplanche, will invite readers into a more ambivalent, vexed, and challenging tradition of thinking about queerness, sexuality, and what it means to be "driven" by a sexuality that is not our own.

Narrow vs. Enlarged Sexuality

Isolation of Sex From Interpsychic-Ethical Context

To those outside of queer theory, it might seem as though all of queer theory is proclaiming the physical and political supremacy of sex, but in fact, one of the discourse's founding coordinates is a famous interview given in 1981, "Friendship as a way of Life" (1997), in which Michel Foucault, the great genealogist of sexuality, flatly rejects the commonsense assumption that non-normative sex is hated because of the particular kinds of physical pleasure it represents. Describing a scene of "two young men meeting in the street, seducing each other with a look, grabbing each other's asses and getting each other off in a quarter of an hour," he says he knows this "neat image of homosexuality" is what people are supposedly afraid of, but actually, he says, "to imagine a sexual act that doesn't conform to law or nature is not what disturbs people. But that individuals are beginning to love one another – there's the problem" (1997, p. 137). Foucault's astonishing argument that what makes homosexuality "disturbing" is "the homosexual mode of life, much more than the sexual act itself" (1997, p. 136) is a scandalous proclamation from an icon of queer thought, particularly insofar as it unabashedly diminishes a popular trope in queer communities that the fear of sexual activities between members of the same sex is what underlies homophobia. Eschewing this rather intuitive notion, Foucault asserts that the relational aspect of homosexuality might be more threatening than any physical–genital activity a couple engages in. Why? Because whereas the intimacy between members of a heterosexual dyad can eventually result in marriage and reproduction, the two men who "are beginning to love one another" are relating outside the normative conventions of established society. Their love has no roadmap, no endpoint, no safe or definitive trajectory.

This provocative interview has cast an exceptionally long shadow over queer theory, such that, for a generation of queer thinkers, reading these sentences was like being told by the grandfather of queer theory that sex is only radical if it is put to certain use. Not only is the equation between what's "radical" and "prohibited" categorically disturbed,[7] but sex becomes radical because of the *relating* it enables, a relating which potentiates an entirely new "mode of life." The queer critic Leo Bersani, in particular, has perhaps made the most of this provocation, dedicating his vast oeuvre to identifying the specific features of sexual activity that make it radical. What Bersani finds is that sex has the potential to "shatter" the ego's control and this "shattering" of ego mastery provides a foundation for a new kind of relating he calls "impersonal narcissism" in which one experiences their universality through the erasure of acquisitive selfhood. In a sense, if sex shatters the ego's sense of mastery, then having sex effectively trains the individual to tolerate a loss of mastery so that they can learn to relate to others from a psychic place of not-knowing and not-needing-to-know (1986, 2008, 2009).

As Bersani shows, it is not nearly sufficient to *have* sex and hope that the sex cures the ego of its mastery. For sex to be psychologically, relationally, and politically meaningful, it needs to be cultivated as a spiritual practice in relation to impersonal others. That is, even though sex is an embodied, individual experience, it is not an activity or encounter that is isolated from relationships to other people even if what sex accomplishes is a new way of relating to them. There is, in other words, no such thing as "just" sex in the way Dean demands because even when sex is "shattering," powerful, and utterly disorganizing, this matters to us because of the ethical effects it potentiates and enables.

Sex as Strictly Genital

Whenever I teach queer theory, and specifically texts that trouble the direct correlation between sexuality and sex, invariably some students ask me why – if sexuality is not limited to sex – then should "sex" be the word we use at all? After all, if sexuality is equally applicable to abstractions that are beyond the strict purview of bodily sex – affectivity, attachment, futurity, negativity, relationality, sovereignty – then why bother calling it sexuality, why not call it desire, sensation, eros, or being? This is a complicated question to answer because it requires making two correlated claims: first, that bodily sex is a unique experience of sensation, undoing, pleasure, and a loss of control coalescing in intense and destabilizing ways, and second, that while genital sex is exemplary of this kind of experience, genitality is not the only form this experience can take. This is what Sedgwick is saying when in the passage quoted at the outset, she distinguishes between "'having sex'" and being "sexual" (1999, p. 44), but to get here one needs to have a definition of sexuality that is "enlarged" in both its scope and range of available expressions.

Within contemporary psychoanalysis, Ruth Stein has provided an immensely influential account of sexuality's development that explains the individual's capacity to derive pleasure from a panoply of situations that would otherwise be unpleasurable. Written while queer theory (as a discipline) was still emerging, Stein's, "The Poignant, the Excessive and the Enigmatic in Sexuality" (1998) asks: what makes sexuality so uniquely alluring, and answers, "sexualization." What does she mean by this? Drawing on Laplanche, Stein explains that it "is the ability of the infant and the child to deal with the painful gap between him and the 'excessive' adult and/or the influx of stimuli and sensations through sexualization" (1998, p. 265) that renders adults particularly susceptible to sexual activity. In a sense, adults have sex because it replicates a series of maneuvers that were developed in infancy to manage overwhelming stimulations.

We could hypothesize that such a disposition to sexualization exists from very early on, from the first time the infant shifts its attention from drawing in sustenance (ex. nourishment) to enjoying and repeating the poignant pleasure of body zones and surfaces (Freud, 1905; Laplanche, 1976, 2016). It seems that the human organism has the capacity to deal with the excess influx of stimuli and the experience of a gap between the infant/child's identifications with a more mature ('excessive') adult and his own limited structures and resources through sexualization. In other words, sexualization is a capacity, a positive achievement, not only a pathological and/or defensive operation (Stein, 1998, p. 266).

Situating these ideas in a robust tradition of speculations about what makes sex compelling – what I call a phenomenological quest to document and specify the effects of sex on the mind-body (Marquis de Sade, Georges Bataille, Jean Genet, Leo Bersani)[8] – Stein develops a theoretical schema that continues to inform psychoanalytic templates of sexuality today. Indeed, although infrequently acknowledged, most current efforts to queer psychoanalysis generally follow Stein's theoretical template: (1) by showing that the infant cannot help but *sexualize* its own unpleasure; (2) by demonstrating that this sexualization forms the bedrock of adult "perversion;" (3) in arguing that perverse sexuality can be psychologically transformative.

And yet, while Stein is arguing that sexualization is a skill developed in infancy and re-experienced in adult sexuality, this does not mean that genital sex is the *only* or even purest format for this re-experience. That is, just because genital sex can be traced to infantile experiences of sexualization does not mean that sexualization is restricted to genital activities. On the contrary, it would seem that the opposite is true: the individual's capacity to sexualize means that *anything* can be experienced sexually, appropriate or not. This is what Laplanche means when he defines "enlarged" sexuality in the following way:

1. A sexuality that absolutely goes beyond genitality, and even beyond sexual difference; 2. A sexuality that is related to fantasy; 3. A sexuality that is extremely mobile as to its aim and object; and 4. (a point on which I myself lay great emphasis) a sexuality that has its own 'economic' regime in the Freudian sense of the term, its own principle of functioning, which is not a systematic

tendency towards discharge, but a specific tendency towards the increase of tension and the pursuit of excitation. In short, it is a sexuality that exists before or beyond sex or the sexed, and which may perhaps encompass genitality but only under the very specific modality of the phallic (2011, p. 142).

As Stein explains, "human sexuality responds to and expresses the need for magic" and it represents "a quest and the desire for the lost object, which is not necessarily a particular, real object, nor is it any object relative to the drive. Such a lost object is… the lost object of continuity" (1998, p. 266). Thinking about sexualization as the infant's capacity to derive pleasure from excessive stimuli, and sexuality as the desire for lost continuity with the other, allows us to see how sexuality is indissociable from its relation to other objects, and from the regulatory economy of the individual psyche. As Atlas and Benjamin remind us, "many forms of sexuality" are "actions the individual takes to soothe or regulate the self, rather than primarily to engage or elicit responses from the other. In this context, sexual discharge means using the body to solve the problem of mental excess, that is, emotional content which cannot be held in the dialogically created mental space is experience as physiological arousal and resolved at that level" (Atlas & Benjamin, 2014, p. 11). The complaint that psychoanalysis hates or ignores sex when it talks about trauma, desire, or relationality falls into the unfortunate trap of presuming genital sex is somehow dissociable from a more complex regulatory, fantasmatic, and intersubjective context. Such a blindspot may be unproblematic for queer theorists who mainly address sex as a theoretical abstraction, but in clinical work, the view that shattering sex is always an expression of pure sexuality is simplistic and impoverished because it leaves us with no way to interpret when sex is defensive, pathological, or dysfunctional. Genital sex may conform to the rhetorical clarity of yes/no, happening/not happening, but "enlarged" sexuality involves fantasy and otherness and is infinitely more complex, contradictory, and compromised, as a result.

Sex is Perverse

The third component of this chapter's critique focuses on what kind of sex is being hailed as inherently radical. According to Laplanche, any model of sexuality that reduces it to genitality and reinscribes the trajectory of an instinctual economy inadvertently returns us to a "Ptolemaic" version of psychoanalysis that is unable to grasp the distinctive economy of "enlarged" sexuality (Laplanche, 1999). Put another way, Laplanche wants to distinguish between (1) the economy of instinct, which is motivated to seek satisfaction through discharge, and (2) the economy of drive, which is motivated to pursue increased excitation without resulting in discharge/relaxation. And he wants to make sure that "enlarged" sexuality operates within the economy of "drive": the objects and experiences that we are "driven" to pursue are not "instinctual" and not satisfiable as such. But if, according to the narrow view of sexuality, genital sex is the only legitimate site of sexuality, then it cannot just be *any* kind of sex either, because normal sex is instinctual sex. For sex to be radical, it has to be "perverse" sex that violates boundaries, destabilizes the ego, and transgresses the norms of mastery, control, and normativity. In other words, for genital sex to abide by the economy of drive rather than instinct, it has to seek excitation rather than discharge, the implication being that only certain kinds of sexual behavior (that seek to increase tension) are worthy of being considered sexual experiences.

Consider, for instance, the fact that ordinary sex often falls into the "instinctual" economy Laplanche describes: tension seeks discharge and then achieves relaxation. This is the kind of sex most people are having a lot of the time. Or as Stein notes, "eroticism is outside of ordinary life," "so extraordinary," "so much beyond the pale" (1998, p. 258), that it cannot be easily integrated into biological and emotional existence. The particular features of these exquisite sexual experiences include violence, the violation of boundaries, shattering, disruptiveness, force, and overwhelm, and as such, they cannot be replaced or conflated with the ordinary instinctual economy of tension and discharge. Crucially, this means that eroticism and sex are not identical; if you merely "have sex" the way Sedgwick describes – vanilla sex, with the lights on, with the same person you have been married to for 25 years, after the shower – you are hardly experiencing the kind of eroticism that Bataille, Stein, and Bersani describe. The result of defining sexuality so narrowly is that it cannot recognize sexuality in anything other than perverse experiences.

Stein is grappling with how to capture what makes certain sexual experiences so overwhelming, exotic, terrifying, and profound, and her descriptions resonate with what it feels like to desire and momentarily attain "continuity with the lost object" (1998, p. 266). But if genital sex is the only format in which to experience the extraordinariness of sexuality, then we are inadvertently limiting sex to a category of individual experiences that are, by definition, perverse, deviant, and structurally at odds with the norms. Such a position is deeply problematic, not least because, as queer theorists have more recently noted, norms are themselves social constructions that exist in dynamic relation to anti-normative goals. As Robyn Wiegman and Elizabeth Wilson point out in their influential essay, "Queer Theory without Antinormativity," "the claim that sexuality has been repressed is caught in spirals of power-knowledge-pleasure that make such a claim an enactment of norms (rather than a transgression of them)," meaning that we cannot determine what constitutes a violation of norms without constructing the norm in the first place. Therefore, "even as it allies itself with Foucault, queer theory has maintained an attachment to the politics of oppositionality (against, against, against) that form the infrastructure of the repressive hypothesis" (2015, p. 12), invariably turning queer theory into advocacy for "radical" sex without acknowledging that judgment about what is or is not radical hinges on the false stability of "norms" and "normal" sex.

It is precisely because sexuality is not limited to any particular desire, orientation, or bodily act that Bersani said it was not the task of queer theory to defend the inherent radicalism of specific sexual activities (1986, 2008, 2009). Similarly, and with respect to our clinical work, we might wonder who is being helped by a model of "radical" genital sex as the only kind of sexuality there is? Beyond the de-pathologization of perversion, and a correlating openness toward some peoples' exotic, violent, unnerving encounters, the absolute insistence that sex is "radical" and extraordinary, or it is hated, deprives us of a vital theoretical concept for understanding our patient's inner lives. Are we to understand that patients who do *not* have extraordinary and shattering genital sex ought to be pathologized for being covertly defensive in their hatred of sex? Are we to believe that patients who experience the heat and pulse and rush of sexuality in relationships that are not oriented genitally, are not being psychologically shattered, unraveled, undone? The problem is not only that a reliance on anti-normativity as a reliable metric of authentic queerness always depends on a fantasy of what the norm is, but that restricting sexual experience to such a narrow definition of perversion invalidates an animating insight of psychoanalysis since its inception: that sexuality inheres and disrupts the putative normalcy of everyday life, that it is not localized to the bedroom, dungeon, or street corner, that it is not isolated to the body, or genitality alone. Is it not precisely this unwieldiness that renders our patients so susceptible to encountering their sexuality where they least expected to find it? And is not the challenge of psychoanalysis to listen for the sound this "drivenness" makes, especially when our patients cannot or do not want to hear it?

Eros and "Enlarged" Sexuality

Now, while Laplanche mounts a vigorous critique of "narrow" instinctual sex, he is less clear or definitive about what constitutes an alternative "enlarged" sexuality. Interestingly, there is another post-Freudian philosopher and psychoanalyst who, like Laplanche, spent his lifetime trying to conceptualize erotic life, but whereas Laplanche emphasized the centrality of "sexuality" without describing it, Hans Loewald described how eros drove psychic-interpersonal life without exactly naming it. As Jonathan Lear, one of Loewald's most careful interlocutors, explains, "although Freud thinks of the death drive as going "beyond the pleasure principle," Loewald sees that it is really eros which represents something new in psychoanalytic thinking" (1999, p. 135).[9] Approaching drives from a different angle but sounding quite a lot like Laplanche, Lear shows that Freud dramatically altered his ideas on sexuality as the only viable way to retain its link to the drive. As Freud writes in 1924, "what psycho-analysis calls sexuality was by no means identical with impulsion towards a union of the two sexes or towards producing a pleasure sensation in the genitals" (1924, p. 218). Not only was sexuality irreducible to genitality or pleasure, but for drive to have any meaning beyond a mere synonym for instinct, it needed to behave differently than a mere biological impulse or need; for drive to be drive, it needs to name a developmental force that is outer-directed and impelled toward differentiation. In other words, if drive is just another word for "inner stimuli seeking discharge" then it is not any kind of drive at all because the pressure to release energy is biological, instinctual, and rudimentary, as Laplanche would say. For sexuality to have any meaning as a "drive," the concept of a "drive" must change entirely. That is why Loewald reformulates the relationship between the ego and reality to situate the drive as a force that is always seeking *differentiation* rather than release. But, how does he account for this activity?

According to Loewald, the mother and infant start out as a "unitary whole" that gradually "differentiate into distinct parts" (1951, p. 11). Or as he famously put it, "mother and baby do not get together and develop a relationship, but the baby is born, becomes detached from the mother, and thus a relatedness between two parts that originally were one becomes possible" (1951, p. 11). What this means is that there is something *in the baby* that seeks out differentiation from the "unitary wholeness" of original mother–child relating. While Freud routinely characterized the emergence from mother–infant wholeness into hostile reality as an unwanted and unwelcome intrusion, Loewald sees the infant as *driven* toward development and growth. It is not to say there is not anxiety or pain in this emergence, but just that reality is not hostile so much as already there – inside the mother–infant dyad – from the outset. According to Loewald, "the ego mediates, unifies, integrates because it is of its essence to maintain, on more and more complex levels of differentiation and objectivation of reality, the original unity" (1951, p. 11). In other words, the infant is impelled to seek out "more and more complex levels of differentiation" even as this differentiation is painful and eruptive because there is something in the infant – Loewald calls it eros – which puts pressure on the mind for growth.

In Stephen Mitchell's hugely influential gloss on this account, he explains that whereas Freud believed human conflict resulted from the clash between inborn drive and external prohibitions, "there was, for Loewald, something fundamentally wrong with this vision" (2000, p. 35). What did Loewald believe Freud had so thoroughly gotten wrong? "In the beginning, Loewald says over and over, is not the impulse; in the beginning is the field in which all individuals are embedded. Experience does not proceed, as Freud believed, from inside outward, from the id's impulse, through the ego, into negotiation with the outside world. Experience initially moves from outside inward, from an increasingly differentiated unity of which the individual is a part to the development of the individual through an internalization of those external patterns" (Mitchell, 2000, p. 35). Here the essential difference from Freud lies in Loewald's emphatic refusal to believe in drive as some kind of primordial impulse; the infant is not a separate entity with her own mysterious sexual urges which she is driven to express, but is, instead, one part of an undifferentiated environment motivated to differentiate from the unitary whole.[10] Therefore, what Loewald's concept of eros accomplishes is the total reformulation of drive as a force with its own "economic regime" (Laplanche, 2011, p. 142) irreducible to the tension–discharge sequence of instinctual pleasure. That is, the infant is not propelled toward differentiation because she has something inside of her (sexual desire) that she feels pressured to express; rather, the infant is driven to differentiate herself because eros pushes her to move toward greater and greater levels of psychological complexity and sophistication. As Mitchell observes, "one of the central psychoanalytic questions has always been 'why do we seek objects?'". There have been many different answers: pleasure, safety, attachment, recognition, and so on. In Loewald's perspective, the question actually does not make sense. It presumes "we" and "objects" are separate phenomena" (2000, p. 40).

Sexuality and Others

This chapter has sought to complicate the dynamic between queer theory and psychoanalysis by demonstrating that the popular assumption that queer theory represents the celebration of radical sex and concomitant call for a radical assault on normativity is both misguided and misleading. For while queer theory unapologetically names sex and sexuality as the center of its analytic, the field hardly corroborates the flawed "repressive hypothesis," which states that sex is socially repressed and liberation can release it. Instead, what the insistent interest in relationality reveals is that queer theory is immensely and intensely critical of sex's emancipatory potential, that rather than a guarantor of genitality's importance, queer theory has long been focused on sexuality *beyond* sex and pleasure, and on "new relational modes" that challenge the economy of instinct. And yet, as I have shown in detail elsewhere, so far queer theory has limited conceptual resources for developing a new paradigm of relationality that moves beyond the most well-known ideas of Freud and Lacan.[11] Psychoanalysis, by contrast, is uniquely positioned to think deeply and creatively about relationality because not only are there vast theoretical resources within psychoanalysis, but the demand to work on questions of relationality – both in the patient's life and within the treatment dyad – are fundamental to clinical practice. In this vein, I want to briefly suggest that when it comes to looking for examples of eros/"enlarged" sexuality (terms I use here interchangeably), we need look no further than the frequency with which our patients are attracted to damaging relationships.

Today, it is not at all uncommon to hear patients talk about "toxic relationships," a phrase referring to relationships – often romantic, although not necessarily – in which they are attracted and attached to someone who threatens their capacity for flourishing.[12] Not only are "toxic relationships" an explicit challenge to the pleasure principle – the idea that individuals seek to minimize pain and maximize pleasure – but the predominant explanation – that early trauma causes an individual to seek out trauma later – cannot explain the role of transformation in this masochistic sequence.[13] As Mitchell observed, "one of the most interesting unsolved problems in psychoanalytic theorizing" is "*why* are the residues of early object relations so persistent and resistant to change? It is just this feature of human psychology that makes our work so difficult, that necessitates such long stretches of time. Freud could describe it, but he couldn't really explain it" (2000, p. 44). Interestingly, most of contemporary psychoanalysis cannot really explain it either since the reliance on early trauma as the signal cause for damaging relationships leaves out many patients who strain to draw the link between their early childhoods and adult compulsions. In my work as a clinician, I regularly listen as patients lament their object choices and complain about their own judgment – "what do I see in him?" they ask me often, "why am I doing this to myself?" they want to know.

While the problem of "toxic relationships" requires its own excurses, for now it will suffice to say that "enlarged" sexuality offers an account of the drive toward higher levels of differentiation that we feel compelled toward *regardless* of how bad or good it feels. Without sufficient space to lay out all the steps, I merely wager here that what one is desperately attracted to is an opportunity for integration via regression and differentiation. This is not genital experience insofar as it is not motivated toward a particular outcome but is instead organized by the economy of drive, excitation, and desire. As Lear reminds us, "we tend to think we already know what human sexuality is; the only question is what counts as instances of it. It is against this assumption that Freud's claim that infants have a sexual life looks outrageous[14]... [but] what Freud is discovering is not simply new items that fall under the concept of sexuality; he is discovering that the concept of sexuality must itself shift. Indeed, in our life with the concept we've become stuck, rigidly insisting that only *this* can be sexual!" (2003, p. 149). Against this tendency, what if we defined erotophobia as the fear of sexuality and consequent belief in *psychic self-begetting*. If, as Laplanche insists, the "economy" determines sexuality and not the object or the means, then we might be afraid of sexuality because it challenges our fantasy of self-sufficiency, and no single sexual practice or identity inures us to this painful fact.

After all, if Freud can be his own Ptolemy then surely queers can be *erotophobic*; which is to say, maybe, despite the temptation to be inoculated, immunity to erotophobia is neither a worthwhile nor realistic goal. Maybe queer theory teaches us the value of surrendering to eros, helping us to see that we want people who are "bad" for us because we sense, unconsciously, that some kinds of bad might actually be good for us, where good means we are vitalized and closer to erotic life. What if good and bad did not depend on proximity to pleasure, but potentiality for growth, where growth was not necessarily "better" in the moralistic sense, but in Loewald's psychoanalytic sense as differentiated. What if we are not suffering from the hatred of sex, but the fear of sexuality, not the hatred of unbinding, but the terror of the others we might yet become.

Notes

1 It would be impossible to provide a comprehensive genealogy of queer theory here, but it is important to say that the question of the relation between sex and sexuality is at its center, see especially, Foucault (1990, 1997), Rubin (2011), Sedgwick (1985, 1999), Bersani (1986, 2008, 2009).
2 See *Queer Theory: An Introduction* (1996) by Annamarie Jagose.
3 See the full description here: https://division39springmeeting.net/conference-info-1.
4 Until very recently, queer theory and psychoanalysis have been "frenemies" rather than friends. As Tim Dean and Christopher Lane announce in the opening of their 2001 book,

Homosexuality & Psychoanalysis, "until quite recently, the relationship between homosexuality and psychoanalysis was wholly adversarial" (2001, p. 3). Not only was the APA complicit with the pathologization of non-normative sexualities – waiting until 1973 to remove homosexuality from its list of mental disorders – but "psychoanalytic attitudes towards homosexuality as a 'developmental arrest' (Segal, 1990, p. 253), bisexuality as an immature regression to fantasy (Rapoport 2009) and transsexuality as a marker of a psychotic structure (Millott, 1990), have resulted in uneasy and suspicious reactions from those involved in sexuality studies (Dean and Lane 2001)" (Giffney and Watson, 2017, p. 28). In addition to these historic insults, there is an irreconcilable tension between queer theory's commitment to the deconstruction of developmental paradigms and psychoanalysis' adherence to frameworks of 'normal' mental growth. That is, whereas "queer theorists believe that there is no 'normal' teleology of sexual development, insisting that desire and pleasure are both fluid and historically contingent," clinicians who are tasked with identifying disorders rely on some evaluative framework for "healthy" psycho-sexual development (Giffney and Watson, 2017, p. 30). As such, the hostile relationship between queer theory and psychoanalysis is not merely the anomalous result of discrete historical rifts, but a feature of the ideological irreconcilability between a discourse that problematizes identity and structuration, and a clinical practice concerned with integration and self-continuity. Or as Bersani liked to famously say, he worked on "Fr-oucault," the fraught and "agitated" nexus of Freud and Foucault (2004, p. 133). Since Dean and Lane's 2001 call for a rapprochement between queer theory and psychoanalysis, we are living in, what might be called, the 'golden era' of "queer psychoanalysis." Not only are queer critics less suspicious of psychoanalytic formulations and less hostile to the clinical establishment, but on the other side, psychoanalysis has gradually transformed itself from a discipline that once pathologized aberrant sexualities to one that now puts sex, gender, and desire at the forefront of the field.

5   Laplanche uses the word "enlarged" to refer to the kind of sexuality that is not reducible to genital sexuality. The editors of *Freud and the Sexual* write, "Laplanche invents a neologism in French by transforming the German component adjective *Sexual*—into a free-standing noun, in pointed contrast with the standard French term *sexuel*. . . This is an attempt to register terminologically the difference between the enlarged Freudian notion of sexuality (le sexual) and the common sense or traditional notion of a genital sexuality (le sexuel). This terminological innovation can't really be captured in English as the German term Sexual coincides exactly with the spelling of the standard English term 'sexual,' rather than contrasting with it as in French. The translators have chosen to signal Laplanche's neologism by italicizing *sexual*—pronouncing with a long 'a': ahl]."

6   See *Freud and the Sexual* (2011) by Jean Laplanche.

7   Queer theory refers to a body of work that emerged in the 1990s within and outside academic departments and that can be located at the nexus of academic research and political activism. Attempting to define queer theory, Annamarie Jagose writes that, "broadly speaking, queer describes those gestures or analytical models which dramatize incoherencies in the allegedly stable relations between chromosomal sex, gender, and sexual desire" (1996, p. 3). Later in the text, Jagose expands upon this definition further: "Clearly, there is no generally acceptable definition of queer; indeed, many of the common understandings of the term contradict each other irresolvably. Nevertheless, the inflection of queer that has proved most disruptive to received understandings of identity, community and politics is the one that problematizes normative consolidations of sex, gender and sexuality – and that, consequently, is critical of all those versions of identity, community and politics that are believed to evolve 'naturally' from such consolidations. By refusing to crystallize in any specific form, queer maintains a relation of resistance to whatever constitutes the normal" (Jagose, 1996, p. 99).

8 Perhaps Stein's interpretation of Bersani is limited by the fact that she focuses exclusively on a single text by Bersani, *The Freudian Body* (1986), when in fact his oeuvre was vast and multifaceted.

9 As Lear explains, "Ironically, just as Freud formulates this truly fundamental opposition, he defines a drive as 'an urge inherent in organic life to restore an earlier stage of things.' This definition, as Loewald points out, harks back to the constancy principle. But by this definition, eros does not even count as a drive! Only the death drive, a tendency in every linking organism toward decomposition, would strictly speaking be a drive" (1999, p. 135).

10 Mitchell writes: "If experience begins in a boundaryless unity, Loewald reasoned, mind, at its fundamental levels, cannot be composed of body-based impulses emerging from the individual and clashing with the external world. The very experience of being an individual mind and an individual body distinct from other minds and bodies – all this is secondary development, a reorganization" (2000, p. 36).

11 My book *Homo Psyche: On Queer Theory and Erotophobia* (2021) offers an extended critique of how relationality is worked on in contemporary queer theory.

12 I wrote an article on "toxic relationships" for the *Los Angeles Review of Books* (LARB [Ashtor, 2020]). See also *Cruel Optimism* (2011) by Lauren Berlant.

13 The question of masochism in toxic relationships is a much broader topic which I will explore in greater depth in the upcoming *Masochism: A Contemporary Introduction* (under contract).

14 Lear has a footnote here which reads: "Anecdotally, I have found that those who are made angry by Freud's claim of infantile sexuality are often holding onto a fixed conception of sexuality and see him as attributing that to infants. Freud is then suspected of taking too much pleasure in debunking illusions about childhood. His project then looks objectionably reductionist. For his part, Freud is clear that we cannot attribute sexuality to children without altering what we mean by sexuality" (2003, p. 149)

Bibliography

Ashtor, G. (2019). "Sex *Instead* of Shattering: A Critical Exploration of Bersani and Laplanche" *Studies in Gender and Sexuality, 20*(4), 249–262.

Ashtor, G. (2020, December 20). "Toxic Relationships in the Affective Age." *Los Angeles Review of Books*.

Ashtor, G. (2021). *Exigent Psychoanalysis: The Interventions of Jean Laplanche*. New York: Routledge.

Ashtor, G. (2021). *Homo Psyche: On Queer Theory and Erotophobia*. New York: Fordham University Press.

Atlas, G. & Benjamin, J. (2014). "The 'Too-Muchness' of Excitement: Sexuality in Light of Excess, Attachment and Affect Regulation." *IJP Open, 1*(28), 1–35.

Berlant, L. (2011). *Cruel Optimism*. Durham: Duke University Press.

Berlant, L. and Edelman, L. (2014). *Sex, or the Unbearable*. Durham: Duke University Press.

Berlant, L. & Edelman, L. (2015). "Sex, and the Unbearable: A Response to Tim Dean." *American Literary History, 27*(3), 625–629.

Bersani, L. (1986). *The Freudian Body: Psychoanalysis and Art*. New York: Columbia University Press.

Bersani, L. & Dutoit, U. (2004). *Forms of Being: Cinema, Aesthetics, Subjectivity*. London: British Film Institute.

Bersani, L. & Phillips, A. (2008). *Intimacies*. Chicago: University of Chicago Press.

Bersani, L. (2009). *Is the Rectum a Grave? And Other Essays*. Chicago: University of Chicago Press.

Butler, J. (1990). *Gender Trouble: Feminism and the Subversion of Identity*. London: Routledge.

Christinaki, A., Narayanan, A. & Saketopoulou, A. (2023). "Sexuality Beyond Consent: Risk, Race, Traumatophilia: A Conversation Among Artemis Christinaki, Amrita Narayanan, and Avgi Saketopoulou." *Studies in Gender and Sexuality* (24), 322–337.

Davis, O. & Dean, T. (2022). *Hatred of Sex*. Lincoln: University of Nebraska Press.

Dean, T. (2015) "No Sex Please, We're American." *American Literary History*, *27*(3), 614–624.

Dean, T. & Lane, C. (Eds.) (2001). *Homosexuality and Psychoanalysis*. Chicago: University of Chicago Press.

Foucault, M. (1990). *The History of Sexuality. Vol. 1: An Introduction*. Trans. Robert Hurley. New York: Vintage.

Foucault, M. (1997). "Friendship as a Way of Life." Interview by R. de Ceccaty, J. Danet, and J. Le Bitoux. Trans. J. Johnston. In *Ethics, Subjectivity and Truth, Essential Works of Foucault, 1954–1984. Vol. 1.* (Rev. ed.). Ed. Paul Rabinow. New York: New Press.

Freud, S. (1905). "Three Essays on the Theory of Sexuality." *The Complete Standard Edition of the Psychological Works of Sigmund Freud (SE)* VII. London: Hogarth Press. pp. 123–246

Freud, S. (1924). "The Resistance of Psycho-analysis." In *The Standard Edition of the Complete Psychological Works of Sigmund Freud (SE). Vol. XIX.* Ed. J. Strachey. London: Hogarth Press: 213–224.

Giffney, N. & Watson, E. (Eds.) (2017). *Clinical Encounters in Sexuality: Psychoanalytic Practice and Queer Theory*. New York: Punctum.

Huffer, L. (2010). *Mad for Foucault: Rethinking the Foundations of Queer Theory*. New York: Columbia University Press.

Jagose, A. (1996). *Queer Theory: An Introduction*. New York: New York University Press.

Laplanche, J. (1976). *The Life and Death of Psychoanalysis*. Baltimore: Johns Hopkins University Press.

Laplanche, J. (1999) "Masochism and the General Theory of Seduction." In *Essays on Otherness*. Trans. J. Fletcher. London: Routledge: 198.

Laplanche, J. (2011). *Freud and the Sexual*. Trans. J. House. New York: The Unconscious in Translation.

Laplanche, J. (2016). *New Foundations for Psychoanalysis*. Trans. J. House. New York: The Unconscious in Translation.

Lear, J. (1999). *Open Minded: Working out the Logic of the Soul*. Cambridge: Harvard University Press.

Lear, J. (2003). *Therapeutic Action: An Earnest Plea for Irony*. New York: Routledge.

Loewald, H. (1951). "Ego and Reality" (1951). In *Essential Loewald: Collected Papers and Monographs*. New Haven: Yale University Press.

Millot, C. (1990). Horsexe: Essay on Transsexuality, trans. Kenneth Hylton. New York: Autonomedia.

Mitchell, S.A. (2000). *Relationality: From Attachment to Intersubjectivity*. New York: Routledge.

Pellegrini, A. (2023). "No Sex Please, We're Psychoanalysts." In *Reading with Muriel Dimen/Writing with Muriel Dimen*. Ed. S. Hartman. New York: Routledge.

Rubin, G.S. (2011). *Deviations: A Gayle Rubin Reader*. Durham: Duke University Press.

Sedgwick, E.K. (1985). *Between Men: English Literature and Male Homosocial Desire.* New York: Columbia University Press.

Sedgwick, E.K. (1999). *A Dialogue on Love.* Boston: Beacon.

Segal, H. (1990) "Hanna Segal interviewed by Jacqueline Rose." In Hanna Segal, *Yesterday, Today and Tomorrow* (2007). Edited by Nicola Abel-Hirsch. London and New York: Routledge. pp. 237–57.

Society for Psychoanalysis and Psychoanalytic Psychology (SPPP), American Psychological Association (APA) Division 39 (2024). *2025 Spring Meeting Information.* https://division39springmeeting.net/conference-info-1.

Stein, R. (1998). "The Poignant, the Excessive and the Enigmatic in Sexuality." *International Journal of Psychoanalysis (79),* 253–268.

Tuhkanen, M. (Ed.) (2014). *Leo Bersani: Queer Theory and Beyond.* New York: SUNY.

Wiegman, R. & Wilson, E. (2015). "Queer Theory Without Antinormativity." *Differences, 26*(1), pp. 1–25.

Chapter 11

Freud Would Not Be Queer Without Us

An Autotheory on Psychoanalysis as Queer Praxis

Molly Merson

As I write this chapter, I have a dream. In this dream, I have to pee, but I cannot find a working toilet. I see many toilet-shaped objects around, but either none of them are accessible or none of them are connected to pipes, so the water simply sloshes around in the bowl, going nowhere. As I am looking around a room with big, beautiful windows and dealing with a bowl full of water that my dream-mind attempts to reason into a toilet, a woman walks in asking for a bottle of wine called *Afterwardsness.* "It is a rare wine," she says. "A special wine." I felt a sense of recognition – I thought I was the only one who liked this kind of wine. She seemed to know a great deal about how special the wine is. It is a blend of riesling and kerner grapes, she said. In my hypnopompic waking afterwards, the words linger and morph into *reasoning* and *kemmer.* I slowly come back to consciousness, wondering about the timing of this dream.

As I wake, I wonder what a dream toilet could mean. I wonder about the primal scene. I wonder about stages of sexuality and development. Then I think: wait a minute – this is not merely a dream about finding a receptacle to evacuate bodily contents into. Perhaps this dream is about my own psychic kemmer-somer cycle (LeGuin, 1969),[1] as a being constantly in process of being and becoming, reasoning and reflecting, ending and adapting, morphing and regenerating. A queer life is one in which I make use of myself, my community, and my experiences in ways I could not have in the past; libidinal, constantly in motion, oscillating between irrelevant and wholly relevant, "both/neither" (Hansbury, 2011). The sexual, whether in relation to an object or not, is the libidinal energy of being alive, in the way transition *is* trans* and trans* *is* transition (Reading & Pivnick, 2023). Just as gender, sexuality, kinship, identity, and being/becoming are not inherently static or definitive, but have become marked as such by a social realm that cannot tolerate ambiguity, encountering a living queerness in oneself opens up the possibility of looking forward and making a future life, as it also makes a past possible, imaginable, and thinkable. Through a kind of Freudian (1897) *nachtraglich,* or deferred action, or Laplanche's (2017) *après-coup,* a subsequent, retrospective, belated, re-working of an experience becomes possible. There is potential to revise our relationship with the unimaginable myths and stories that we adhere to, unconsciously and consciously, and that have assembled ways of living and meaning-making. In this

DOI: 10.4324/9781032624129-12

re-working, something previously unthinkable opens into kaleidoscopic and imaginable possibilities of living, doing, and meaning-making.

I did not know I was queer until I was much older – queers around me usually knew I was queer, but I did not seem to. The more I thought about gender, the more it seemed to me that I was a masculine person performing some aspects of femme life because femaleness, whatever that meant, seemed to fit the expectations of those around me. It also fit the shape of my body most easily, and fit the shape of how I could think about gender and selfhood. Pretending gender in this way just made certain aspects of life easier. Of course, pretending also made the actual living of my life harder, as I buried parts of myself deeper into my unconscious, which would often and only emerge in waves of tremendous pain that had no thinkable source and a protracted disbelief at this fractured doppelgänger I saw in the mirror. I was practicing the social bid to alienate myself from myself.

Fortunately, this was precisely the moment psychoanalysis found its way to me, via Lacan's (1968) essay *The Mirror-Phase as Formative of the Function of the I*. In it, Lacan distinguishes the moment when a subject recognizes themself as a different subject to the outside world than they experience themself internally. As I read this in my very first college course, I immediately entered that mirror. Something in me shattered and expanded. In a moment, I saw myself seeing myself as the child seeing himself in the mirror, being seen by Lacan, and discussed by our class. The multitude of simultaneous reflections, and locating myself somewhere in the matrix, struck open an affective contact with the ways I had never been accurately recognized, and had yet been required to replicate and repeat that which was in the mirror for the benefit of a culture that amplified the gender binary through obedience to Whiteness, tact, and power-over. In that moment I understood that I had never realized that it could be possible to see myself seeing myself, and in doing so, recognize myself as both a replication of my environmental gaze and as a subject to myself. A lifelong strange sensation and uncanny doppelgänger experience started to make sense, both as a fiction to protect me and as a reality that had shaped me the more I had invested my own libidinal energies and idealizations into it. It was a sadomasochistic bind that I had not even realized I invested in, relied upon, and also hated.

From this tormented place, I found Freud. Confused about the prohibitions I felt and enacted upon myself regarding what I have come to understand as my queerness, I carried forward certain sadistic and annihilatory constraints from my social milieu which I levied against myself and others. I dutifully upheld the linear trajectory of controls and prohibitions levied against me by a rules-oriented, white family system which replicated and was reinforced by the greater carceral system. Some of this I could find reflected in Freud's writing, and much of it I could not.

I was unsure of Freud, as so many feminists are, and my initial encounters with his work were tentative. So, when I first read Freud's "Three Essays on the Theaory of Sexuality" (1905), I could not tell if I loved it, hated it, or if I just did not understand it. I could understand that he was writing about his (limited) understanding of sexuality, "bisexuality," homosexuality, and what seemed like a linear order to arousal and sexual organization. And his description of masturbation and polymorphous perversity was exciting, interesting, and shocking but not bawdy; still, a little sterile and white lab-coated, even though some of it resonated with me, somewhere in me. While Freud was more matter-of-fact about sex than my parents or school had ever been with me, there was nothing particularly erotic or compelling about these essays for me. What was he really saying about pleasure? Was sex really just about reproduction? Was he taking the party out of the body, or the body out of the party, or trying to linearize something messy, ecstatic, fractally kaleidoscopic? In re-reading these essays today, I find them surprisingly erotic, curious, playful, and even kinda kinky.

But Freud, wishing to control psychoanalysis while he was alive, had positioned himself as an authority on psychoanalytic thinking and praxis (Carter, 2023). Thus, psychoanalysis was, and still is, rife with replications of authority, projection, alienation, and idealized transferences to authority figures, which makes it inherently uncomfortable to take up his theories when one does not feel clear about (or has become alienated from) one's own mind and body. I was so dislocated from myself that I could not parse whether I was uncomfortable with Freud because I was uncomfortable with sexuality and my own body, or because I was uncomfortable about these century-old theories that seemed out of place in a time of HIV, anti-trans and anti-gay legislation, State-regulated "life" beginning at conception, and the emergent and expansive thinking being generated through contemporary queer and black theory. But, I gave it a shot: I thought I might be able to think about my sexuality and gender and body through Freud.[2]

This, of course, was an extreme challenge. If this is what linear progression or sexuality and erogenous development is *supposed* to be, what if I do not fit into it? Or, what if I have learned how to fit into these parameters *too well*, and have done so by leaving pieces of myself behind in order to move through the world a little more smoothly, perhaps with less shame?

What if my sexuality and gender has adapted like a seed to its environment, knowing when to germinate based on temperature and time and sunlight in the environment?

What if I already know what it means to be queer in the way the desert is queer, the way the plants open themselves to drink in and exhale for a few moments a day in the liminal twilight, transpiring again for a few short moments in the coolest part of the morning, and then spending all the waking moments of a human mammal in a show of spikes, scales, fuzz, and sometimes the most luminous flower in the heat of the sun? The barrel cactus full of juice, the cholla with its jumping spikes, are material adaptations that are as queer as the Earth and all its multitudinous permutations.

The question of how to think about Freud, and psychoanalysis, when I think about sexuality and embodiment in this way, is at first confusing, and then revelatory: where are the moments of Freud's own breath, his moments of transpiration when the rest of the desert sleeps, where his queerness emerges? How might my queer reading of Freud shape and define, in a kind of deferred action, what he was expressing over a hundred years ago? Is this queer reading a psychoanalysis in itself, a way of dreaming myself into being (Ogden, 2004)? Maybe I would never find myself in Freud, after all, but maybe I could do something else.

Several years ago, I thought that the "something else" could be psychoanalytic training, so I applied and was accepted to an institutional psychoanalytic training program. I say that as though it is the easiest thing in the world to do. It is not. In fact, I often experience it as yet another hierarchical space encouraging splitting, alienation, and dissociation, often acting as a mirror image of the sociopolitical milieu in which it nests. I frequently have a hard time squaring the hierarchies, bo-dylessness, and forced Oedipalization of Institutional political fantasy – for example, what constitutes "analysis" for the purposes of having been officially trained as an analyst and thus legitimized – with the warm, deep, complex engagements of a good supervision[3] and rich clinical cases that are invited and facilitated through the institutional space. But Institutional psychoanalysis is not the same thing as *psychoanalysis*. I have come to recognize over the past near decade of analytic training that, though the institutional myths may wish us to believe otherwise, psy-choanalysis is – as, I suppose, are most living things – both a singular discipline and a bundle of contradictions, and thus cannot be held captive inside institutes. In some cases, these contradictions are quite egregious, such as the positioning of institutional knowledge as exclusive and definitive of psychoanalysis, and the repetitive and ongoing racist, homo-and transphobic, classist, ableist, and elitist enactments within text, theory, and interpersonal interactions, as documented, re-futed, queered, cripped, and challenged by so many scholars and clinicians who choose to reside or are forced outside of institutionalized training spaces. How have psychoanalysts created a psychoanalysis that is so *rejecting* of multitudes of being? This is so obviously untenable. Psychoanalysis bids us open to unknown, and potentially unknowable or im/mutable, aspects of ourselves; and yet, I often find in the praxis and imaginations of many who claim to represent and practice psychoanalysis a rigid insistence on psychoanalysis in a vacuum and only one path as the correct one, demanding to be acknowledged as "universal." This is short-sighted at best. As if psychoanalysis could stay bound up on the straight and narrow path! And as if psychoanalysis is an object to be blanketed over culture, psyche, society, and history.

Psychoanalysis is a remarkably transformative practice when it reminds us that there is no universal path because there is no universal human – at least, beyond various supremacist myths and aspirations. All these disparate representations of psychoanalysis[4] suggest seemingly irreconcilable differences, some exposing and some reinforcing the ways in which white cisheteronormativity limits imagina-tion and subjectivity, and how subjectivity can be experienced as moving between relativistic and static states such that we are all influenced by our environments, our projections, and our introjections. All of this said, psychoanalysis *is* specific and differentiated *because* it is a living, intimate framework used to facilitate being and becoming, oscillating in the matrix of action, reflection, culture, and theory. Embodying this bundle of contradictions, psychoanalysis is at times singular and diffuse, specific and exponential. Some attempts at defining psychoanalysis often suggest that it is a tool to open minds, which is quite a seduction for someone like me. But often, institutional psychoanalytic spaces that have the power to define psychoanalysis struggle to articulate and enact a consistent vision for a workable, engaged openness that invites multidimensionality alongside specificity. This includes how psychoanalysis conceptualizes or fails to conceptualize, acknowledges or fails to acknowledge, its entanglements in racial, economic, power, and gender- and culture-bound subjectivities and experiences.

When theorizing psychoanalysis through a colonial, supremacist lens, it appears to claim itself as a universal representation of the "human" condition. However, much like commentary on the Anthropocene (Yusoff, 2018) and queer ecology (Morton, 2010), we find that there is no "human" condition but rather conditions of economics, politics, and positionality that shape the options of the human imagination, and the human imagination in turn shapes the conditions of its environment. This is where, while I cannot square these contradictions, I can queer them. In order to survive the training process, psychoanalytic training required me to tap into the queerness that I had left behind in the desert, under the cholla, hiding away, spiked and dry. I had to be there, 40 years ago under the cacti, amidst the sand and rock, within my earliest memories of my childhood, while also being here, in the classroom, contending with bits of invisible affect, with no place to land but inside me. I needed to remember my queer self, to invite that part of me in, to give me back my mind, to give me back my body. I needed to resurrect, to animate, to re-constellate my queer self, whom I had abandoned in the desert.

Ahmed (2018) teaches me many things, including that queers queer society. But what does society do to queer life? Maybe I could not square the institute because the institute was trying to square me. We are meant to progress at a certain pace and jump through hoops, legible and documentable, in order to graduate and join the replication of institutional psychoanalysis. In similar ways, white cisgender heteronormativity retains and renews its capability of moving through time and space, redefining itself in ways that allow it to gain further power; it does so by jettisoning the affective detritus onto the Other. Specifically, I think of the difficulties that individuals and groups often have with adapting to change. These difficulties get localized onto the queer body and in State interpellations of queer life, as though the queer/trans* Other is the cause of social pain, rather than the receptacle for it.[5] However, queer is as queer does, and queer stays doing: queering power seems less, to me, of a grasp at static, immovable, and complete power-over, and more of an ability to play with power, however seriously, bodily, and irreversibly. While queer does not need the heteronormative to define itself, the dominant is often defined and maintained by its Other. In order to keep this balance and maintain its existence, the queer *and* cisheteronormative individual and society is bidden to disavow, repress, or reject further any of their own organic connections to queer life or the undercommons,[6] except in the ways that are legible to normative society and useful for it to continue to identify itself against. I had thought that I needed to do that, too, in order to stay alive. But it was, in fact, killing me.

Here, I feel my rage. My rage shapes something. Articulating my rage here commits me once again to life.

My rage brings a reverie: *I'm pruning fruit trees with my father, who is telling me how his father used to prune them. Take off the central leader to about three feet high. Do not cut above any buds that will create downward-growing branches. Make a vase shape that is reachable from your height when you are reaching as tall as you can reach.*

These are lessons in social organizing and mutual aid as much as they are lessons about trees. If the central leader is cut, the branches grow larger and more capable, and the roots dig deeper. Perhaps effective mutual aid requires no central leader, but multiple parts working towards living with what we can make, including dissident critiques of Whitewashed notions of wholeness. While he teaches me the way of fruit trees, my father admits that his father had often not followed his own advice, and only those brave and able to climb a ladder could reach the highest fruit. Well, them, and the birds. I have always wondered about pruning fruit trees, or pruning anything, for that matter. Who has the authority to prune, to shape the life of a tree or at least the direction in which it grows? I have learned from Kimmerer (2013) that some plants need animals, including human animals, as a part of the right-enough conditions for growing and flourishing. I suppose my father has tried to figure out how to make and shape a life given the conditions of his own life, just as I have, with only pieces and parts that demand that the only two choices we have are to prune hard or watch the tree unwield itself – while the focus still remains on bred, hybridized, grafted European fruit trees and their surplus response to human intervention. I think of the ways he, and I, and many of us, do this under capitalism and the Christian manifest destiny foundations of the American settler colony. We prune our psyches and our movement hard to make a living, and party hard outside the view of the boss; we restrict ourselves during this life to be promised the blessings of the next life; we compromise and compress our vitality and transformation in ways that reinforce the status quo.

I feel sympathy for the younger me who felt and knew my gender as fully as I felt and knew the way the desert smelled after a rain, deep in my bones and in my dreams, whose knowing became pruned at the wrong spot, not conducive to growth. For me, my central leader was cut, but so were my branches. Masochism seemed the only way forward in response to this required pruning of my psychic limbs. I tried in different ways, but I could not actually prune my own body, so I pruned my psyche, and acquiesced to never speak my dreams aloud into this world.

These fruit trees are a colonial endeavor. I read once in a *National Geographic* that Indigenous communities would regard the honeybee as the harbinger of the end of Native ecologies and plant stewardship, as the buzzy fuzzy little import was necessary to pollenate these European trees. I read today that the Israeli settlers would, and still will, cut down ancient Palestinian olive trees and plant fast-growing pine trees in their place. It echoes the way European settlers massacred the buffalo and the carrier pigeon of Turtle Island, planted their own fruit trees and pushed out the serviceberry and acorn, a further move toward establishing dominance and erasing a culturally rooted history. But, it seems that even so, the olive trees, steadfast and determined, with deepest roots that could not be burned out nor dug up, split right through the pine trees, growing through them, their ancestral libidinal energy reclaiming their presence in the light. It reminds me that we can keep ourselves alive, relevant, and connected, by making life underground. We become the mycelium and the springtails that move it, commuting nutrients between each other's roots, strengthening each other, making beautiful life.

I have spent much of my adult life (problematically) trying to figure out how to make and shape a life that is simultaneously loyal to and unlearning, or learning differently from, my immigrant settler ancestors and their rigid legacies of authority. This loyalty is a treacherous bond, and often propels me into immense pain. My libidinal investments in the promise of attaining an ultimate endpoint that will concretize my sense of ever-receding happiness is a longing to be deeply connected to my environment, but devastatingly linked to a capitalist framework. It is both a paradoxical and an impossible task: paradoxical in that pouring more concrete is not going to help me or any other living being on this planet; and impossible, because when my planetary environment is expressing symptoms of disaster, the bliss I receive from the Earth becomes tinged with tragedy. I wonder – how to unbind my longing from the capitalist imaginary?

These are the moments I come back to the trees. There are small buds on some of them right now, and I wonder how many flowers will survive the coming rainstorm. I cannot control the rain. If I could, I would be generous with it. It is the structures that fail us, not the rainstorms. I pay my respects to the trees, knowing they are me and I am them. We do not control each other, but we offer each other something we both need, forging connection outside the bondage of control.

I can feel how an indiscriminate pruning has affected my life. Some people in my life only had a sense for control as the way of relationship. Because of this and other reasons, some of my branches were pruned too hard, some never got enough sun, and some grew too thick, too visible, sunburnt. Constantly under scrutiny, the best I could do was hide my graft point – the point of a grafted tree most easily sunburnt – in the underbelly outside the normative view, and let the parts of my body and mind that stood out become co-opted into my identity by the heated gaze of my surround. I grew up in the heat of the desert sun, a place that seems desolate and empty if we are moving too quickly and from far away, but expands delightfully, teeming with secret life, the closer and slower we get. The normative, superficial view sees only the spines of the desert cacti and never the day-long bloom, only the sand and cragged rock and never the lizard quick to retreat to the rock's crevice upon feeling the pounding of my footsteps. This is my way of knowing. It is a knowing, on a cellular level, of the heat and the cool, and all the movement in the desert, as in my relational life. As such, I always forged psychic companionship with that which could not be seen, living in the shadows cast by the surface glare. As I grew older, I continued in-between, caught between a longing for a commune with the pulsing of more-than-human life, and a forever glaring parental companion that prevented full surrender to the shade. This shade always held a queer life that could have been.

Cactus roots are different from fruit tree roots. They spread out far and wide on the surface of the Earth, still hidden, but adapted well to the faint taste of rain and dew. My knowing is of these roots, too, even though for a long time I constantly and violently self-erased my knowing. This is not the kind of thing people talk about. What I mean is, I have not really talked about it much. Yes, even in psychoanalysis. Or maybe I have forgotten.

When I was young, I played a game with myself. It did not really have a name, but I played this game like this: *Forget what you have learned, forget the links you have made, so that you will always have to re-learn it, and then you will never get bored, always re-encountering something old as new.* I easily made links where others did not usually see them, and then some part of me would attack these and other links and pieces of threads that could be made into links, constantly doing and undoing, making myself and being unmade by the mismatched bodies, psyches, and imaginations around me. I guess one could say I performed a mixture of Bion's (1962, Chapter 28) – K and a sprinkling of some Buddhist principles. However, the real task of this action was to preserve the sanctity of the status quo. Here is where my loyalty shows up: I was precocious and earnest, I felt excited about life and growth and all its potentials. This is also my lived experience of my relationship to gender, sexuality, and my erotic (Lorde, 1984/2007) self: to be fully and deeply in love with life and all its sensations. However, my experience of the sensation, no matter the joy, was so overwhelming at times that I did not know what to do with it. Too much, too much. So, this game had the effect of preventing me from having to *do* anything with what I had learned and with what made me come alive. I would stop at the too much. Redirect. Forget. Repress. Return. Redirect. Perhaps my own existence felt challenged to the brink of erasure, so I did the same to myself – my own battle with what Sheehi & Sheehi call "colonial extractive introjects" (2020, p. 7). What was hidden that my family tried to forget, and where did they learn how to do that? I think some quiet, wise part of me suspected that my joyful contact with this sensory world and the psychic and affective links I was making would likely challenge my existence in the face of a limiting and frustrating family and social system. I did not realize that making links was my way of making a self, though these links were often pruned at the wrong spot. *Too many downward facing branches.*

Cacti do not need pruning, but they do have remarkable regenerative skills. If a paddle falls off, it roots itself where it lands. Always rooting, even when displaced.

I did manage to find a way of surviving, if not circumventing, this system while remaining inside it, an attempt at self-preservation in raging against the machine. I believed I depended on the status quo and did not want to destroy it. Somehow, though, I could rationalize its destruction of me. *Too many branches, too unweildy, rein it in.* Obediently, I continued the task of assembling my own prison of normativity with the bricks and bars that my D.A.R.E.-infused[7] high school offered, while smoking cigarettes, wearing a spiky belt, and listening to Dead Kennedys on cassette tape. This is when my behavior began to deteriorate. I did not maintain my shape. I was not performing the appropriate suburban role anymore, at least not until Hot Topic became a staple at the local mall.

Yes, I refused conformity on a certain level; but in retrospect my refusal was in the service of a conservative, neoliberal stance, merely scratching at an itch that I quite desperately, and quite unconsciously, wanted to alleviate but could not actually find the origin of. Or, if I did find it, the reality was too much to bear, so I erased it, hid it again in the shadows with the rest of my truths.

Meanwhile, I continued to carry around the irritants my family and social norms had bestowed upon me, thinking my allergic reaction was my problem rather than an appropriate response to punitive introjects. My gender presentation and anarchist interrogation of normative culture became an opposition to the sharp and violent edges between "human" and "nature," the psychic world-shaping inherited by a family who inherited their own violent rigidity from a desperate need to conform to the logistical and carceral necessity of becoming and remaining White, middle-class, straight, and private. This irritant was still inside me, no matter how much I fought back. While my re/presentation was all I could hold on to, I still did not feel like I could trust myself. I did not know my body. My body had been buried in another dimension, and with it I had left my integrity, my relationality, my willingness to surrender to uncertainty. I did not know it then, but I needed psychoanalysis to offer me a chance to fall apart and into someone I had been slowly assembling, via repression, underground.

I do not wish to malign rebellion and refusal, for in it we find and make something to keep us alive. As Stryker notes, "my exclusion from human community fuels a deep and abiding rage in me that I, like [Frankenstein's] monster, direct against the conditions in which I must struggle to exist" (1994/2022, p. 245). I would always choose joy over the fight, but as there was little joy to be found in conformity, I found joy in the fight itself and the connections it brought me with other exiled folks. Some part of me, at the time, implored me to accept my *becoming* as a bondage, like an espaliered apple tree, tied to the wall surrounding the gated community in which I lived. I had to encounter the bound tree in order to see how it had been shaped, and thus that trees could be shaped. In doing so, I began to build a relationship with a different kind of environmental gaze, located in the Earth, pulsating with Earth rhythms.

Today, if you ask me what is my gender and sexuality, and if I trust that you can play with me, I might respond: I am the dirt and the microbes that live in it and the tree that grows from it and the rock that shed millions of years of dust to make the minerals in the soil. I am a tree. A tree is genderless, yet with shape. My shape can come from haircuts and clothing, binding garments or loose kaftans, muscularity from weightlifting and outdoor labor or softness from sitting, and the precision of polish or the markings of dirt under my fingernails. My shape is an expression of an interiority which flows more like a river than sits like an identity. My shape is an ecotone, a collision of multiple landscapes and moments on a non-linear timeline.

My pronoun is redwoods, mycelium, they, we. Whatever you may see of me is a combination of the multitudes of which I consist, and your own expectation, projection, and your own unbearable affect. It is a queer life that need only name itself as such when met with the edges of an internalized and socially held material and psychic prison, this carceral state of mind that I consistently encounter within myself and other people. I try and remember this about other people when I meet them. We are all trapped by our introjects and our own – and others' – projections. We are trapped by what we have come to make and believe are the edges of things. We are also all more than we seem, and more than we know of ourselves. The river finds a way forward, under, over, through, skyward.

Psychoanalysis, too, tries to remind us of this, or at least it can depending on who is using it and for what purpose. The unconscious' roots require us to use our multitude of senses to encounter their existence. The use of psychoanalysis is to encounter that which roots beneath the surface. Freud seemed to know this well, though his articulation of it still, in my opinion, requires a queer analysis. Though he was the first to use the word "psycho-analysis," Freud did not invent it; rather, this praxis is a living being that breathes through dreams,[8] through Earth-based practices, and is cultivated through openness to the queer and the uncanny. Psychoanalysis is more embodied, tactile, vital, rooted than a fragment of an analysis of a case. With psychoanalysis, those of us who depend on vision to move through the world may unburden ourselves from needing to "see" and set our reliance on sight aside. Sight, while helpful, cedes to touch; now, the tactile feeling of one's hands on the body of the trunk as one pushes on the tree to test its root system, or tugs slightly on the seedling to check if it has rooted, becomes primary. This is not to suggest clinicians use touch when practicing psychoanalysis; rather, it is to illustrate that psychoanalysis similarly offers access to another sensory system, one that relies on more than vision to develop a relationship with the parts underneath and underground. *Psychoanalysis is a sensory system in itself.* It is a full-body experience, even if you are not in the same room. Psychoanalysis is how breath connects with light connects with the hair on your arms standing and falling, or the smallest muscle in your neck or gut tensing, your mind at once porous, dense, open, and clamped down; all these senses and more, some of which can be registered and some of which cannot, except in dreams, communicate something of a moment and all the history of moments that have led up to, and inform, this communication of love and hate and other transferences.

Like roots, psychoanalysis finds as its source of nourishment that which is not always reliant on the light of day and the wonders of chlorophyll. In fact, the unconscious material we encounter in psychoanalysis often thrives on staying mostly out of the light. The unconscious, made up of repressed material, is both the soil and the root, one nourishing or depleting the other. The deeper it digs the more intricate it becomes, binding us deeper in ways we cannot always name. Sometimes, what we repress may rob us entirely of our ability to feel, to think, to become. In these moments, we become our most deadened and rote performers, representatives of a life not lived. Perhaps in these moments we become more reliant on the branches than on the roots – for if we cannot feel them, do they even exist to us? Do we exist if someone else can see them? We become reliant upon the other to see us, but the other cannot fully see us, so they make us up and into what they project. Nourishment becomes conflated with obedience. It becomes easier, then, to cut ourselves off from this nourishment, attacking linking (Bion, 1959) between meaning-making and between each other, because the link itself is felt as the attack, because the link-maker, whether an introject or the real person, cannot register us at the deepest level of our soul.

But there is a way that what we unconsciously repress takes on a life of its own. This can be what brings someone to analysis – the unconscious is so full, or so emptied (Alhanati, 2004), that before we can have any way of knowing which are the roots and which are the branches, we spend time in the mud. In the beginning, "[b]irth and killing, light and darkness, would have to go hand in hand" (Alhanati, 2004, p. 772). When we are not legible to a dominating other, sometimes we are killed off, but sometimes we do not die; rather, we create life in and of the shadows cast by the other's projections, in and of the mud, in ways and places where thinking is not required to be legible, linear, linked, or measurable by the dominant other. We become vibrant *in spite of* authoritative, legitimating, and often violent epistemophilic compulsions to know us, create us, and "presume to know what is in the heart and mind of another person" (Alexandra Woods, email correspondence, October 23, 2023). These sites of transformation, *sumud* (Sheehi & Sheehi, 2020), and *living otherwise* (Lewis in Jackson, 2023; Taylor, 2023) are impenetrable to the demands of a logic and power structure that would keep bodies and minds orderly, legible, and restricted. How would someone digging a hole with an excavator to build a pool or a settlement apartment complex ever see the microbes, the tiny insects, the fungi, the minerals of the ground in which they dig, let alone mentalize (Fonagy, 1991) the beings they have displaced?

My queer self lives inside and outside at the same time. We are "seen" and registered as a passport and genitals and coloration and kink while also unseen, except to each other, made in context, made in longing. We make life outside and inside. We make music from and into an existence that does not require a label as validation. We exist as a truth on our own, between one another, in relationship with one another. We compost each other and negate each other and exceed each other and come back to each other because at the end of the day, it is a small world, and we all have to breathe. We remind each other that while submitting to a dominant and legible ideology may offer some juridical legitimacy, oppressive systems require recitation and repetition of myths, and require our unflinching belief in these myths, to keep itself in control of the narrative. We remind each other, please do not lose your flinch. Let your heart crack open every time.

Oppressive systems require, and thus attempt to make, the mud and the shadow lifeless, negated, and unchanging. This is not vitality. But these systems bid us to recite the lines, aiming to make all of us think that the mud is, in fact, dead, or maybe alive but in the "good ways," and good for your skin if you pay for it. Capitalism aims to seduce us through the neoliberal belief that monetizing and individualizing our liberation and care will resolve these existential anxieties once and for all. I am an anxious person, but I have come to realize that my anxieties are also my connection to a world that is falling apart endlessly. I grieve endlessly. And then I go back to the dirt. I go back to the bugs and the fungi who incite in me a joy, an ecstatic arrangement made out of putting ourselves back together, and weaving roots of a life in the shadows. I become we, and we look for sustenance, for what sustains us, in a queer life that negotiates the sun, roots into the Earth, and extends into a network of relatedness even, and especially, when the central leader has been cut.

I am thinking back to the dream I introduced in the beginning of this chapter. I am thinking about the toilets, and the water, and about feelings and bodies and thoughts that have nowhere to go; unable to dream themselves into being, they slosh and stagnate or become something else. As a young person, what felt alive to me – that my gender and my body always felt different from how everyone else responded to me – became unworkable when external social demands became a plugged drain, a hostile blockade. This made any idea of transition, vitality, queer use (Ahmed, 2018), or movement impossible. My dream toilets going nowhere have earned their place in my unconscious and lived life as representations of isolation and alienation I have felt when searching my surroundings for a way to move in emergent relationship to what is possible. The gift of infantile mutability and polymorphousness stagnated the more I responded to social prohibitions, which developed into introjected prohibitions, on the free-flowing entanglements between my psyche, body, imagination, materiality, and libido. Curious queries or imaginative explorations about the *why* of the world seemed to collapse reflective space in my privatized milieu. In the dream, the person who comes to me offers here-and-now reflective capability, and transformation of toilet water into wine. I feel seen, recognized in this transformation and reflection. This reflective space was rarely afforded or encountered in my formative years, though it is a staple of a psychoanalytic encounter.

Though Freud purports to not feel the "oceanic feeling" of spiritual experience (1930, p. 64), I now recognize that my initial feelings about Freud's writing came to me as a tidal wave: in the moment of first reading him, it felt to me he opened as many psychic doors for me as he shut; and at the end, I found myself wondering, imagining, recognizing the ways he challenged me to remain bodily in the face of transmuting his words into something workable for me. I would like to think that Freud would feel both infuriated and delighted by psychoanalysis' countless queer provocations (see Dean, 2003; Semerene, 2015; Hansbury & Saketopoulou, 2022; Saketopoulou & Pellegrini, 2023; and many others). Himself a human of many contradictions, I imagine him dipping in and out of queer imaginings – a scientist who at times presents his theory through the lens of biological evolution and evidence-based scientism, as well as a philosopher and storyteller who is willing to "queer-y" and question the assumptions of his colleagues and himself. Queering Freud, as so many have done, means opening up to a retrospective re-working of theory without erasing its context. I am not here talking about Freud and his own sexuality or gender or erotics, but I am naming that his attempt at articulating the language, art, and science of psychoanalysis is queer in and of itself: iterative, emergent and new, sexually organized, and grappling with desire, death, the Earth, and the ever-transmutational context of what it is to live.

Notes

1 Kemmer here refers to the sexuality of the characters of Ursula K. LeGuin's fictional world in *The Left Hand of Darkness* (1969). The gender and thus sexuality of the inhabitants of Hearth are mutable and not static except during the time of *kemmer*, when they mate; to *vow kemmering* means to take a partner for life. This novel also includes a character's self-exile in the ice, not dissimilar to the monster in Mary Shelley's *Frankenstein*, who becomes exiled from a society which has made him a monster, a society which is thus too monstrous for him to survive (2018). Susan Stryker (2022) also writes of trans* experience in the metaphor of Frankenstein and his monster.
2 While I wish I had been introduced to the writings and theorizing of queer psychoanalysts before Freud, gay and lesbian clinicians were only just being allowed entry into psychoanalytic institutes (in 1991), and it was only in 1973 that the DSM had finally been revised to no longer include homosexuality as a disorder.
3 "Good supervision" is not always available in institutes, as they tend to only allow supervisors who have graduated from their program, thus limiting the theoretical and representational pool to known and legible entities.
4 There are some who are dubiously claiming that any kind of social justice or critical theory has no place in psychoanalysis, so again, not all psychoanalysts agree on what psychoanalysis really is.
5 I have learned a tremendous amount from Black theorists, scholars, and artists about the ways in which the Black Other has been positioned as a receptacle for white fantasy and sadism. I wish to avoid equating queerness with Blackness because these identifications are distinct – I can always move through the world with Whiteness no matter my gender and sexuality – and also intertwine in specific bodies and lives which I have not lived.
6 Here I use this term as Harney and Moten describe it, as an assemblage of that which exists outside and inside institutional spaces where learning happens that is not directly beneficial to, or claimable by, the institution itself (2013).
7 D.A.R.E To Keep Kids Off Drugs (Drug Abuse Resistance Education) was founded in 1983 and "is a police officer-led series of classroom lessons that teaches children from kindergarten through 12th grade how to resist peer pressure and live productive drug and violence-free lives" (from dare.org).
8 In Graeber & Wengrow's text *The Dawn of Everything*, they point to documentation of the communal dream practices of the Wendat of Turtle Island: "…in dreams, such secret desires are communicated in a kind of indirect, symbolic language, difficult to understand, and that the Wendat therefore spend a great deal of time trying to decipher the meaning of one another's dreams, or consulting specialists. All this might seem like an oddly clumsy projection of Freudian theory, but for one thing. The text is from 1649… precisely 250 years before the appearance of the first edition of Freud's *The Interpretation of Dreams* (1899)…. [and further,] realizing the desires of the dreamer, either literally or symbolically, could involve mobilizing an entire community." (2021, p. 455).

Bibliography

Ahmed, S. (November 18, 2018). "Queer Use." *Feministkilljoys*. https://feministkilljoys.com/2018/11/08/queer-use/.

Alhanati, S. (2004). "To Die and So To Grow." *Psychoanalytic Review*, *91*(6), 759–778.

Bion, W.R. (1959). "Attacks on Linking." *International Journal of Psychoanalysis*, *40*, 308–315.

Bion, W.R. (1962). *Learning from Experience*. London: Classic Books.

Carter, C.J. (November 16, 2023) "Fascism in Psychoanalysis, and Antifascist Psychoanalysis." [Video]. *YouTube*. https://youtu.be/nny_r5w-0cY?si=yIWna77jL8yoKrur.

Dare. (n.d.). *About Dare*. https://dare.org/about/#MissionVision.

Dean, T. (2003). "Lacan and Queer Theory." In J-M. Rabaté (Ed.) *The Cambridge Companion to Lacan*. Cambridge: Cambridge University Press. pp. 238–52.

Fonagy, P. (1991). "Thinking About Thinking: Some Clinical and Theoretical Considerations in Treatment of a Borderline Patient." *International Journal of Psychoanalysis*, *72*(4), 639–656.

Freud, S. (1897). "Letter 75, Extracts from the Fliess Papers." In J. Strachey (Ed.) *The Standard Edition of the Complete Psychological Works of Sigmund Freud* (*SE* I). London: Hogarth Press. pp. 268–271.

Freud, S. (1905). "Three Essays on the Theory of Sexuality." In J. Strachey (Ed.) *The Standard Edition of the Complete Psychological Works of Sigmund Freud* (*SE* VII). London: Hogarth Press. pp. 123–246.

Freud, S. (1930). "Civilization and its Discontents." In J. Strachey (Ed.) *The Standard Edition of the Complete Psychological Works of Sigmund Freud* (*SE* XX1). London: Hogarth Press. pp. 57–146.

Graeber, D. & Wengrow, D. (2021). *The Dawn of Everything: A New History of Humanity*. New York: Farrar, Straus and Giroux.

Hansbury, G. (2011). "King Kong & Goldilocks: Imagining Transmasculinities through the Trans–Trans Dyad." *Psychoanalytic Dialogues*, *21*(2), 210–220.

Hansbury, G. & Saketopoulou, A. (2022). "Sissy Dance $1: The More and More of Gender." *Psychoanalytic Review*, *109*(3), 227–256.

Harney, S. & Moten, F. (2013). *The Undercommons: Fugitive Planning & Black Study*. London: Minor Compositions.

Jackson, C. (2022). "The Big Interview: Gail Lewis." *Therapy Today*. https://www.bacp.co.uk/bacp-journals/therapy-today/2022/june-2022/the-big-issue/.

Kimmerer, R. (2013). *Braiding Sweetgrass: Indigenous Wisdom, Scientific Knowledge and the Teachings of Plants*. Minneapolis: Milkweed Editions.

Lacan, J. (1968). "The Mirror-Phase as Formative of the Function of the I." *New Left Review*, *51*, 71–77.

Laplanche, J. (2017). *Après-coup*. J. House (Ed.) & L. Thurston (Trans.). New York: The Unconscious in Translation.

LeGuin, U.K. (1969). *The Left Hand of Darkness*. New York: Ace Books.

Lorde, A. (2007). "Uses of the Erotic: The Erotic as Power." In *Sister Outsider*. Emeryville, CA: Ten Speed Press. pp. 53–59. (Original work published in 1984.)

Morton, T. (2010). "Guest Column: Queer Ecology." *pmla*, *125*(2), 273–282.

Ogden, T. H. (2004). "This Art of Psychoanalysis: Dreaming Undreamt Dreams and Interrupted Cries." *International Journal of Psychoanalysis, 85,* 857–877.

Reading, R & Pivnick, B. (June 4, 2022). "Exposing Transphobic Legacies, Embracing Trans Life." [Audio Podcast episode]. In *Couched*. https://couchedpodcast.org/exposing-transphobic-legacies-embracing-trans-life/.

Saketopoulou, A. & Pellegrini, A. (2023). *Gender Without Identity*. New York: The Unconscious in Translation.

Semerene, D. (2015, April 5). "Forget Theory: In Praise of Psychoanalysis' Queerness." *Academia.edu.* https://www.academia.edu/11804526/Forget_Theory_In_Praise_of_Psychoanalysis_Queerness?email_work_card=title.

Sheehi, L. & Sheehi, S. (2020). *Psychoanalysis Under Occupation: Practicing Resistance in Palestine.* London: Routledge.

Shelley, M. (2018). *Frankenstein: The 1818 Text.* New York: Penguin Classics.

Stryker, S. (2022). "My Words to Victor Frankenstein Above the Village of Chamounix: Performing Transgender Rage." In S. Stryker & D. McCarthy (Eds.) *The Transgender Studies Reader Remix.* London: Routledge. pp. 67–79. (Original article published 1994.)

Taylor, F. (2023). *Unruly Therapeutic: Black Feminist Writings and Practices in Living Room.* New York: Norton Press.

Yusoff, K. (2018). *A Billion Black Anthropocenes or None.* Minneapolis: University of Minnesota Press.

Chapter 12

Credo
So Our Lives Glide On[1]

Ken Corbett

As I set about to contemplate a set of psychoanalytic beliefs, I was reminded of one of my favorite passages in English literature, from George Eliot's novel, *Felix Holt The Radical*: "So our lives glide on: the river ends we don't know where, and the sea begins, and then there is no more jumping ashore" (1995/1866, p. 219).

There are too many tributaries in a human life to jump ashore and give an orderly psychoanalytic account. There is too much to hear. There are too many modes of exchange, conscious and unconscious. There are too many voices, objects, and states of being clamoring for an audience. Mental processes are emergent and non-linear; so too, is any analysis. Analyst and patient emerge, spill over, and emerge again. Unique idioms flow and overflow every analysis.

The same can be said about psychoanalytic beliefs: they evolve, circulate, and flow. Psychoanalytic believing, therefore, must flow onto an open field that affords the necessary consideration of dependent, coexisting, and even contradictory facts. An ordered catalogue of beliefs would be a jumping ashore without dripping the surfeit of the psychoanalytic enterprise.

Hence, contemplating a set of psychoanalytic beliefs must be an act of ongoing revision, with an eye toward how our lives glide on. Or more to the point, how they do not glide on, and how psychoanalysis offers the creative potential for change.

The Social Frame

I believe in foregrounding the social as it shapes our minds and frames our practices. I begin with the social so that it does not become an afterthought, divorced from the psychological. Studying social theory and philosophy led me to psychoanalysis. Reading Foucault, Marcuse, and Ricouer in my first semester of graduate school led me to Freud. Reading Chodorow in that same semester led me to Klein, which led me to Winnicott.[2] Reading Butler in my second year of graduate school led me to Derrida, Lacan, Sedgwick, and back to Freud. Some might look upon my route as circuitous, but I enjoyed and continue to enjoy the circulation.

The social is not outside the door; it operates within, always within. I believe that we, the humans, are always and already socially and historically constituted (even before birth), and reconstituted through "normative anxiety as it seeks to regulate

DOI: 10.4324/9781032624129-13

and define that which is normal, qua healthy" (Corbett, 2011, p. 442). Normative constitution is not, however, an unremitting prototype. Norms are configured through variance, and thereby open to discontinuity and mobility. Similarly, cultural orders are open to rupture and expansion; yes, we live in a here and now, but there is also a there and then. Reckoning with the social frame, to the extent that we have, has allowed us to look toward a wider arc of livable lives; ideality is not reserved for the more normative among us. Psyches need not be fenced in the same old cage.

By foregrounding the social, we stay on our toes, revising our beliefs and expanding our borders. 21st century clinical psychoanalysis surely has as much to do with feminism, queer theory, critical race studies, disability studies, and social philosophy as it does with Freudian tenets, postwar British object-relations theory, American ego psychology, or Relational theory. Arguably, much of the most influential work undertaken in psychoanalysis in the last half-century has been in the spaces between psychoanalysis and social theory. The gray-haired guardians have had to listen to those rattling the gate, as the rattlers have sought to become speaking subjects in a discourse that too readily spoke for or, more to the point, *about* them.[3]

Without this social frame, we are left with no social demarcation for the clinical scene of address. We are left with a "neutral" analyst, who appears as if they magically live outside of social forces. By thinking the social as it circulates within, we are better prepared to address countertransference, and to recognize if counter-anxiety is being repeated through normative presumption, and reactive pathologization.

At stake here is nothing less than how we measure the wellbeing of our fellow citizens, and how that being is employed to confer a life that is seen to matter. Who counts as a citizen? Who counts as a patient? Who counts as an analyst? And how does that identity follow on conventions of membership that construct psychoanalytic institutions? How do we rethink our psychoanalytic beliefs and ethics as we begin to consider who has been left out of the frame? How do we rethink our modes of care, including the social configuration of the clinical setting? How do we rethink the curricula that undergird psychoanalytic educations to include a social education that serves to perplex our psychoanalytic beliefs?[4]

Mental Freedom

I believe in the useful potential of mental freedom, and establishing a therapeutic frame in which that freedom can be risked, lived, and named. I am guided by Freud's bipartite model of mental freedom (1915): (1) *Freedom is the unconscious made conscious* through the organizing authority of the reality principle. In this frame, the unconscious is made manifest and given to the patient through an analyst's knowing interpretations. (2) *Freedom is the lifting of resistance to the unconscious.* In this frame the unconscious manifests, one might say breathes, through states of being and becoming. The pivot is no longer interpretation, but one of bringing patients to the creativity of playing and experiencing a new set of objects.[5]

I derive great pleasure in joining patients in the mental freedom found in play-ing and dreaming, even when the water grows dark with the blood of ghosts and the bile of bad objects. But I do not immediately jump into these streams; I wait. Patients anxiously defend against the establishment of transitional spaces that fos-ter the lifting of resistances to unconscious processes. There is a delicate balance between waiting for a patient to arrive, and helping them experience their fears in so doing.

I strive to stay one step behind and lean into what I think of as an instructive uncertainty, a mode of unknowing. The position of constructive uncertainty is not equivalent to withholding or holding back, as it has sometimes been construed; it is, rather, an active, if not quite affirmative *something*: a containing-searching, a potential, and a mode of mutuality that may or may not be simultaneous.

I am not so much concerned with the content of what is being thought per se, or the interpersonal conversation as pace. I am more concerned with ferreting out shifts between affects and thoughts as these shifts do or do not allow for construct-ing and sustaining transitional space. It is within these shifts or crevices that I can comment on the interference. I do so in order to push at the boundaries of what can be experienced, along with that which Michael Parsons calls, "the *sud-den* pleasure of discovering an unexpected freedom of exploration" (1999, p. 871, emphasis added). I believe that the unforeseen discovery should be in the realm of the patient's experience, and not as a matter of my rushing forward with too much naming and knowing. I move into the crevices and keep my observations brief. I often speak in the voice of hypothesis. Such observations are offered in an effort to help patients as they experience and come to name their own anxieties, histories of trauma, personality structures, fears of breakdown, primitive agonies, bad objects, and so on. It is equally important to listen for the structural social histories that in-terweave a patient's capacities to play and dream. How do matters of race, gender, sexuality, disability, and class inform a patient's experience of mental freedom, along with their experience of the setting? How does the despair and disrepair of the social imaginary thwart us all?

My first patients were two three-year-old boys. I worked with them daily for three years, within a therapeutic nursery. I learned that children are rarely (almost never) looking for someone with a lot to say. I find this also to be true with adults, with whom I now primarily work. Too much talking is akin to wind drag, and slows the patient down. In other words, I learned how to move into transitional spaces without talking such spaces out of their potential. The importance that I place on the work of transitional spaces follows on from the potential mental freedom to be found therein: aliveness, illusion, states of being, and the creation of the other.

Famously, Winnicott proposed that mothers adapt to an infant's needs, and that mothers, "when good enough, give the infant the *illusion* that there is an external reality that corresponds to the infant's own capacity to create" (2017, Vol. 9, p. 275, emphasis in original). A mother is made, then found. And the reality of such finding is not simply frustrating or limiting, but enriching as it provides relief. Part of that relief unfolds through holding the loving and hating that together make a mother and a baby.

I find enormous satisfaction in moving with patients between illusion and reality: being made, then found in an intermediate area of experiencing. I am often confused, both unwittingly and with intent. Hour by hour, I feel myself to be enveloped in a polyphonic field, and I struggle to get my mind into and around the excess. Adding to my confusion, I often court it, indulge it, and mine it to see where it may lead. In other words, I strive to keep transitional experiencing in play, as per Winnicott:

> The third part of the life of a human being, a part that we cannot ignore, is an intermediate area of *experiencing*, to which inner reality and external life both contribute. It is an area that is not challenged, because no claim is made on its behalf except that it shall exist as a resting-place for the individual engaged in the perpetual task of keeping inner and outer reality separate yet interrelated (2017, Vol. 9, p. 267).

The resting "*experiencing*" to which Winnicott refers is "*illusory experience*" (2017, Vol. 9, p. 267, emphasis in original). We rest, we might say repair, through illusion. Who among us has not laid our head down? We also grow through the interchange of illusion and reality, including our capacity to move from merged objects to separate others upon whom we still depend, as we move into our dense and intense social worlds.

Further, I believe that mental freedom comes to life through the eroticism of coming into existence. In this light, I am keen to track the eros that brings transitional spaces to life. Much can be understood through the contemplation of the infantile sexual as it defends against or expands experiencing. Infantile sexuality, as I see it, does not instinctively drive forth as a pre-coded expression of the body's needs; rather, it is an emerging outcome as infants are summoned into existence by the intimate and primary penetrations of parental preoccupation and care. Parental devotion not only potentiates biological life, it also inflects, enlivens, and disrupts object-relational life through libidinal turbulence.[6]

Attending to this primordial undoing, and the ways in which libido overrides relations and the self, aids us in understanding the relational troubles that generally bring patients into treatment. Importantly, I think that it also keeps us aware, to the extent that we can stay aware, of the rogue character of unconscious processes. It humbles us and stumbles us (in just the right way) as we seek to learn how the infantile sexual colors and creates therapeutic exchange. To what degree is the exchange ego-syntonic, or is it freighted by resistant residue that awaits further experiencing and integration?

I struggle to capture the hue and cast of patients' experiencing. How does their aliveness or deadness carry the parenting and parental unconscious transfers that brought them into being? How do they sustain and link associations, psychically-somatically-socially? How might those links be freighted by trauma and primitive agonies? How has their access to experiencing – "the third part of life" (Winnicott, 2017, Vol. 9, p. 267) – and the rest of illusion shaped their personalities and modes of defense? How are they thus formed or "unformed," as per Alvarez (1998)? How might dissociation or depersonalization leave a patient blank to that which happened, but has yet to be experienced? How do their unique idioms shape the setting and the gradual construction of a transitional area in which we can work? How does their idiom join with mine to find the language of our exchange?

I believe it is best to be multilingual when helping a patient move into "an intermediate area of experiencing" (between inner reality and external life, between them and them, between them and me, between us and world). Sometimes I speak relational, sometimes I speak interpersonal, sometimes I speak within the dream, but almost always I speak those languages within the frame of play.

Playing

I believe that therapeutic action rests on returning to the past not yet experienced, and the aliveness not yet found. I privilege playing as my preferred mode of transit and returning (Corbett, 2017). Consider Winnicott's deceptively simple dictum, offered in "Playing: A Theoretical Statement": "Psychotherapy has to do with two people playing together" (2017, Vol. 9, p. 44). Winnicott is not describing one person playing while another looks on. He is not describing one person playing while the other person comments on the action. The two people are proximal or combined in present progressive action: playing together.

Winnicott is privileging the transitive hospitality of playing as psychotherapeutic action that serves to build therapeutic space and potential. Following upon his dictum about playing, Winnicott drew a distinction between play, play content, and playing:

> In the total theory of the personality, the psychoanalyst has been too busy using play content to look at play content to look at the playing child, and to write about playing as a thing in itself. It is obvious that I am making a significant distinction between the meanings of the noun "play" and the verbal noun "playing." (2017, p. x)

By repeating *play content* ("using play content to look at play content") Winnicott folded obsessive rumination into his critique of what he took to be psychoanalysts' obsessive focus on play content, driven by their diligent quest to find unconscious derivatives and busily interpret. Game over.

Some *thing*, Winnicott tells us, is missing: "playing as a thing in itself." He does not elaborate on this point, beyond describing playing as a "verbal noun." Doing and being are coupled in an intermediate state, in which playing is noumenal, not phenomenal. Playing is inferred through experience and the self-evidence of sense and presence, time and space. Playing is transitory, and thereby open to transitions, potential, unknowing, and being. Game on.

Playing should not, though, be mistaken for lightheartedness. Like fantasy, playing includes many kinds of activities. Play is not playfulness; it is the expansion of experiencing, along with the paradox of depth. As Parson's summarizes, "The play element is not just an occasional aspect of analysis, but functions continuously to sustain a paradoxical reality where things can be real and not real at the same time. This paradox is the framework of psychoanalysis" (1999, p. 871).

Illuminating play's paradox are the ways in which it is as much blood as it is glitter. Grief comes onto the field, and rage brings it to its knees. Envy and competition elbow their way down the field. Paranoid flight runs for the corners, where it lingers and haunts. Sputtering schizoid drones fly overhead dropping cluster bombs. Playing includes long periods of waiting and stillness, spellbound moments that are ungrounded and unchanging. As well, the potential of potential space does not simply jump the shark of the social imaginary's disrepair; more often, it follows on the bereaved inability to imagine.

Finding one's way as the analyst onto the field, and into the action of playing, opens onto a range of languages and modes of exchange from the interpersonal to waking-dreaming. Yet, play is neither a dream nor predominately interpersonal. It is potential, the liminal space created between the material and the psychic. Such alterity affords long periods of contemplation and consideration of a wide variety of affects and thoughts, both within any given hour and in my recollection and rumination after any treatment.

I have a longstanding interest in examining the mutative processes of *playing* (Corbett, 2004, 2009, 2023. I am especially interested in the transformational processes of play, and how the analyst is transformed and transduced while playing. How the analyst transitionally turns into an object to be played, played with, and used. How the analyst *becomes* the analyst through playing the object and coming into contact with the psychic reality of the patient. How the analyst accumulates insight through reverie and contemplation, and eventually joins the patient in association, linking, and reflection.

In keeping with my faith in the work of playing, I pay particular attention to the blurring of material and psychic realities and the undoing of temporal-spatial boundaries. I am especially interested in my experience of transduction and transfiguration as potential sites for reclaiming that which has yet to be found and experienced. I focus on the ways in which play ripens through transductions, with a particular interest in the ways in which patients move to not only psychically, but also physically, create the analyst as a potential object.

I believe that it is through becoming the object, culling the paradoxes found therein, that the analyst eventually gathers their reflections and interpretations. How does the transitional space compose the object, the analyst? What time is it? Who traffics the junction, and in what affect states do they arrive? How do I come alive or fall into deadness? How does my own inner world and transference-countertransference bring me forward or hold me back? How am I transduced, sometimes unaware until it arrives in the potential spaces of enactment? How do I stumble on the field, and why? How do I make room for the hate's constitution and destruction? How do I remain steady, even still, in the face of the unbearable grief that so often arrives? How do I sustain the stable attention that values the loss, while preserving that which is left of what was loved and hated? How much need I say about the ways in which my patients and I have already been re-gathered through the psychic realities with which we have been at one?

I privilege the mutative experiences of being and creating within playing. As Winnicott plainly maintains, "It is good to remember always that playing is itself a therapy" (2017, Vol, 8, p. 310). In other words, the intimacy of playing is itself transformative. Elaborating on this intimacy and primacy, Winnicott situates playing as "a basic form of living," and as such, establishes "the basis of what we do" when we do psychotherapy (2017, Vol. 8, pp. 310–311). Bion similarly looked upon sustained experiences of being at one with the psychic reality of the patient as transformative. Such experience, by Bion's account, eclipses interpretation: "What the patient is saying and what the interpretation is (which you give), is in a sense relatively unimportant" (1967, p. 11). Ogden, reflecting on Bion, clarifies that, "*the analyst and the patient have already been changed by the experience of jointly intuiting the unsettling psychic reality with which they have been at one*" (2015, p. 295, emphasis in original). Reis also elaborates on the joined unconscious relation between the analyst and the patient, and how it "subtends the content of any conscious exchange and provides the basis for a non-rational production of knowledge through non-interpretive mutual intervention, the operation of which represents the very heart of the treatment" (2020, p. 3).

I believe it is the played/joined psychic states of creative repetition that matter most. But at the same time, patients look meaningfully to the analyst to join them as they undertake the hard work of translating and repairing formative archaic influences and determinative relational configurations. I think of this hard work, that has traditionally been called working-through, as a zone wherein patient and analyst find the not yet found: sabotaging objects; necrotic love; malignant relational configurations; failures of recognition; modes of psychic retreat; primitive agonies; atomized objects that roll in like fog to blind and obscure, or gather as clouds that burst into affect storms; sexual intromissions carrying abuse; pathways riven with neglect; frayed and dis-regulated affect states, to name but a few. Working-through comes to life as object-relational patterns and affective states are transferred between patient and analyst, who Green describes as "a potential object inducing transformations" (1997, p. 276).

Within this realm of working through, I look for transformational openings: perhaps melancholia moves toward mourning, leaving room for the rest of illusion; or the hate-driven grip of obsessional patterns loosen, affording the contradictions and chaos of loving; or the dogged drear of neglect cracks just enough to allow for some sustained care. In such moments, other possibilities for recognition emerge:

repressive and oppressive hierarchies are questioned, re-significations and new modes of identity come out, more inclusive relational dispositions are found, and bit by bit more livable lives come to be.[7]

Clinical Coda

A young gender non-binary patient recently told me about their experience in rehearsing for a play. They were playing a policeman "who has a job, and he messes up terribly. So, he kind of has this little angry moment and this is just very fun to do." They reflected a bit on this experience and said, "It is fun getting to forget about who I am in that kind of way – the way people, society pressures you. Like, 'Be yourself!' That's almost more daunting than having something forced upon you."

Could there be, I wondered, a more perfect account of the work of experiencing as it opens through illusion and the play of mental freedom, while also capturing the pushback of normative regulatory anxiety. For my young patient, pretending to be something or someone other than who they are was an improvisational opportunity to shake the chain of material reality and historical consequence. It was a temporal turn from knowing toward an aesthetic experiment in living otherwise.

The ongoing reconsideration of psychoanalytic believing rests on the probity and potential revealed in these aesthetic experiments. It is the analyst's job to listen for those moments of improvisation, and the noise they make on the threshold of the past and the present as they clatter toward the future. It is our job – one might say, our ethical charge – to hone in on those potential spaces as they reveal how life may be otherwise livable. In kind, it is our charge to rethink our psychoanalytic beliefs to include the potentials that are not in our consulting rooms, to include patients who remain outside the setting, and to reach toward modes of practice and care that we cannot yet imagine.

Notes

1 First published in J. Salberg (2022). *Psychoanalytic Credos: Personal and Professional Journeys of Psychoanalysts*. London: Routledge.

2 John Broughton introduced me to these writers in a seminar on personality and culture. I would be remiss to not recognize my debt to the spirit of his pedagogy, and his remarkable generosity as I made my way into what I did not know would become my life's work.

3 I fill this space between psychoanalysts and cultural theorists with a brimming chorus: Lewis Aron, Galit Atlas, Lisa Baraister, Jessica Benjamin, Daniel Butler, Judith Butler, Anne Cheng, Francoise Davoine & Jean-Max Gaudilliere, Muriel Dimen, David Eng & Shinhee Han, Franz Fanon, Michel Foucault, Stephen Frosch, Virginia Goldner, Francisco Gonzàles, Orna Guralnik, Griffin Hansbury, Adrienne Harris, Saidiya Hartman, Stephen Hartman, AB Huber, Annie Lee Jones, Lynne Layton, Kimberly Leary, Julie Levitt, David Marriot, Jade McGleughlin, Robert McRuer, Fred Moten, José Muñoz, Ann Pellegrini, Jaqueline Rose, Eyal Rozmarin, Gayle Rubin, Avgi Saketopoulou,

Andrew Samuels, Eve Sedgwick, Gayle Solomon, Warren Spielberg & Kirkland Vaughans, Karen Star, Gillian Straker, and Melanie Suchet.

4 Of particular note is work underway to reconstruct training curricula at the Psychoanalytic Institute of Northern California, and at the New York University Postdoctoral Program in Psychoanalysis and Psychotherapy.

5 See Ogden (2019) for an intriguing discussion of what he terms the "ontological" turn in psychoanalysis, a move toward being and becoming, and a move away from the founding "epistemological" frame of psychoanalysis, based in knowing and interpretation.

6 Cf. Anzieu, 1993; Bick, 1968; Bulter, D., 2019; Laplanche, 1997; Scarfone, 2012; Winnicott, 1956.

7 My thoughts about working through are so overdetermined, (so long in the oven), and rest on reading and re-reading many psychoanalytic theorists. It is impossible to pay due heed to them all. I direct readers to the following writers, to whom I often return on those days (and they are many) when I feel stuck: Alvarez, 1998; Aron, 2001; Benjamin, 1998, 2017; Bick, 1968; Bion, 1967, 1970; Bollas, 1989; Butler, J., 2005, 2006; Bromberg, 2001; Cooper, 2011, 2019; Davies, 2018; Ferro, 2006; Green, 1993, 1997; Grossmark, 2012; Harris, 2009; Levine, 2016; Loewald, 1989; Mitchell, 2003; Ogden, 2012, 2019; Parsons, 1999; Reis, 2020; Seligman, 2014: Stern, 2013a, 2013b: Winnicott, 2017.

Bibliography

Alvarez, A. (1998). "Failures to link: Attacks or defects? Some questions concerning the thinkability of Oedipal and Pre-Oedipal thoughts." *Journal of Child Psychotherapy*, 24: 213–231.

Anzieu, D. (1993). "Autistic phenomena and the skin ego." *Psychoanalytic Inquiry*, 13(1): 42–48.

Aron, L. (2001). *A Meeting of the Minds: Mutuality in Psychoanalysis*. New York: Routledge.

Benjamin, J. (1998). *Like Subject, Love Objects: Essays on Recognition and Sexual Difference*. New Haven: Yale University Press.

Benjamin, J. (2017). *Beyond Doer and Done To: Recognition Theory, Intersubjectivity, and the Third*. New York: Routledge.

Bick, E. (1968). "The experience of the skin in early object-relations." *International Journal of Psycho-Analysis*, 49: 484–486.

Bion, W.R. (1967). *Second Thoughts*. New York: Jason Aronson.

Bion, W.R. (1970). *Attention and Interpretation*. London: Tavistock Publications.

Bollas, C. (1989). *The Shadow of the Object: Psychoanalysis of the Unthought Known*. New York: Columbia University Press.

Bulter, D. (2019). "Riding instincts, even to die." *Studies in Gender and Sexuality*, 20(2): 106–118.

Butler J. (2005). *Giving An Account of Oneself*. New York: Fordham University Press.

Bulter, J. (2006). *Precarious Life: The Powers of Mourning and Violence*. London: Verso.

Bromberg, P. (2001). *Standing in the Spaces: Essays on Clinical Process, Trauma, and Dissociation*. New York: Psychology Press.

Cooper, S. (2011). *A Disturbance in the Field: Essays in Transference-Countertransference*. New York: Routledge.

Cooper, S. (2019). "A theory of the setting: The transformation of unrepresented experience and play." *International Journal of Psycho-Analysis*, 100(6): 1439–1454.

Corbett, K. (2004). "Cracking in." *Psychoanal. Dial.*, 14(4): 457–474.

Corbett, K. (2009). *Boyhoods: Rethinking Masculinities.* New Haven: Yale University Press.

Corbett, K. (2011). "Gender regulation." *Psychoanalytic Quarterly*, 80(2), 441–459.

Corbett, K. (2017, November). *Transit: Playing the Other.* [Plenary address]. Psychology and the Other Conference, Cambridge, MA, US.

Corbett, K. (2023). "Play changes us: Playing the object, becoming the analyst." *Journal of the American Psychoanalytic Association*, 70(2), 263–282.

Davies, J.M. (2018). "The 'rituals' of the relational perspective: Theoretical shifts and clinical implications." *Psychoanalytic Dialogues*, 28(6): 651–669.

Elliot, G. (1995). *Felix Holt the Radical.* New York: Penguin. (Original work published in 1886).

Ferro, A. (2006). *Psychoanalysis as Therapy and Storytelling.* London: Karnac.

Freud, S. (1915). "Observations on transference-love (further recommendations on the technique of psycho-analysis III)." In J. Strachey (Ed.) *The Standard Edition of the Complete Psychological Works of Sigmund Freud (SE)*, Volume XII (1911–1913). pp. 157–171.

Green, A. (1993). *On Private Madness.* London: Karnac.

Green, A. (1997). "The intuition of the negative in *Playing in Reality.*" *International Journal of Psycho-Analysis*, 78(6): 1071–1084.

Grossmark, R. (2012). "The unobtrusive relational analyst." *Psychoanalytic Dialogues*, 22(6): 629–646.

Harris, A. (2009). *Gender as Soft Assembly.* New York: Routledge.

Laplanche, J. (1997). "The theory of seduction and the problem of the other." *International Journal of Psycho-Analysis*, 78: 653–666.

Levine, L. (2016). "Mutual vulnerability: Intimacy, psychic collisions, and the shards of trauma." *Psychoanalytic Dialogues*, 26(5): 571–579.

Loewald, H. (1989). *Papers on Psychoanalysis.* New Haven: Yale University Press.

Mitchell, S. (1995). *Hope and Dread in Psychoanalysis.* New York: Basic Books.

Mitchell S. (2000). *Relationality: From Attachment to Intersubjectivity.* New York: The Analytic Press.

Mitchell, S. (2003). *Can Love Last?: The Fate of Romance over Time.* W.W. Norton: New York.

Ogden, T. (1997). *Reverie and Interpretation.* New York: Jason Aronson.

Ogden, T. (2012). *Creative Readings: Essays on Seminal Analytic Works.* London: Routledge.

Ogden, T. (2015). "Intuiting the truth of what's happening: On Bion's 'Notes on Memory and Desire.'" *Psychoanalytic Quarterly*, 84, 285–306.

Ogden, T. (2019). "Ontological psychoanalysis or 'What do you want to be when you grow up?'" *Psychoanalytic Quarterly*, LXXXVIII, 661–684.

Parsons, M. (1999). "The logic of play in psychoanalysis." *International Journal of Psycho-Analysis*, 80: 871–884.

Reis, B. (2020). *Creative Repetition and Intersubjectivity: Contemporary Freudian Explorations of Trauma, Memory, and Clinical Process.* London: Routledge.

Scarfone, D. (2012). "Winnicott: Early libido and the deep sexual." *Canadian Journal of Psychoanalysis*, 20(1): 3–16.

Seligman, S. (2014). "Paying attention and feeling puzzled: The analytic mind as an agent of therapeutic change." *Psychoanalytic Dialogues*, 24, 648–662.

Stern, D.B. (2013a). "Field theory in psychoanalysis, Part 1: Harry Stack Sullivan and Madeleine and Willy Baranger." *Psychoanalytic Dialogues*, 23: 630–645.

Stern, D.B. (2013b). "Field theory in psychoanalysis, Part 2: Bionian field theory and contemporary interpersonal/relational theory." *Psychoanalytic Dialogues,* 23: 487–501.

Winnicott, D.W. (1956). "Primary maternal preoccupation." In M. Masud & R. Khan (Eds.) *Through Paediatrics to Psycho-Analysis. International Psycho-Analytical Library,* 100: 1–325. London: The Hogarth Press and the Institute of Psycho-Analysis.

Winnicott, D.W. (1974). "The fear of breakdown." *International Review of Psycho-Analysis,* 1, 103–108.

Winnicott, D.W. (2017). *The Collected Works of D.W. Winnicott (CW).* L. Caldwell & H. Taylor Robinson (Eds.). Oxford: Oxford University Press.

Index

Note: Page numbers followed by "n" denote endnotes.